BONES AND JOINTS

BONES AND JOINTS
A Guide for Students

Eighth Edition

James Harcus
BHSc(Hons) MSc PgCert PgCHE FHEA

Lecturer in Diagnostic Imaging, School of Medicine
University of Leeds, United Kingdom

First edition 1984
Second edition 1992
Third edition 1996
Fourth edition 2002
Fifth edition 2007
Sixth edition 2012
Seventh edition 2018

Notices

Practitioners and researchers must always rely on their own experience and knowledge in evaluating and using any information, methods, compounds or experiments described herein. Because of rapid advances in the medical sciences, in particular, independent verification of diagnoses and drug dosages should be made. To the fullest extent of the law, no responsibility is assumed by Elsevier, authors, editors or contributors for any injury and/or damage to persons or property as a matter of products liability, negligence or otherwise, or from any use or operation of any methods, products, instructions, or ideas contained in the material herein.

ISBN: 9780702084300

Content Strategist: Nicola Lally
Content Project Manager: Ayan Dhar

Printed in India

Last digit is the print number: 9   8   7   6   5   4   3   2

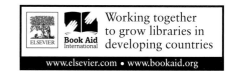

CONTENTS

FOREWORD vi

PREFACE vii

1 BONE 1

2 JOINTS 14

3 FRACTURES 21

4 PATHOLOGY 29

5 UPPER LIMB 63

6 SHOULDER GIRDLE 102

7 LOWER LIMB 127

8 PELVIC GIRDLE 194

9 THORAX 221

10 VERTEBRAL COLUMN 238

11 THE SKULL 299

GLOSSARY 363

INDEX 373

FOREWORD

I was first approached in the early 1980's to write the first edition of *Bones and Joints*. The first edition was very different from the current book in that it was a replication of my lecture notes with the bones and joints illustrations, drawn by my husband, to accurately reflect the radiographic appearances as seen in departments at the time. Over the years, and in future editions, radiographs were added to the text and by the fourth edition, new imaging modalities were included. In the fifth edition we introduced colour to the layout. PET and SPECT images appeared in the sixth edition and finally by the seventh edition, colour was added to the drawings to aid clarity. It was apparent over the years that the book was used not only by radiography students, but also by other students who were required to study osteology and arthrography as part of their course. In addition, it was used by some medical students and qualified staff as a reference book.

When the time came for this edition, I felt that it was time to hand it over to someone who was currently practicing in radiography to update the text. As a result, this edition includes many updated images to reflect current practice, a revision of the fracture and pathology sections whilst maintaining the clarity of the layout and design and the simple line drawings to enable to students to be able to reproduce the illustrations when revising. More insights have been included to aid understanding and the inclusion of additional images to demonstrate the ossification centres of bones, something which has been lacking in previous editions. Additional online resources have been included to reflect the change in radiography over the years as it has progressed from a diploma to a degree course where a more in depth understanding of the subject is required. This edition fully reflects the changes that have occurred over the years and should continue to be a useful aid to learning.

Chris Gunn

PREFACE

With a clinical background in image interpretation, I have always maintained that a thorough understanding of the underlying anatomy on a medical image is imperative to visualising and interpreting pathology. This is why I am honoured to have been asked to author the new edition of this classic textbook, which has been a core resource for students for many years.

Whilst this new edition is based upon the successful format of the previous seven editions, and I have deliberately not deviated too far from the previous versions, I have looked to update a number of aspects to hopefully further explain difficult concepts and support them with a range of appropriate images.

The essence of this book remains the same; to present the subject of anatomy and arthrology of the skeleton in a concise and systematic way and then apply it to practice by discussing common fractures and pathologies that will be encountered. It is not designed to be an exhaustive resource but more of a succinct guide to the key principles of the topics and for use in three main ways:

1. To support a programme of study by covering the key aspects of osteology and arthology and then focussing on individual skeletal regions.

2. For revision purposes. The accompanying online resources help to support the illustrations and content in the book when preparing for exams.

3. As a reference book and source of information both as a student and graduate health professional.

In Chapters 1 and 2 the fundamentals of the structure and development of bones and joints are introduced to support understanding of the following chapters. Chapters 3 and 4 briefly outline some key concepts in the pathophysiology and appearance of fractures and pathologies. The remaining chapters systematically outline each part of the skeletal system using labelled illustrations and radiological images to support learning and revision. Common fractures and pathologies are also explained with the support of medical images.

Development of medical terminology is important, so relevant terms are introduced early in text and used throughout. An extensive glossary aims to provide a quick reference guide for the terms used in the book.

Despite the relatively succinct nature of the content, there is a lot of information to take in! For that reason, where there are important or commonly misunderstood concepts, the 'Insights' within each chapter aim to highlight and explain some of these. Many of these concepts are those which I enforce in my teaching to students so I am grateful to now be able to share some of these to a wider audience.

I must pay gratitude to the author of the previous editions, Chris Gunn, and all other previous contributors for providing me with such a sound and successful format with in which to work. You have made my job a lot easier! Sincere thanks must go to Helen and Millie whose support during those writing days throughout lockdown was invaluable in keeping me motivated.

James Harcus
Lecturer in Diagnostic Imaging,
University of Leeds

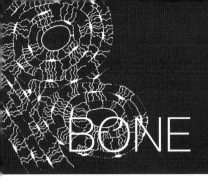

BONE

1

CHAPTER CONTENTS

Function of Bone	1	Types of Bone	8
Structure of Bone	1	'Normal' Radiographic Bone	
Development of Bone	5	Appearances	9
Ossification	5	Terminology	11

Despite being a fairly simple looking inert structure — bone, like any other organ, is a complex, vascular, highly innervated living tissue that is continuously being turned over. Throughout life, bone is being built and broken down. The study of bones is called *osteology*.

FUNCTION OF BONE

Bone has a number of key functions:
- **supports** the body weight and soft tissues; acts as an attachment site.
- enables **movement** as levers for muscles.
- **protects** organs, e.g., the brain.
- **stores** calcium, phosphorus, and other important minerals for the balance of body homeostasis. Also, a store for fatty (*adipose*) tissue within the yellow bone marrow.
- **produces** blood cells from the red bone marrow stored within it.

STRUCTURE OF BONE

Bone is a type of connective tissue in which mature bone cells (*osteocytes*) are enclosed in an intercellular network (*matrix*) of *organic* collagenous protein fibres, called *osteoid*, and a harder *inorganic* mineralised component.

In the process of bone production, bone-forming *osteoblast cells* secrete the collagenous organic osteoid, which is then hardened when mineral salts are deposited within it to form the mineralised, or calcified, inorganic matrix.

In a typical mature bone, the organic osteoid forms approximately one-third of the matrix and gives resilience and a degree of flexibility. The inorganic mineral salts (mainly a calcium and phosphate substance called *hydroxyapatite*) form the remaining two-thirds and provide the strength, hardness and weight bearing capabilities of the bone.

Within this bone matrix are four types of cells. They all have a role in bone development, growth, maintenance, and repair.

Osteogenic cells – stem cells that are found within the inner aspect of the periosteum, the endosteum and in the communicating channels between the units of bone. These cells divide to form osteoblasts.

Osteoblasts – *bone-building* cells secrete the osteoid, collagen, and other components that build the organic matrix. They then start the process of calcification for the inorganic mineral matrix in the spaces between the collagen fibres.

Osteocytes – mature bone cells that maintain the normal cellular activity of bone, such as the exchange of nutrients. They are formed from osteoblasts when they become trapped within their matrix and can no longer secrete the osteoid.

Osteoclasts – *bone-consuming* cells. These large cells are made of many monocytes (type of white blood cell) that release strong enzymes to dissolve the bone matrix. They are mainly found within the endosteum on the inside of the bone.

Throughout life, there is a constant balance (homeostasis) of bone formation and resorption by the osteoblasts and osteoclasts, a process called *remodelling*.

There are two main types of bone: *compact* (dense) and *cancellous* (spongy). Compact bone forms the surface layer, or *cortex*, of mature bones and cancellous bone forms the interior aspect. The skeleton comprises approximately 80% compact and 20% cancellous bone.

Compact bone

This type of bone is very hard and strong. It is found mainly in the shaft (*diaphysis*) of long bones, where a strong tubular structure is required and forms the outer layer (*cortex*) of all bones. It consists of a number of cylindrical structures or units called *Haversian systems* (or *osteons*) (Figs. 1.1, 1.2). The mature bone cells (*osteocytes*) sit in spaces (*lacunae*) between concentric rings of bone (*lamellae*). A network of channels run between the lacunae spaces to provide nutrients to the osteocyte cells and ensure bone homeostasis. Each system comprises:

A central Haversian canal – which contains nerves and blood, and lymphatic vessels.

Lamellae – concentric rings/layers of bone around the Haversian canal.

Lacunae – spaces between the lamellae containing osteocytes (mature bone cells).

Canaliculi – channels carrying nutrient fluid; connect the lacunae and communicate with the central Haversian canal.

Fig. 1.1 Transverse section of bone (microscopic).

A – Haversian canal
B – Canaliculi
C – Circumferential lamella
D – Interstitial lamella
E – Lacuna
F – Lamella.

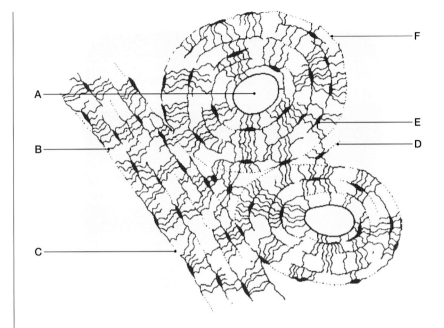

Fig. 1.2 Longitudinal section of bone (microscopic).

1 – Haversian canal
2 – Volkmann's canal
3 – Lacuna
4 – Canaliculi.

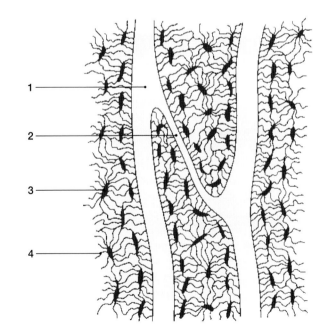

Between the individual Haversian systems are:
Interstitial lamellae – layers of bone that fill the space between adjacent Haversian systems.
Volkmann's canals – join the various Haversian canals between different systems and contain nerves and blood and lymphatic vessels.

Enclosing the Haversian systems both externally and internally are:
Circumferential lamellae – rings of bone tissue around the internal and external surfaces of the bone; communicate with the Haversian systems via canaliculi.
Periosteum – an external membrane that surrounds the compact bone, except at the articular joint surfaces where it is covered by articular hyaline cartilage. The inner layer of this membrane is vascular and cellular and essential in providing nutrition, growth and repair of the bone. The outer layer is tough and fibrous and blends with tendons and ligaments for attachment.
Endosteum – a vascular internal membrane that lines the medullary cavity. Its role is in providing nutrition and the growth and repair of bones.

Cancellous bone

This type of bone, also called *spongy bone*, is found in the parts of bones where lightness, strength and increased surface area are required. It is found mainly within the ends of long bones and in the middle of other types of bone. The structure is similar to compact bone but does not contain true Haversian systems. Rings of lamellae are arranged in an irregular lattice of thin columns of bone called *trabeculae*. These trabeculae provide the internal support structure of bone and are aligned along the direction of forces to provide tensile and compressive strength. Spaces between the trabeculae reduce the overall weight of the bone and also contain bone marrow.

Bone marrow

The medullary cavity of long bones and the spaces between the trabeculae of cancellous bone are filled with bone marrow. At birth, this is red bone marrow, which produces red and white blood cells in a process called *haematopoiesis*.

In adults, active red bone marrow is found only in the following:
- proximal (upper) femora
- vertebrae
- scapulae
- sternum
- ribs
- clavicles
- diploë of skull bones
- hip bones

Elsewhere in the skeleton, the red bone marrow becomes inactive yellow marrow and is predominantly a storage site for fatty (adipose) tissue.

Blood supply

As living tissue, bones require nutrients and are highly vascular structures. The blood to the bone supplies:

- bone tissue (matrix)
- bone cells
- bone marrow
- epiphyseal (growth plate) cartilage
- periosteum and endosteum

There are several distinct points where the large blood vessels enter the bone. In long bones, large *nutrient arteries* enter through the periosteum into the diaphysis (shaft) of the bone through obliquely orientated holes, called the *nutrient foramina*. These usually point away from the dominant growing end of the bone. The nutrient artery then divides into distal (lower) and proximal (upper) branches that supply most bone. Additional numerous smaller metaphyseal and epiphyseal arteries enter at the ends of bones to supply these respective regions.

The arterial blood feeds the bone and then drains into veins which leave the bone following their accompanying arteries. Blood vessels are particularly prevalent where bones contain red bone marrow. Blood vessels do not enter or exit the bone at surfaces covered by articular hyaline cartilage.

Nerve supply

Nerves are widely distributed in the periosteum, and nerve fibres accompany the arteries into the bone via the nutrient foramen.

 INSIGHT

The abundance of nerves in the periosteum explains the pain associated with a fracture. The vascular nature of bones is also important to allow fracture repair.

DEVELOPMENT OF BONE

The shape of an embryo's skeleton is entirely made up of fibrous connective tissue membranes (*mesenchyme*) and *hyaline cartilage*. After the sixth week *in utero*, this tissue starts to turn to bone through a process called *ossification*. Some bones develop from rods of cartilage (intracartilaginous), such as the bones that form the limbs, the trunk, and the skull base. Some bones develop from membranes (intramembranous), such as bones of the vault of the skull, the face and the clavicle. Some bones develop in tendons (intratendinous); these are sesamoid bones such as the patella and fabella.

Ossification

Ossification is the formation of bone from connective tissue and requires:

- adequate calcium, phosphorus and other minerals in the blood to form the mineral component of the inorganic bone matrix.

- a supply of vitamins such as A, C and D are important as they have specific roles in the activity of bone cells, the production of proteins like collagen, and the ability to absorb calcium.

 INSIGHT

Hydroxyapatite, chemical symbol $Ca_5(PO_4)_3$, is the main mineral salt of bone and tooth enamel. It provides strength and hardness and comprises up to two-thirds of the weight of the skeleton. Calcium, as a major component, is essential to the health and strength of bone and, when found in excess or deficiency, is a cause of bone disease. Calcium is also essential to a number of other systems and processes in the body, such as blood cell production, blood clotting, and nerve conduction. Therefore, it is required by the body in large amounts and can be stored in bones and released into the blood as required.

Growth and turnover of the bone are influenced by the following hormones:
Parathormone/Parathyroid hormone (from the parathyroid glands)–increases the level of calcium in the blood by increasing the rate of bone resorption by osteoclasts.
Calcitonin (from the thyroid gland)–works in opposition to parathormone to help decrease the level of calcium in the blood by reducing the rate of bone resorption by inhibiting osteoclast activity.
Growth hormone (from the anterior lobe of the pituitary gland)–influences growth and replacement of bone tissue.
Thyroxine (from the thyroid gland)–influences normal physical development by acting on the rate of bone turnover.
Testosterone (in males) and oestrogen (in females)–influences normal skeletal growth, especially at puberty.

Weight bearing and exercise are also important to stimulate bone growth and maintain its strength; general ill health inhibits it.

Intracartilaginous ossification
The process by which most bone formation occurs, e.g., in long bone (Fig. 1.3), is where ossification occurs within a hyaline cartilage model of the bone. *Ossification centres* are the sites (or parts) within a bone where this process occurs before finally fusing together in skeletal maturity. Ossification occurs within these sites at specific ages of development, although this varies from person to person.

Primary centre of ossification
This appears in the middle of the *diaphysis* (diaphysis means 'through the growth'). *Osteoblasts* appear, and the matrix of bone tissue is laid down.
Osteoclasts 'destroy' (or resorb) the bone and therefore mould the bone into the required shape through a process called '*remodelling*'. Osteoclasts are also responsible for forming the *medullary canals* and *sinuses* within the bone.
The primary ossification centre spreads from the middle of the diaphysis towards the epiphyseal (growth) plates at the ends of the bone.

Fig. 1.3 Section through a developing long bone.

A – Diaphysis (shaft)
B – Epiphysis
C – Epiphyseal plate
D – Metaphysis
E – Medullary cavity
F – Periosteum
G – Endosteum
H – Articular hyaline cartilage.

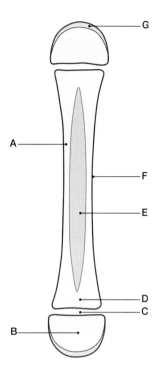

At the same time as the diaphysis is being formed, bone is being built up around the outside of the diaphysis and later forms the *periosteum*. The bone width increases and is then maintained by the bone formation and turnover in the sub-periosteal and endosteal surfaces of the bone.

Secondary centres of ossification

These appear at the ends of the bone and form the *epiphyses* (singular *epiphysis*, meaning 'upon the growth'). The epiphysis is separated from the diaphysis by a thin layer of cartilage called the *epiphyseal plate (or physeal plate or physis)*. The epiphyses in long bones typically form the surface of an adjacent joint.

Some secondary ossification centres form a distinct projection or bony protuberance where a ligament or tendon may attach, and these are specifically called an *apophysis*, or *apophyses* (plural).

Growth

Growth in the length of a bone occurs during childhood by the production of bone within the epiphyseal plate. It occurs at the side of the epiphyseal plate nearest the diaphysis, which is called the *metaphysis* (meaning 'between the growth'). Cartilage cells *(chondrocytes)* within the epiphyseal plate are produced and *hypertrophy* (enlarge). They then calcify and, in turn, ossify to form new bone. This continuous process causes the bone to lengthen.

Fusion
The fusion of the epiphysis with the metaphysis and diaphysis occurs when the bone reaches the desired size. A typical long bone can take up to 20 years to reach fusion, and full skeletal maturity does not occur until approximately 25 years.

Intramembranous ossification
This occurs in a connective tissue membrane (*mesenchyme*) where it does not turn to hyaline cartilage first (e.g. in the vault of the skull in a developing foetus). At the point of ossification, *osteogenic* (bone-forming) fibres and osteoblasts appear in the connective tissue to produce the bone matrix. Ossification spreads from the centre of the bone outwards.

TYPES OF BONE

The adult skeleton consists of 206 individual bones split into two divisions. The *axial* skeleton consists of 80 bones in the centre of the body and includes the bones of the head, thoracic cage, and spine. The *appendicular* skeleton (126 bones) is attached to the axial skeleton and comprises the bones of the upper and lower limbs and the girdles (shoulder and pelvis), which attach them to the axial skeleton. There are five principal types of bone based upon their shape.

Long bones (Fig. 1.3)

Long bones are considered 'typical' in structure. They are longer than wide and consist of a shaft (*diaphysis*) of compact bone with a central medullary cavity. The expanded ends (made of the epiphysis and metaphysis) are formed by cancellous bone covered with a layer of compact bone.

Examples include
- humerus
- radius
- ulna
- femur
- tibia
- fibula
- phalanges
- metatarsals
- metacarpals

Short bones (cuboidal shape)

These are formed by cancellous bone with a thin covering of compact bone, offering strength but with limited movement.

Examples include
- carpal bones, in the wrist
- tarsal bones, in the foot

Flat bones

These have a thin layer of cancellous bone enclosed in two thin layers of compact bone and are found where protection for underlying organs or extensive muscle attachment is required.

Examples include

- scapulae
- ribs
- vault of the skull

Irregular bones

These types of bone are complex in shape and are composed of cancellous bone surrounded by a thin layer of compact bone. They often have many bony projections to allow attachment for soft tissue structures like ligaments and tendons.

Examples include

- vertebrae
- facial bones
- hip bones

Sesamoid bones

These develop in tendons, usually near a joint, and their main function is to protect the tendon from wear as it moves over the bony surface and improve the mechanical efficiency of certain joints. Besides the kneecap (patella), the number of sesamoids varies from person to person, particularly in the hands and feet. Some are more common than others.

'NORMAL' RADIOGRAPHIC BONE APPEARANCES (FIGS. 1.4, 1.5, 1.6)

Cortex–compact bone; denser than the cancellous bone and medullary cavity and, therefore, absorbs more X-rays producing a reasonably solid sclerotic (white) line around the periphery of the bone.

Medullary cavity–is less dense than the cortex and appears slightly more radiolucent (darker).

Cancellous bone–the trabeculae, which are the support structure of the cancellous bone, have the appearance of very fine sclerotic (white) lines throughout the inside of the bone.

Epiphyseal plate–as this is formed by cartilage, it is radiolucent and therefore invisible, so care must be taken not to confuse it with a fracture. It has the appearance of a radiolucent (dark) line with two fairly smooth regular margins, extending to the periphery of the bone and situated near the ends, between the metaphysis and epiphysis.

Fused epiphyseal plate–usually appears during the teenage years and occurs as a very thin sclerotic line along the site of the old epiphyseal plate. These lines are no longer visible with age, although they persist in some people (particularly in the distal radius and tibia bones).

Joint cavity–this contains articular hyaline cartilage and synovial fluid and is radiolucent (and therefore not demonstrated).

Fig. 1.4 Normal bone appearances: left wrist (paediatric). (From STATdx © Elsevier 2022).

A – Joint cavity/space
B – Compact bone/cortex
C – Medullary cavity
D – Epiphysis
E – Epiphyseal (growth) plate
F – Metaphysis.

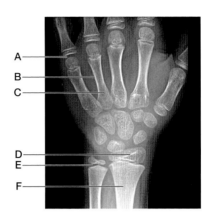

Fig. 1.5 Normal bone appearances: right ankle. (From STATdx © Elsevier 2022).

A – Compact bone/cortex
B – Medullary cavity
C – Cancellous bone
D – Fused epiphyseal plate.

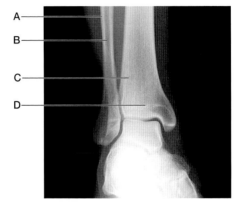

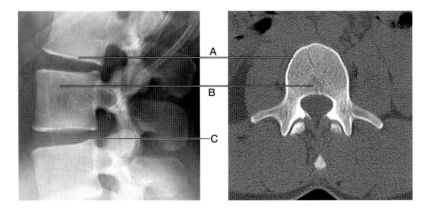

Fig. 1.6 Radiograph and CT of a lumbar vertebra. (From STATdx © Elsevier 2022).

A – Compact bone/cortex
B – Cancellous bone
C – Intervertebral disc (joint) space.

TERMINOLOGY

 INSIGHT

Learning these terms will enable the reader to work out the names of different parts of a bone and start describing where injuries and pathologic conditions occur. It is important to learn and use appropriate terminology. These terms will be used throughout this book so use the lists below to refer back to; try and get used to using them. They are also all detailed in the glossary.

The names of most parts of a bone can be built up logically from a combination of some of the following:

- an adjective derived from either:
  - the name of the bone, or
  - the bone with which they articulate, or
  - part of the bone with which they articulate.
- a prefix (not always needed); locates where within a bone. When used, they come before the adjective.
- a descriptive term – see following lists (elevations, projections, holes and depressions).

Even the most complex anatomical and pathological terms are built up of a combination of smaller parts.

Examples are

Subscapular fossa–a depression below the scapula (literally; below scapula depression).

Trochlear notch–a large groove that articulates with the trochlea.

Radial fossa–a depression that receives the head of the radius.

Supracondylar ridge–a ridge above a condyle (literally, above condyle ridge).

Elevations and projections

These protrude from the bone and are normally soft tissue attachment points or form part of a joint.

Auricular–ear-shaped.

Condyle–a smooth, rounded elevation often covered with articular hyaline cartilage (forms part of a joint surface).

Crest–a sharp ridge.

Epicondyle–an elevation above/upon a condyle.

Facet–a smooth area, usually covered with articular hyaline cartilage (another type of joint surface).

Hamulus–a hook-like projection.

Lamina–a thin plate.

Line–a long, low, narrow ridge.

Process–a localised projection.

Spine–an elongated process.

Squamous–thin, flat, like a scale.

Trochanter–a large rounded elevation (specifically in the femur).

Trochlea–a pulley-shaped surface.
Tubercle–a small rounded elevation.
Tuberosity–a large rounded elevation (specifically in the humerus).

Holes or depressions
These normally contain and protect soft tissue structures like nerves and tendons.
Canal–a bony tunnel.
Fissure–a narrow slit.
Foramen–(plural *foramina*) a hole.
Fossa–(plural *fossae*) a wide depression or hollow.
Groove–an uncovered passage.
Meatus–a narrow passage.
Notch–a large groove.
Sulcus–a groove or furrow.

Prefixes
Demi–half
Epi–above/upon
Infra–below
Inter–between
Intra–within
Sub–beneath
Supra–above

Descriptive terms

 INSIGHT

When using descriptive terms or prefixes to describe the location, movement, or displacement of the body (or a fracture), always refer back to the standard anatomical position. This is someone:
- standing erect, front of the body facing forwards.
- head level, eyes looking forwards.
- arms by the side, palms facing forwards.
- feet flat on the floor.

Anterior–nearer the front of the body
Distal–further away, the lower end of a bone
Dorsal–the back surface of the body
External–outside
Inferior–below
Internal–inside
Lateral–away from the midline of the body
Medial–nearer the midline of the body
Posterior–nearer the back of the body

Proximal–closer to; the upper end of a bone
Superior–above
Ventral/Volar–nearer the front of the body

Terms associated with teeth
Buccal/labial–adjacent to the cheeks/lips
Cusps–rounded projections
Distal–towards the back of the mouth
Lingual/glossal–next to the tongue
Mesial–towards the front or the midline
Occlusal–biting edge

 INSIGHT

The body can be divided into a series of planes, and these are used when referring to the different 'slices' used in cross-sectional imaging such as computed tomography and magnetic resonance imaging:
- ***median sagittal plane (MSP)***–dividing the body into left and right sides directly down the middle.
- ***sagittal plane***–either side of the median sagittal plane, dividing the body into left and right.
- ***coronal plane***–90 degrees to a sagittal plane, dividing the body into anterior and posterior (front and back).
- ***axial (or transverse) plane***–divides the body horizontally; top and bottom.

JOINTS

2

CHAPTER CONTENTS

Synovial Joints (Diarthroses)	14
Features of a typical	
synovial joint	14
Accessory joint structures	15
Movements of the joints	16
Types of synovial joints	17
Fibrous Joints	18
Types of fibrous joints	18
Cartilaginous Joints	19
Types of cartilaginous joints	19
Cartilage	20

A joint is formed either where two or more bones meet or where a bone meets cartilage or a tooth. Both its structure and intended function determine the type of joint; some joints are freely moveable, others completely rigid but very strong. Joints, also known as *arthroses* (singular *arthrosis*), can be classified as being solid (*fibrous* or *cartilaginous*) where the bones are firmly fixed together by connective tissue or cartilage, or *synovial* where there is a space between the bones that allows more movement. The study of joints is called *arthrology*.

SYNOVIAL JOINTS (DIARTHROSES)

Features of a typical synovial joint (Fig. 2.1)

The most common types of joints found in the body are classified as synovial joints. As well as connecting the articulating bones, their function is to provide movement–*diarthroses* (moveable joint).

All synovial joints have a broadly similar structure. The surfaces of the articulating bones are covered in a layer of articular hyaline cartilage with a space in between the bones called the *synovial cavity*. The cavity is filled with a small amount of lubricant called *synovial fluid*. Enclosing the cavity is a tough outer *fibrous capsule* lined with a *synovial membrane* that secretes the synovial fluid.

Articular (hyaline) cartilage–covers the bone's articular surfaces to provide a smooth, reduced friction surface. It is predominantly *hyaline cartilage*; a flexible blue-white substance where *chondrocytes* (cartilage cells) are interspersed in a network of fine collagen fibres.

Fibrous capsule–outermost layer surrounding the joint cavity. It is made of tough, dense connective tissue connecting the bones by blending with their periosteum. It allows free movement but adds joint strength by resisting the

Fig. 2.1 Typical synovial joint (coronal section).

A – Fibrous capsule
B – Synovial membrane
C – Articular hyaline cartilage
D – Synovial cavity/fluid
E – Bone

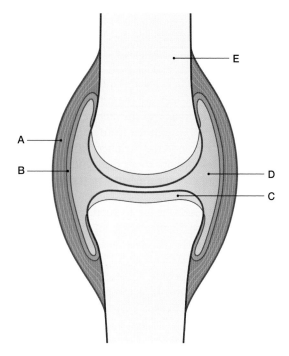

bones being pulled apart; *capsular ligaments* are thickened bundles of the capsule which help perform this role.

Synovial membrane–lines the inner surface of the fibrous capsule and bone surfaces, except where articular hyaline cartilage is found. Secretes the synovial fluid into the joint cavity.

Synovial fluid–fills the joint. A viscous, clear/white fluid that looks like egg white. It acts as a lubricant and shock absorber, becoming more viscous when put under pressure. It also provides nutrients to the avascular articular cartilage and removes joint debris formed from 'wear and tear.'

Nerves–correspond to muscles moving the joint; act to pass pain signals and information on movement and stretch at the joint

Blood vessels–supply all tissues of the joint except the articular cartilage, which is nourished by the synovial fluid. Normally several different blood vessels encapsulate and converge around the joint to form the arterial supply and venous drainage

Accessory joint structures

As well as the typical features of a synovial joint, there are accessory structures that are found in and around certain synovial joints. Specific examples will be encountered as each joint is looked at in turn in subsequent chapters.

Accessory ligaments–strengthen the joint by resisting tension stresses. Separate to those found as part of the fibrous capsule, these bands of very strong fibrous tissue help hold bones together, e.g., the cruciate ligaments in the knee.

Tendons–attachment of muscles to the periosteum of bones. A direct continuation of the dense, tough connective tissue within muscles. Transmit the force of muscle contractions to the bone to initiate movement.

Articular discs–pads of *fibrocartilage* (stronger than hyaline cartilage) that sit in between the ends of the bones and attach to the fibrous capsule. Their shape increase the congruity of the articulating bones and also acts as a shock absorber, e.g., the meniscus in the knee (See Chapter 7; Figs 7.37, 7.38)

Labrum–similar to articular discs, these are rings of fibrocartilage that surround the periphery of an articular bone surface to increase the congruity of the bones, e.g., the glenoid labrum in the shoulder (See Chapter 6; Fig. 6.13) or acetabular labrum in the hip joint (See Chapter 8; Fig. 8.17).

Articular fat pads–collections of fatty (adipose) tissue that help cushion and protect the joint structures. Examples are found in joints such as the elbow (See Chapter 5; Fig. 5.20).

Bursae–(singular *bursa*) fluid-filled sacs of synovial membrane found around joints where there is increased friction, such as between bony protuberances and the skin or between tendons and bones. They help to reduce friction which may lead to pain and tissue damage. Examples include within the knee joint (See Chapter 7; Fig. 7.39).

Tendon sheaths–similar in structure and function to bursae. Surround some tendons where there is an increased amount of friction; such as where tendons cross (e.g., in the wrist) or where they pass through or over a bone feature

 INSIGHT

The bone structure of synovial joints is inherently very weak; the strength comes mainly from the supporting soft tissue structures.

Movements of the joints

Flexion – bending the joint; decreasing the angle between the bones.
Extension – straightening the joint; increasing the angle between the bones.
Abduction – to move away from the midline, usually a limb.
Adduction – to move towards the midline, usually a limb.
Internal rotation – to turn inwards.
External rotation – to turn outwards.
Circumduction – a combination of the above movements.
Gliding – one articular surface sliding smoothly over another.

Other specific movements relating to the movement of the skeletal system.
Pronation – rotating the arm internally, so the palm faces posteriorly, or the foot by rotating the plantar aspect (sole) laterally.
Supination – rotating the arm externally, so the palm faces anteriorly, or the foot by rotating the plantar aspect is rotated medially.

Inversion – turning internally (commonly the foot/ankle).
Eversion – turning externally (commonly the foot/ankle).
Valgus – abnormal angulation at a joint where the distal bone is angled laterally.
Varus – abnormal angulation at a joint where the distal bone is angled medially.

Types of synovial joints

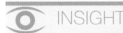 INSIGHT

Though the structures of many synovial joints are similar, it is the range of movements that the joint has that determines the type of joint.

Synovial hinge joints

Uniaxial joints (movement around one axis). The convex surface of one bone fits in a concave surface of the other; acts like the hinge on a door.
Movements – flexion and extension.
Examples – elbow joint, interphalangeal joints in the digits

Synovial bicondylar joints

Biaxial joints (movement around two axes at 90° to each other) but only minimal movement in one of the planes (rotation usually) compared to the other. Similar to a hinge joint, two rounded condyles on one bone articulate with a flat or slightly concave surface on the other.
Movements – flexion, extension and rotation.
Examples – knee joint, temporomandibular joint (TMJ) of the jaw

Synovial ellipsoid (condyloid) joints

Biaxial joints. One rounded convex bone surface articulates with a concave depression on the other.
Movements – flexion, extension, abduction and adduction.
Examples – Wrist (radio-carpal) joint, metacarpophalangeal joints, metatarsophalangeal joints, atlanto-occipital joint

Synovial saddle joints

Biaxial joints (with additional small amount of rotation). Similar to an ellipsoid joint with more rotation. One elongated convex bone surface sits in an opposing concave depression. Like sitting on a saddle, movement can be forwards and backwards, side-to-side, and rotation in the saddle.
Movements – flexion, extension, abduction, adduction and a degree of axial rotation.
Examples – first (thumb) carpometacarpal joint, calcaneocuboid joint sternoclavicular joint, ankle joint

Synovial pivot joints

Uniaxial joints. A projection or 'peg' of bone that sits within a bony ring (or part bone, part ligament) surrounding it. Like a pencil in a pencil sharpener.
Movements – rotation only.
Examples – superior radioulnar joint, inferior radioulnar joint, atlantoaxial joint (the odontoid process in the arch of the atlas)

Synovial ball and socket joints

Multiaxial joints (movement around more than two axes). A ball-shaped articular surface within a concave surface; like a golf ball sitting on a tee
Movements – flexion, extension, abduction, adduction, rotation and circumduction.
Examples – hip joint, shoulder joint

Synovial plane joints

Non-axial (sliding only). Two flat (or slightly curved) surfaces which move over each other.
Movements – gliding only.
Examples – sacroiliac joint, superior tibiofibular joint, cubonavicular joint, tarsometatarsal joints, acromioclavicular joints, second to fifth carpometacarpal joints, costovertebral and vertebral facet joints

FIBROUS JOINTS

These joints usually have either no movement *(synarthroses)* or minimal movement *(amphiathroses)*. The bones are strongly joined together by dense fibrous connective tissue.

Types of fibrous joints

Sutures

Bones of the skull vault are linked by a thin band of connective tissue called the *sutural ligament*. Irregular interlocking 'teeth' of the bones add to the strength (see Chapter 11; Fig. 11.5). Since there is virtually no movement, sutures are classed as synarthroses. Some sutures persist into adulthood, whilst others fuse completely and are called *synostoses* (fusion of two bones).
Movements – limited movement up to about the age of 20, then the joints become fixed. This allows for the growth of the brain in childhood.
Examples – limited to joints between bones of the skull vault.

Gomphoses

Singular *gomphosis*. Literally meaning 'bolt', the teeth are held firmly into their socket in the mandible and maxilla by strong connective tissue called the

periodontal ligament (see Chapter 11; Fig. 11.55). Since there is no virtually no movement, they are classed as synarthroses.
Movements – minimal.
Examples – between the teeth and the maxilla/mandible

Syndesmoses

Singular *syndesmosis*. The bones are typically further apart and held together with either a fibrous band (ligament) or sheet (*interosseous membrane*). Whilst strongly holding the bones together, they allow some movement, so they are classed as *amphiarthroses*.
Movements – variable but minimal.
Examples – inferior tibiofibular joint, middle tibiofibular and radioulnar joints

CARTILAGINOUS JOINTS

Like fibrous joints, they lack a synovial cavity and bones are joined by a layer or disc of either hyaline or fibrocartilage. There are two types; primary, or *synchondroses*, which are usually temporary, and secondary, or *symphyses*, which are usually permanent throughout life.

Types of cartilaginous joints

Synchondroses

Singular *synchondrosis*. Bones are directly connected by a plate of *hyaline* cartilage. Includes the epiphyseal plates in immature bones. Generally, these joints are temporary, offer no movement (*synarthroses*), and completely fuse with skeletal maturity, so they become *synostosis* (like sutures) and completely rigid.
Movements – absent or minimal (synarthroses).
Examples – first sternocostal joints, epiphyseal plates - the joint between the metaphysis and epiphysis of a growing long bone

Symphyses

Singular *symphysis*. The ends of the bone are covered with a layer of articular hyaline cartilage, separated by a disc of fibrocartilage and supported by surrounding ligaments. These only occur in the midline of the body. Most are permanent throughout life.
Movements – variable but minimal (amphiarthroses).
Examples – joints between the vertebral bodies (intervertebral discs), sacrococcygeal joint (sometimes fuses), symphysis pubis, manubriosternal joint (often fuses)

CARTILAGE

Cartilage comprises *chondrocytes* (cartilage cells) interspersed in a network, or matrix, of collagen, elastic fibres, and a rubbery substance called *chondroitin*. There are three types of cartilage, their different properties dependent on the relative structure of this matrix:

Hyaline cartilage – most abundant but least strong; smooth, bluish-white appearance. Provides friction-free movement and provides strength and structure. Examples include

- articular surfaces of bones in synovial and cartilaginous joints.
- the cartilage model of the skeleton of the embryo.
- anterior part of ribs.
- the airways of the respiratory system.

Fibrocartilage – Strongest of the three types of cartilage. Provides strength and rigidity between bones. Examples include

- Cartilaginous joints, e.g. symphysis pubis and intervertebral discs
- Articular discs of synovial joints, e.g. the menisci of the knee
- Labrum of synovial joints, e.g. of the hip and shoulder

Elastic cartilage – Not associated with joints. Provides strength, flexibility and shape to structures. Examples include

- The external ear
- The epiglottis in the larynx

FRACTURES

3

CHAPTER CONTENTS

Fractures	21	Fracture Healing	26
Types of Fracture	22	Joint/Soft Tissue Injuries	27
Orthopaedic Management		Describing Traumatic Injuries	28
of Fractures	23		

Trauma to the skeleton from an external force might be sufficient to cause damage to a bone, joint, soft tissues, or a combination of these. Injuries might include the fracture of a bone, dislocation of a joint, or rupture of ligaments, tendons, or muscles. The injuries caused will be reliant on a large number of factors, including the *mechanism of injury* (what happened to the body at the time of injury), where the force was applied, and the age and health of the individual. *Patterns of injury* (or what typically occurs) can be used to predict the likely injuries that will occur according to such factors, and a good clinical history is essential for this reason.

 INSIGHT

When reviewing radiological images relating to trauma, it is important to remember that imaging is performed after the event and cannot see the full effect of the forces that happened at the time of injury. Knowing the mechanism of injury can help picture what happened. It is also important to consider what we cannot see, such as the soft tissues.

FRACTURES

A fracture is any abnormal 'break' in bone continuity and may be complete or partial (incomplete), displaced or non-displaced. It may be gross and clearly visible on imaging, microscopic, or not visible on imaging at all (referred to as *occult*).

Causes

Fractures are caused either through an *abnormal force on normal bone* or a *normal force on abnormal bone* (because of the underlying pathologic condition), by any of the following:

- Direct trauma to the area
- Indirect trauma away from the area (usually rotational / twisting)
- Repetitive strain (stress fracture)
- Underlying pathologic condition (pathological fracture, e.g. bone tumour, osteoporosis).

TYPES OF FRACTURE

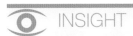 INSIGHT

Understanding the type of fracture helps to understand the mechanism of injury (and predict other injuries) and is also important in the prognosis and management of the fracture.

Simple (closed) fracture – the skin surface is intact, so there is no communication between the fracture and the body surface.
Compound (open) fracture – the skin surface is broken, and there is direct communication between the external environment and the bone fragments; therefore, there is a risk of bone infection (*osteomyelitis*).

Fractures are usually named after the orientation of the fracture lines. The direction of the forces has an effect on the type of fracture caused:

Transverse: horizontally across the bone (across the short axis)
Longitudinal: vertically within a bone (along its long axis)
Oblique: obliquely/diagonally along the bone
Spiral: spiralling up the bone, usually caused by a twisting movement
Comminuted: composed of a number of fragments of bone (more than two parts)
Impacted: when one section of the bone is pushed into another
Compression: the bone is crushed; usually occurs in the vertebral bodies or calcaneum
Depressed: when the bone has been hit by a sharp object and pushed in; usually in the skull
Avulsion: when a fragment of bone is pulled off by a tendon or ligament
Intra-articular: where the fracture extends into the articular surface of a joint. This is an important cause of future complications such as osteoarthritis.
Greenstick: an incomplete fracture; occurs in younger children. Imagine bending a green/young stick, it bends and splinters rather than snaps in two.

Pathological: caused by any underlying pathologic condition or disease process which weakens the bone.

Subsequent chapters will provide examples of fractures associated with specific bones.

 INSIGHT

Children's bones tend to be softer, more flexible and 'bendy' than mature bones because they contain a relatively higher proportion of organic collagen (osteoid) matrix than inorganic (mineral) material. This is why there are different *patterns of injury* between children and adults.

ORTHOPAEDIC MANAGEMENT OF FRACTURES

Diagnosis

Signs and symptoms of a fracture may include the following:
- Pain and local tenderness
- Soft tissue swelling and bruising (*ecchymosis*)
- Deformity, e.g., angulation, rotation, or shortening of a limb
- Abnormal movement and *crepitus* (grating or cracking)

Diagnosis is usually confirmed radiographically, and the following are assessed:
- The number and location of fracture fragments
- The amount and direction of movement (displacement)
- The presence of other unsuspected injury or underlying pathologic condition
- Evidence of soft tissue injury or foreign bodies

These aspects are required as part of a description of the findings (such as a clinical report or preliminary image evaluation; a 'comment'). Other forms of imaging may be required to fully evaluate the extent of these aspects and guide management.

 INSIGHT

When reviewing radiological images, it is important to apply a *systematic approach* and scrutinise all parts of the images through a *'satisfaction of search'* to avoid missing abnormalities. If one abnormality is identified, look for more.

The three principles of fracture management are *reduction, immobilisation,* and *rehabilitation*.

Reduction

The aim of reduction is to realign the bones to as near the normal position as possible, thereby promoting faster healing. The earlier this is done, the better for ease and to reduce complications. It is also required to prevent neurovascular compromise of affected parts in certain severely displaced injuries.

Methods available include the following:

Closed manipulation: where the bones are 'manoeuvred' back into position. May be performed under an anaesthetic or with analgesia

Open reduction: a surgical operation where the bones are manipulated directly

Mechanical traction: historically used for fractures of the femur, particularly where the contraction of strong muscles prevents manipulation. A weight is attached to apply tension, which counteracts the muscular pull, slowly aligning the bones. It is now less commonly used with the advent of more advanced reduction techniques.

Immobilisation

This ensures that the manipulated fragments of bone maintain their alignment; it therefore encourages faster healing as fractures heal better when there is minimal movement between fragments. Immobilisation may not be required if the fracture is inherently stable (and not likely to move) but does help to reduce pain.

Methods available include the following:

Casts: usually used after closed manipulation. Provides a rigid, hard, protective cover. Plaster of Paris casts are now more commonly replaced with synthetic materials and devices.

Splints: numerous types available; can be made of aluminium, plastic or polystyrene; tend to be used for hand/finger injuries

External fixation: a fixation device with pins is inserted into the bones to stabilise the fracture from the outside without the need for an operation. Often temporarily applied on unstable fractures where other investigations or treatment is required before more permanent fixation. Ilizarov frames are more permanent external devices used for very complex leg fractures.

Open reduction internal fixation (ORIF): Screws and plates (Fig. 3.1), pins/wires, or intramedullary nails (Fig. 3.2) inserted during open reduction to internally stabilise the bone fragments. Used in unstable or comminuted fractures and when other methods are difficult to apply (e.g., for the neck of the femur)

Rehabilitation

This takes place as soon as reduction and immobilisation allow, to *preserve function* and *promote healing* as normal forces are necessary for good bone health. This is especially important with areas of high functional demand like the hands and fingers and can heavily impact patient outcomes. This typically involves physiotherapy and exercises.

Fig. 3.1 Early radiographic signs of provisional callous (arrowed): left foot. This is a metatarsal stress (March) fracture in a patient with osteoporosis (note reduced bone density). Screws from a previous ORIF in the tarsal bones are also evident. (From STATdx © Elsevier)

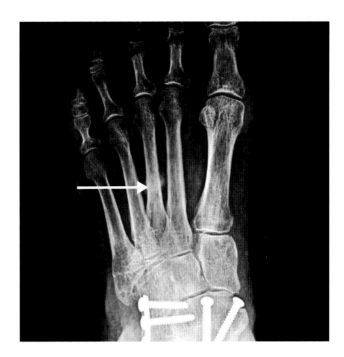

Fig. 3.2 Late radiographic signs of a femoral fracture healing (arrowed). There is prominent dense sclerotic callous and remodelling of the medullary cavity. This fracture has been treated with an intramedullary nail. (From STATdx © Elsevier)

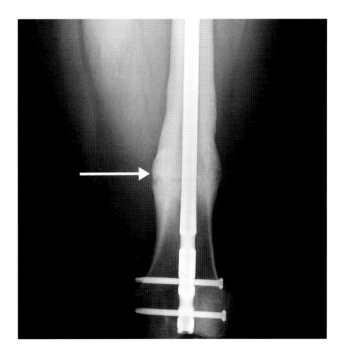

FRACTURE HEALING

Starts immediately after the fracture has occurred through a series of overlapping stages. Sometimes referred to as reaction (days), repair (weeks), remodelling (months).

1. A collection of blood (*haematoma*) and a clot is formed owing to damaged blood vessels in the medullary canal, cortex and periosteum.
2. Within 24 h, the haematoma is converted into vascularised, *fibroblastic* (fibrous building) *granulation* (inflammatory) connective tissue. Osteoclasts and white blood cells remove the dead bone at the ends of the fracture site.
3. After approximately seven days, cartilage and osteoid (organic bone) tissue are laid down by the chondroblasts and osteoblasts, forming an irregular, immature new bone matrix called provisional callous (or *woven bone*).
4. Provisional callous is converted into 'normal' cortical bone containing *Haversian systems* over a period of weeks.
5. After a period of weeks to months, the bone is remodelled by osteoclasts and osteoblasts to regain its original shape and restore the medullary cavity.

Radiographically, stages three to five will progress around the fracture from faint 'hazy' provisional callous (Fig. 3.1) to more prominent dense sclerotic callous (Fig. 3.2) and finally more normal bone.

Factors influencing the rate of healing

The rate of healing varies from individual to individual. While most fractures heal well, some display *delayed union* or *non-union*. The following factors may influence the rate of fracture healing and whether these complications occur:

Malunion: occurs because of poor reduction where the fracture fragments are not well aligned and may not unite and cause a residual deformity or even disability

Infection: common with compound (open) fractures. Infection within the bone (osteomyelitis) can be very difficult to treat.

Foreign bodies: if present, they may introduce infection or come between the fracture fragments preventing healing. Soft tissue (e.g., muscle or ligaments) overlying the fragments will have a similar effect.

Bone fragments: multiple small bone fragments will delay healing if they are not removed by the body's own inflammatory response or through appropriate treatment.

Poor immobilisation: movement at the fracture site may prevent healing and new bone formation.

Age: generally, the older the person, the longer the healing owing to a decreased blood supply and slower metabolic rates. Paediatric fractures tend to heal faster and with better remodelling because of rapid bone turnover.

Fractures involving epiphyseal (growth) plates, however, may affect the growth of that bone.

Blood supply: bone turnover and repair requires an adequate blood supply. Interruption to this blood supply, such as rupture of the blood vessels caused by injury, can cause non-union and death of the bone, *osteonecrosis* (discussed in Chapter 4). Some bones (e.g., scaphoid and head of the femur) are more prone to this because of their unique blood supply.

General health/diet – bone repair requires the same nutrients (e.g., calcium), resources and stresses (e.g., exercise) as in normal bone. Other underlying health conditions, dietary deficiencies, or drugs may influence fracture healing and bone health generally.

JOINT/SOFT TISSUE INJURIES

Joints are also prone to injury from external forces in the same way bones are. Unless the bones of a joint are fractured, then joint abnormalities are more difficult to visualise radiographically (on computed tomography (CT) or X-ray) as most soft tissue structures are radiolucent or lack inherent contrast. While individual structures such as ligaments, tendons, and muscles may not be seen, there are indirect signs of joint injury. Some of the types of joint injury and soft tissue signs include the following:

Dislocation: complete loss of apposition/alignment of the articular surfaces of the bones. Referred to as fracture-dislocation if there is also a fracture present

Subluxation: incomplete loss of apposition/alignment of the articular surfaces of the bones (partial dislocation)

Diastasis: widening of the joint space; the articular surfaces are pulled apart

Effusion: increase in the amount of fluid within the joint cavity. If blood, then it is referred to as haemarthrosis. Visualised by increased soft tissue opacity in the joint cavity (e.g. in the knee) or by displacement of soft tissue planes or fat pads (e.g., in the elbow, See Chapter 5; Fig. 5.6)

Lipohaemarthrosis: similar to effusion/haemarthrosis but contains fat (lipo-) and blood (haem-) within the joint capsule, indicative of a definite intra-articular fracture. Demonstrated as a horizontal line, most common in the knee (See Chapter 7; Fig. 7.23)

Soft tissue and sometimes occult bone injury, while not readily visible on radiographs or CT, can be better visualised using magnetic resonance imaging and, in many cases, ultrasound.

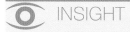 INSIGHT

It is important when dealing with dislocations that associated bone fracture is considered. Imaging both pre- and post-reduction of a dislocation is important to look for bony fragments caused both by the injury or subsequent manipulation, particularly within the joint cavity.

DESCRIBING TRAUMATIC INJURIES

When describing an injury or abnormality, then classification systems (e.g., Salter Harris) and eponyms (e.g., Colle's fracture) can be used. However, these can be used inaccurately or provide confusion and ambiguity. It is important to describe the important features clearly and concisely using appropriate anatomical and medical terminology. Consider the following:

WHAT is the abnormality? (e.g., transverse fracture, dislocation)

WHERE is the abnormality; which bone or joint, which part of the bone? (e.g., neck of humerus, acromio-clavicular joint)

HOW is it displaced; how much and which way? (e.g., undisplaced, minimal displacement; anteriorly, laterally)

 INSIGHT

Getting used to describing fractures, rather than relying on eponyms, is useful for developing anatomical knowledge and terminology.

When describing the direction of displacement, it is the convention to describe the movement of the more distal part (i.e., the bit that is not attached) in relation to the rest of the body (i.e., the bit that is still attached) and the normal anatomical position

PATHOLOGY

4

CHAPTER CONTENTS

Changes Caused by		Causes (Types) of Pathologic	
The Pathologic Condition	29	Conditions	39
Loss of bone density —		Neoplasms (tumours)	40
Osteopaenia	30	Metabolic disease	51
Focal bone destruction	33	Endocrine	51
Increase in bone density —		Infections	56
Osteosclerosis	33	Arthritis	57
New bone growth	37		

Pathology is the study of disease. This chapter only aims to introduce and cover some of the more common types of diseases that will be encountered and can be detected radiologically, particularly on radiographs. Radiographs and images from other modalities have been included to demonstrate some pathologic conditions. However, these are often advanced examples, and it should be remembered that early signs may not be as obvious (or not at all); it may take a change in bone density of 30%-50% to be visible on radiographs.

Pathology seen in bones and joints may be considered by the changes they cause *(pathophysiology)* or by the type, or underlying cause *(aetiology)*, of the pathologic condition. Both will be discussed briefly in this chapter.

CHANGES CAUSED BY THE PATHOLOGIC CONDITION

 INSIGHT

'Before you can know what is abnormal, you must first know what is normal'.

Identifying abnormalities on images relies on us knowing what 'normal' is supposed to look like. Understanding the normal appearances, including those related to age and normal variants, gives us a reference point to spot when things are abnormal. Having a good understanding of the anatomy and 'normal' images helps to build this appreciation of normal.

When considering bone pathologic conditions on radiological images, density, size, location, and shape are all very important considerations. When looking for evidence of pathologic conditions (including fractures), the radiographic appearances of what can be seen may be classed as whether the bone appears too black (more radiolucent or *osteolytic*) or too white (more radiopaque or *sclerotic*).

Loss of bone density — *Osteopaenia*

Literally means 'bone poverty.' This is usually a decrease in the amount of calcium (and other minerals) present in the bone, either in that, the proportion of calcium (to other components) is reduced, or there is just less bone tissue generally. The loss of calcium means the bone becomes less dense in structure and appears more radiolucent, or 'darker,' on a radiograph. This may be an overall loss of density or be specific to particular areas of bone. Pathologies that cause a reduction in bone density may be referred to as *destructive diseases*.

Reduced bone density is termed *osteopaenia* and is a descriptive appearance rather than a specific disease or condition. It may be caused by a range of different pathologic types, but when generalised is most commonly associated with pathologies that affect bone metabolism and turnover, either because of a reduction in the mineral content or the altered balance of osteoblast and osteoclast activity resulting in an overall decrease in bone.

Osteoporosis (Figs. 4.1, 4.2)
Osteoporosis means 'porous bones.' It is a deficiency in the bone matrix because of a reduction in bone formation, due to which the bones fracture easily. The bone composition (and proportion of calcium) is normal; there is just less bone, the cortical bone becomes thinned, and cancellous bone loses trabeculae. Osteoporosis is the most common cause of osteopaenia, particularly in older people. It is normally asymptomatic and may be detected incidentally or when a fragility fracture (commonly vertebral bodies, neck of femur, and wrist) occurs because of weakened bone.

Causes
The causes are extensive; they include the following: increasing age (senile osteoporosis); post-menopausal (reduced oestrogen levels affect bone metabolism); overuse of steroids; and disuse (Fig. 4.1), for example, because of immobilisation following fracture (if activity returns, the bone returns to normal)

Radiological signs
The affected bone appears more radiolucent; the larger primary trabeculae may appear more prominent as smaller secondary trabeculae are reduced first. Cortices are thinned. Fragility fractures are most common in the spine (wedge compression fractures Fig. 4.2). The diagnosis of osteoporosis cannot be made on radiographs but by *dual-energy X-ray absorptiometry* (DXA/DEXA)

Osteomalacia and rickets (Figs. 4.3, 4.4)
An overall decrease in bone mineralisation. Unlike osteoporosis, the amount of bone tissues is similar; it is just of poorer quality and is softer

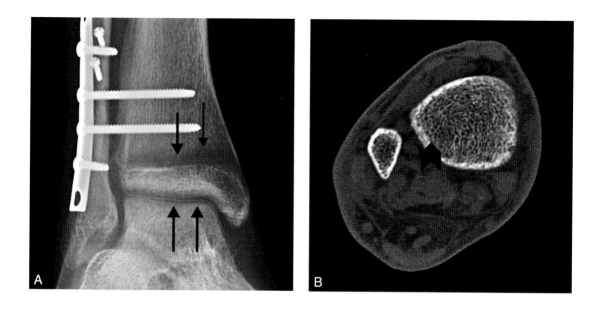

Fig. 4.1 Localised 'disuse' osteoporosis. AP mortise projection (A) and axial CT (B) of the ankle. Reduced bone density can be seen as horizontal lucent bands (arrows) and small lucencies within the bone (arrowhead). (From STATdx © Elsevier 2022)

Fig. 4.2 Osteoporotic vertebral body fracture (arrow). Sagittal CT (A) and lateral radiograph (B). Note loss of body height compared to those above and below and reduced cancellous bone density compared to the outer cortex. (From STATdx © Elsevier 2022)

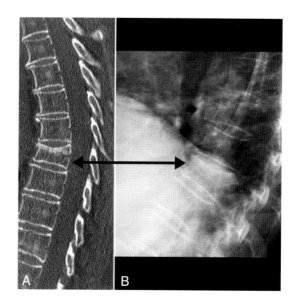

Fig. 4.3 Osteomalacia; left femur. Faint horizontal lucency (arrow), typical of a *Looser's zone*. The bone density appears normal, though radiographs are not sensitive until the bone loss is significant. (From STATdx © Elsevier 2022)

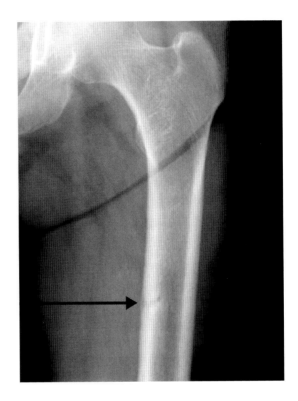

Fig. 4.4 Rickets; right knee. Widened epiphyseal plate (arrows) and splayed metaphyses (arrowhead) (From STATdx © Elsevier 2022)

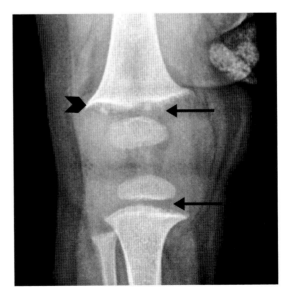

because of reduced mineral content. Though practically identical, in mature skeletons, this is called *osteomalacia*, and in immature skeletons, it is called *rickets*, where it involves the epiphyseal plates and will affect bone growth.

Causes
Causes include diet low in calcium, phosphorous, or vitamin D (or because of lack of sunlight); malabsorption syndromes (e.g., coeliac disease, Crohn's disease); renal disease.

Radiological signs
Osteomalacia (Fig. 4.3): ill-defined narrow lucent bands of decalcification 2–3 mm wide called *Looser's zones* or '*pseudo (false) fractures*'.
Rickets (Fig. 4.4): widening of the growth plates and 'splaying' of the metaphyses, particularly of the long bones.

Focal bone destruction

A focal area of reduced bone density is called an *osteolytic* (or just lytic) lesion and is often associated with bone tumours (benign or malignant), aggressive destructive pathologies such as *osteomyelitis* (bone infection), or erosive diseases like *rheumatoid arthritis*. Bone destruction associated with such pathologies is caused by the 'destruction' or replacement of normal bone. The more clearly defined the area of destruction is, then, generally, the less aggressive and slower growing the disease.

Increase in bone density — *Osteosclerosis*

This is usually an increase in the amount of calcium present or an increase in the amount of bone generally, resulting in the bone becoming denser in structure. The bone becomes more radiopaque and therefore appears *sclerotic*, or 'whiter' on the radiograph. It is caused by pathologies that either result in an increase in the relative mineral matrix of the bone or by an imbalance in osteoblast and osteoclast activity resulting in an abundance of bone formation. Pathologies that cause an increase in bone are *additive diseases*.

Paget's disease (Figs 4.5, 4.6, 11.25)
A metabolic disorder that causes abnormal bone remodelling leading to thickening and osteosclerosis. It has several progressive phases: first, bone resorption (active phase caused by increased osteoclast activity); then irregular coarse cortical and cancellous bone formation (mixed osteoclast and osteoblast activity); and finally, bone sclerosis (excessive osteoblast activity). More common in older males, this disease causes bone pain and limb deformities but may also be asymptomatic and is often identified as an incidental finding on imaging. It most commonly affects the skull, femora, tibiae, lumbar spine and pelvis.

Fig. 4.5 Paget disease; lateral tibia (A) and lumbar spine (B) projections. Lytic active stage (arrows) surrounded by bone enlargement, coarse irregular trabeculae and sclerosis (arrowheads) (From STATdx © Elsevier 2022)

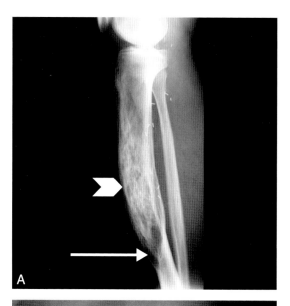

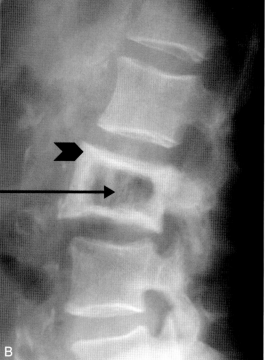

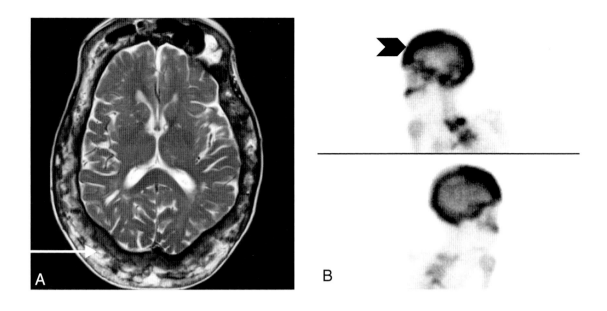

Fig. 4.6 Paget disease; axial T2 MRI head (A) and bone scintigraphy scan (B). Thickened sclerotic skull vault (arrow) and increased isotope uptake (arrowhead). (From STATdx © Elsevier 2022)

Causes
The causes are uncertain but thought to include an inflammatory response caused by viral disease or genetic causes.

Radiological signs
The signs are dependent on stage: early lytic (lucent) regions followed by coarsened trabecular pattern, cortical thickening and sclerosis, bone enlargement and bowing of affected long bones.

Osteonecrosis (Figs. 4.7, 4.8)
Osteonecrosis means bone death, and it is otherwise known as *avascular necrosis* because of a poor or interrupted blood supply, often a consequence of a fracture involving the blood vessels. It is more commonly seen in bones mostly covered by cartilage (e.g. femoral head, talus). After the area of affected bone tissue dies, there is increased osteoblastic activity, which aims to repair the bone and causes osteosclerosis. As the bones are weakened, the bone structure may collapse completely.

Similar appearances may be seen in immature skeletons associated with the ossification growth centres, called *osteochondrosis*.

Different bones normally have specific eponyms when affected (e.g. Legg-Calve-Perthes disease of the femoral head (Fig. 4.7), Kienbock's disease of the lunate).

Fig. 4.7 Idiopathic osteonecrosis of the right hip (Legg-Calve-Perthes disease). Pelvis radiograph (A) and coronal T1W MRI (B). There is evidence of osteosclerosis and collapse of the femoral head (arrow) compared to the left. (From STATdx © Elsevier 2022)

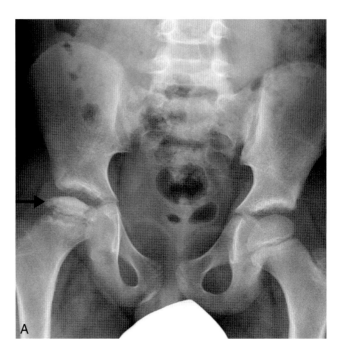

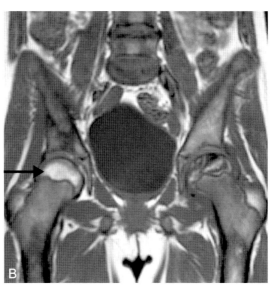

Causes

The causes are extensive and include trauma, where the blood supply to the bone is interrupted (most common in the femoral head and scaphoid); steroid and alcohol use; and idiopathic (no known cause).

Fig. 4.8 Early osteonecrosis. Coronal T2W MRI wrist showing hyperintense bone marrow oedema (arrow). (From STATdx © Elsevier 2022)

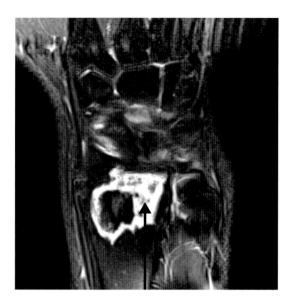

Radiological signs

The radiological signs include early lucency in subchondral bone (crescent sign) followed by increased sclerosis, collapse, and fragmentation of bone. Magnetic resonance imaging (MRI) is more sensitive to early diagnosis than radiographs.

New bone growth

Whilst a number of bone pathologic conditions result in the removal of bone, others cause the formation of new bone through the calcification and ossification of soft tissues or new bone growths. Some of these types of bone 'addition' include:

- **Exostosis**: also known as *osteoma*, these are additional bone growths that grow from the surface of a bone. They may be *sessile* (broad-base) or *pedunculated* (on a stalk, like a mushroom (Fig. 4.13)).
- **Osteophytes**; 'bone spurs' that grow adjacent to a joint surface, usually result from hyaline cartilage damage in degenerative joint disease; *osteoarthritis* (Figs. 4.32, 4.33).
- **Ensthesophytes**; similar in appearance to osteophytes but is ossification of the insertion (*enthesis*) of a ligament or tendon on a bone. May be degenerative or caused by inflammatory pathologic conditions.
- **Syndesmophytes**; similar in appearance to osteophytes and enthesophytes but are specifically calcification or ossification of ligaments and intervertebral discs of the spine. Associated with inflammatory disease of the spine.
- **Ankylosis**; bony fusion of the bones of a joint, normally because of longstanding significant inflammation.

Ankylosing spondylitis (Figs. 4.9, 4.10)

This is a longstanding inflammatory condition mainly of the axial skeleton (spine and sacro-iliac joints) leading to ossification of the ligaments and eventually ankylosis (fusion). The disease first presents in young adults. Fusion of the spine means fractures may occur even with minor trauma, like snapping a stick of chalk.

Causes

The causes are mostly genetic and hereditary; it is more common if a specific antigen (something that causes an immune response) called HLA-B27 is present in the body. People with inflammatory bowel disease can also develop a condition similar to ankylosing spondylitis.

Radiological signs

The radiological signs start with fine syndesmophytes around intervertebral spaces and 'squaring' and sclerosis of the vertebral body corners. There is eventual complete fusion of the sacro-iliac joints, spine (bamboo spine, Fig. 4.9) and sometimes other joints.

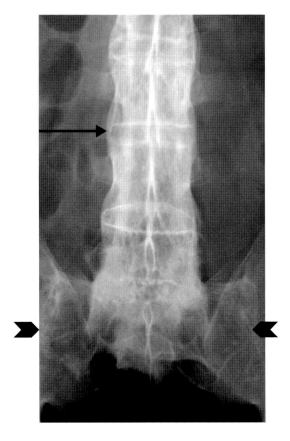

Fig. 4.9 Ankylosing spondylitis; Lumbar spine. Fusion of the vertebral bodies (arrow) – Bamboo spine – and sacro-iliac joints (arrowheads). (From STATdx © Elsevier 2022)

Fig. 4.10 Ankylosing spondylitis; Cervical spine. Fusion of the vertebral bodies (arrow) and facet joints (arrowhead). (From STATdx © Elsevier 2022)

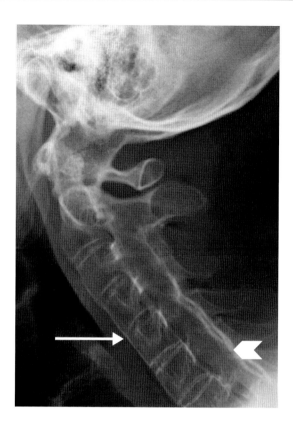

CAUSES (TYPES) OF PATHOLOGIC CONDITIONS

The effects and appearances of bone disease described previously can be caused by pathologies that may be categorised by the underlying cause (a*etiology*). These include those listed here, but sometimes there is overlap and crossover between them. Some of these will be considered in the rest of this chapter.

Traumatic – relating to injury (covered in Chapter 3)

Degenerative – 'wear and tear' because of overuse or ageing; linked to trauma

Neoplastic – relating to tumours (benign or malignant)

Metabolic – relating to metabolism and the action of chemicals and nutrients

Endocrine – relating to the actions of hormones

Inflammatory – relating to inflammation and the body's immune response

Congenital – relating to a condition present at birth; developmental or genetic

Infective – relating to an infection (e.g. osteomyelitis and septic arthritis)

Arthritic – relating to joints (might be caused by any of the categories above).

Neoplasms (tumours)

Neoplasm (meaning new form/shape) is a term used to describe the abnormal growth of tissue. When there is a mass of this tissue, it is called a *tumour*. These may be classed as *benign* (cannot spread or invade other tissues), *in-situ* or potentially malignant (may spread and invade other tissues) and *malignant* (will spread and invade other tissues; *cancer*). When they spread (metastasise), malignant tumours will cause further tumours to grow in other tissues, called *metastases*. A *primary* neoplasm is the original site or tumour. The metastases from the spread are called *secondary* neoplasms/tumours.

Bone tumours may be both benign and malignant; primary and secondary. Whilst there may be some overlap, there are typical radiological appearances that may help to differentiate benign and malignant. Other pathologies like osteomyelitis and Paget's may share similar features to bone neoplasms and can sometimes be difficult to distinguish. The features seen are often related to how fast the pathologic condition grows or how aggressive it is.

Benign/slow-growing (Fig. 4.11):

Typical features include

- **Well defined edge**; clear definition between normal and abnormal bone (*narrow zone of transition*).
- **Cortical outline**; suggests slow-growing as the bone has time to lay down new bone in response.

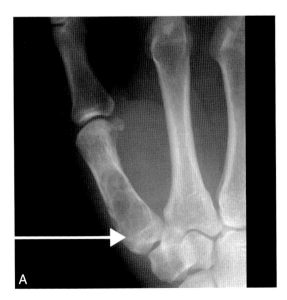
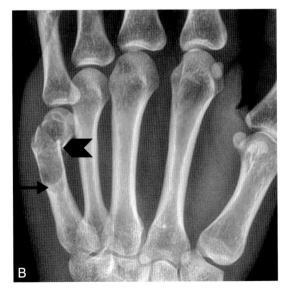

Fig. 4.11 Enchondroma; metacarpals. Features of a benign lesion include a narrow zone of transition (arrow), homogeneous (lucent) texture, and no periosteal reaction. Note the pathological fracture on image B (arrowhead). (From STATdx © Elsevier 2022)

- **No cortical destruction or periosteal reaction**; cortex may be thinned but is intact. Pathological fractures can occur though as a result of weakened bone.
- **No soft tissue mass or swelling**; does not spread to surrounding tissue.
- **Internal texture/density is *homogeneous*** (similar throughout); lytic, or sclerotic. The matrix of neoplasm is all the same.
- **Singular;** tend not to be multiple (though some are).

Malignant/aggressive (Fig. 4.12):

- **Ill-defined edge;** no clear definition between normal and abnormal bone (*wide zone of transition*). The bone may appear 'patchy' (*moth-eaten* or *permeative)* as it spreads within bone.
- **No cortical outline**; suggests faster growing as spread outweighs the ability for new bone to be laid down.
- **Destruction of the cortex and/or periosteal reaction**; caused as the tumour destroys cortex and displaces periosteum as it spreads outside of the bone.
- **May be a soft tissue mass or swelling** as it spreads to (or from) surrounding soft tissues.
- **Internal density/texture is *heterogeneous*** (mixed areas of lucency and sclerosis) because of the irregular spread of the tumour within normal bone.
- May be **multiple** (may also be singular), either because of secondary tumours (metastases) or multiple areas of primary tumour within the bone.

As with other pathologies, radiographs may not always demonstrate all features of bone neoplasms and additional imaging (particularly MRI and computed tomography (CT)), laboratory tests, and biopsies may be required for a full evaluation and definitive diagnosis. Nuclear medicine is useful to evaluate the spread of metastatic disease throughout the skeleton.

Benign tumours
Common examples include the following:

Enchondroma (Fig. 4.11)
Benign tumour of mature hyaline cartilage in the medullary canal. The most common sites are the long bones of the hands and feet (prone to fracture) and other long bones. Sometimes completely lucent, particularly in the hands and feet, or sclerotic (like popcorn) if calcified.

Osteochondroma   (Fig. 4.13)
Produces sessile or pedunculated exostoses (outgrowths) of bone covered in a cartilage 'cap.' Continuation of the cortex and medullary canal and can appear 'mushroom' or 'cauliflower shape.' Mostly occurring at the metaphysis of long bones, they almost always point away from the adjacent joint. Can be numerous; *multiple hereditary exostoses*. Whilst normally benign, the cartilage cap can turn (*differentiate*) into malignant chondrosarcoma, and this is better evaluated on ultrasound or MRI as it usually cannot be seen on radiographs.

Fig. 4.12 Osteosarcoma; distal femur lateral radiograph (A) and MRI (B). Features of a malignant lesion include mixed sclerotic/lucent texture, not clearly defined, periosteal reaction (arrow), cortical destruction of the anterior cortex, multiple deposits (curved arrow), and soft tissue mass (arrowhead). (From STATdx © Elsevier 2022)

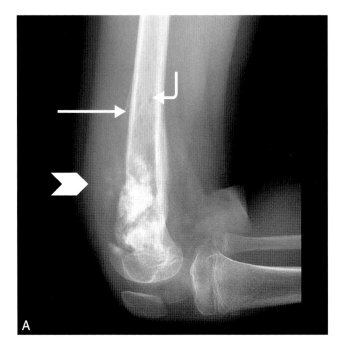

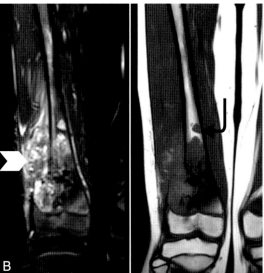

Osteoid osteoma (Fig. 4.14)

Small (<2 cm) tumours of the osteoid (organic) tissue of bone. The tumour is lytic, but dense reactive sclerosis surrounds it, which may obscure the actual tumour on radiographs. Despite being benign, osteomas are very painful, particularly at night. CT is used to evaluate the tumour and guide interventional treatment.

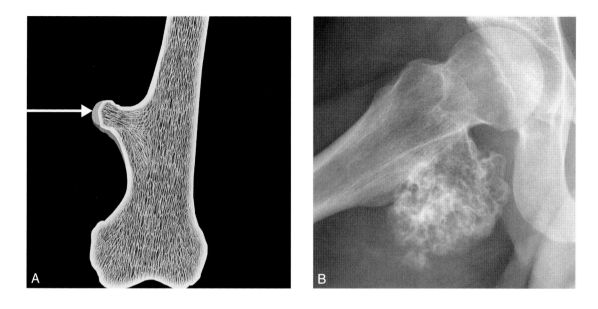

Fig. 4.13 Osteochondroma; distal and proximal femur. The 'stalk' of the exostosis is continuous with the cortex and medullary canal. The cartilage cap (arrow) is not visible radiographically. (From STATdx © Elsevier 2022)

Osteoma

Benign tumour which produces mature, dense bone on the surface of the bone cortex. Appears as well defined sessile (flattened) exostoses of the cortex of the bone. Does not normally communicate with the medullary canal.

Giant cell tumour

Otherwise called osteoclastoma as involves giant osteoclast-like cells. Appear as a well defined lucent area within the epiphysis (usually against the articular surface), particularly around the knee and distal radius. Expands and thins the cortex without breaching it.

Simple (unicameral) bone cysts (Fig. 4.15)

These are cavities arising from within the medullary cavity filled with fluid rather than true neoplasms. Like other benign tumours, they may be asymptomatic and only detected incidentally or if they cause a pathological fracture. Occurring mainly in the metaphyses of long bones (especially the proximal humerus), radiographically, they have the typical appearances of benign tumours.

Malignant tumours

These may be primary neoplasms or secondary metastases. Appearances may be variable according to the type and aggressiveness of the tumour but generally demonstrate the more typical appearances of malignancy previously described.

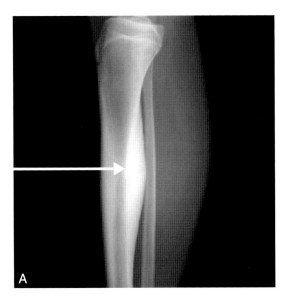
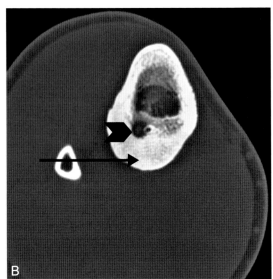

Fig. 4.14 Osteoid osteoma; right tibia. The radiograph (A) demonstrates a dense sclerotic reaction (arrows), but the tumour appears as a lytic central area, called a nidus (arrowhead) on axial CT (B). (From STATdx © Elsevier 2022)

Osteosarcoma (Figs. 4.12, 4.16, 4.17, 4.18)

This is a tumour of osteoblasts (also known as *osteogenic sarcoma*, meaning bone forming tumour of connective tissue); production of irregular osteoid bone tissue is a principal feature.

These tumours can develop in any bone but are predominantly found in the metaphyses of long bones, particularly around the knee. Most primary osteosarcomas occur in young adults and adolescents (most common malignant bone tumour in this age group), but it is also seen in older persons secondary to other diseases such as Paget's disease. Osteosarcomas readily metastasise to the lungs.

Radiological features are variable but demonstrate hallmark features of aggressive lesions, including ill-defined heterogenous texture, cortical destruction, prominent patterns of periosteal reaction, and soft tissue masses and calcifications (Figs. 4.12, 4.16). Whilst radiographs can normally suggest a diagnosis, MRI is useful for full tumour evaluation and involvement of soft tissues (Fig. 4.12), and CT and nuclear medicine can be used to identify lung and bone metastases, respectively (Figs. 4.17, 4.18).

Ewing's sarcoma (Fig. 4.19)

Sometimes difficult to distinguish from osteosarcomas, there are some differentiating features. Ewing's sarcoma tends to occur at younger ages (children and young adolescents) and normally involves the diaphysis of long bones rather than the metaphysis. Ewing's sarcomas do not produce a new

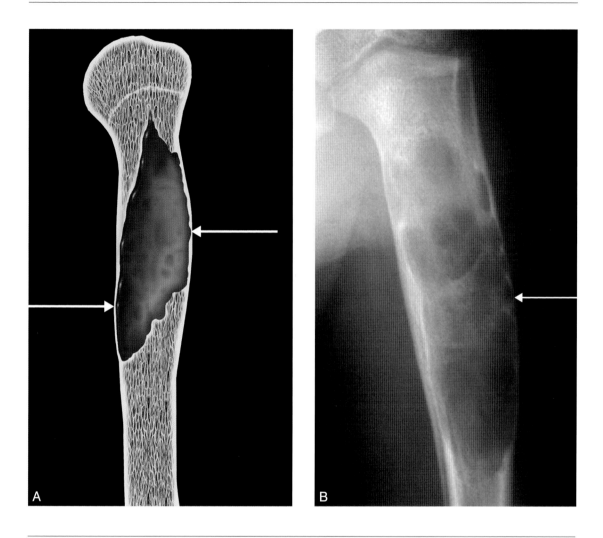

Fig. 4.15 Simple bone cyst; left humerus. Well defined lucent area which thins but does not break the cortex (arrows). (From STATdx © Elsevier 2022)

bone matrix, so radiographically appear more lytic, but there might be normal reactive bone formation if it grows slowly. Periosteal reaction often appears as uninterrupted layers like an onion (known as *lamellar*), a different pattern to that normally seen in osteosarcomas.

Chondrosarcoma

A tumour of hyaline cartilage cells that occur either in otherwise normal bone or secondary to a previously benign enchondroma or osteochondroma. Tend to occur in older people, mostly in the long bones and pelvis. Radiographically they are predominantly lucent with calcification of the tumour. It can be

Fig. 4.16 Osteosarcoma; distal femur. Features of a malignant lesion include ill-defined mixed sclerotic/lytic texture, periosteal reaction (arrow), cortical destruction and calcified soft tissue mass (arrowhead). (From STATdx © Elsevier 2022)

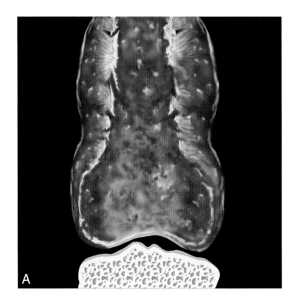

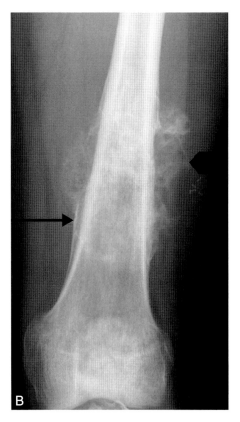

Fig. 4.17 Osteosarcoma; coronal PET/CT image of the distal femur. Focal increased uptake (arrow) within the bone and soft tissue components of the tumour. (From STATdx © Elsevier 2022)

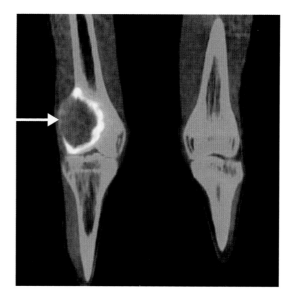

Fig. 4.18 Osteosarcoma metastases; axial chest CT demonstrating multiple lung metastases (arrows). (From STATdx © Elsevier 2022)

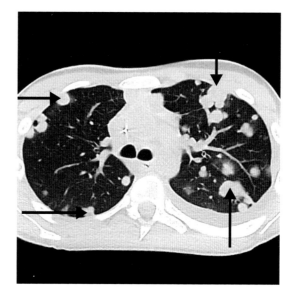

Fig. 4.19 Ewing sarcoma; right femur. Ill-defined lytic lesion with sclerotic bone reaction involving the diaphysis mainly. Onion-skin periosteal reaction (arrow). (From STATdx © Elsevier 2022)

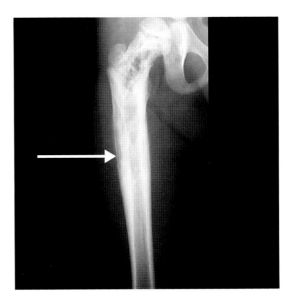

difficult to differentiate from benign enchondroma, so additional imaging is normally necessary.

Multiple myeloma (Myelomatosis) (Fig. 4.20)

This is a tumour of plasma cells in the bone marrow. The most common primary bone tumour affecting older people. Destroys bone tissue and produces multiple, widespread well defined lytic lesions in bones. Common sites are the spine, skull, ribs, pelvis, shoulder girdle and humerus.

Fig. 4.20 Multiple myeloma. Classic multiple, well defined round lytic lesions are seen throughout the skeleton, including the skull. (From STATdx © Elsevier 2022)

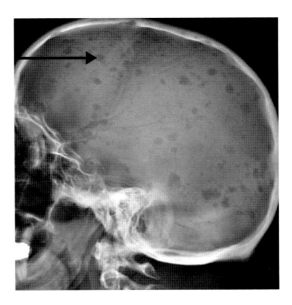

Unlike other widespread skeletal and metastatic diseases, traditional nuclear medicine bone scans are not useful as they cannot identify tumour deposits. Radiographic skeletal survey, full-body MRI, or positron emission tomography (PET)/CT are more widely used.

Secondary bone tumours (Figs. 4.21, 4.22, 4.23)

Metastases are much more common than primary bone tumours. Although up to half of all cancers will eventually spread to the bones, a large proportion come from a primary tumour of the prostate, breast, lung, kidney or thyroid. They produce single or multiple, extremely painful tumours which appear different depending on the primary site (e.g., prostate tends to cause sclerotic lesions whilst lung and kidney tend to produce lytic lesions). Periosteal reaction is less common than in other malignant bone tumours and osteomyelitis (which can mimic malignancy).

Fig. 4.21 Sclerotic metastases from prostate cancer; lumbar spine. All of the visualised vertebrae and ribs are involved. (From STATdx © Elsevier 2022)

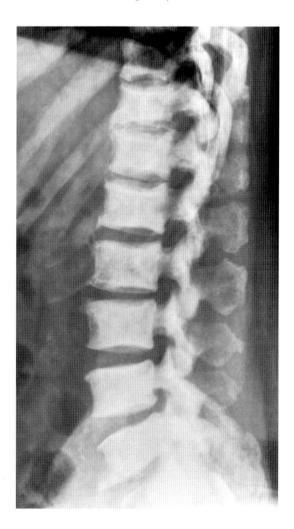

Fig. 4.22 Lytic metastasis from breast cancer; right femur. Note that it lacks many features seen in malignant tumours; it is well defined, and there is no periosteal reaction, though it does destroy the cortex (arrow). (From STATdx © Elsevier 2022)

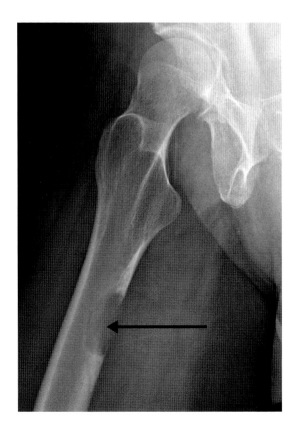

Fig. 4.23 Metastases; bone scan. Multiple metastases can be seen throughout the spine, sternum and pelvis. (From STATdx © Elsevier 2022)

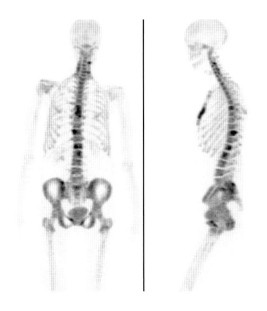

Common sites are where red bone marrow is present, such as the vertebral bodies, proximal ends of large long bones (e.g., femur and humerus), pelvis, ribs, and the skull. Up to 50% of bone mass must be altered to see metastases on radiographs. Nuclear medicine techniques are far more sensitive and can assess the entire skeleton more effectively than other imaging modalities.

Metabolic disease

Bone growth, turnover, maintenance and repair need a continuous supply of certain elements to synthesise the organic osteoid matrix; and mineralisation by calcium and other minerals. It also requires the precise actions of hormones, vitamins, and enzymes to regulate these processes. Any imbalance in bone homeostasis can lead to abnormalities in the skeleton and is called *metabolic bone disease*. Normally the cause is external to the skeleton, and most commonly, these are because of dietary insufficiencies, absorption diseases (e.g., of the kidneys, gastrointestinal tract or liver) and hormonal diseases, though some causes are unknown.

Metabolic diseases cause either an abnormal amount of bone or abnormal bone composition and the radiological changes seen will reflect this. Examples of metabolic bone disease include those already discussed: *osteoporosis, osteomalacia/rickets* and *Paget's*.

The effect of such diseases on the bones can be very significant, and sometimes the underlying cause (e.g. genetics) cannot be treated, but often the changes can be reversed or improved by the use of drugs or dietary supplements.

Vitamin D deficiency

Vitamin D is found in, for example, milk, eggs, fish, liver, and oil and is produced by the body when the skin is exposed to ultraviolet rays from the sun. Vitamin D is essential in allowing the body to absorb calcium and phosphate, the most important components of bone mineralisation. A decrease in the vitamin can result in *osteomalacia* (in adults) or *rickets* (in children).

Vitamin C deficiency

Vitamin C is found in, for example, fresh fruit and vegetables. Vitamin C is essential in collagen production for the organic bone matrix and muscle function. A decrease in the vitamin may result in *scurvy*, which is most common in young children, although it can occur at any age. Radiologically the appearances include reduced bone density (osteopaenia) with splaying, fractures, and sclerosis of the metaphyses (Fig. 4.24).

Endocrine

The action of a number of hormones from various glands are essential in the normal development and homeostasis of bones. Over or under secretion of these hormones can cause a wide range of skeletal changes dependent on when

Fig. 4.24 Scurvy; left tibia/fibula. Features include general osteopaenia, splaying and fractures of the metaphyseal corners (arrowhead) and sclerosis of the metaphyseal line (arrow). (From STATdx © Elsevier 2022)

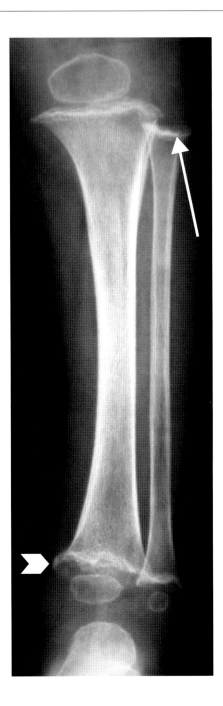

it occurs; either in developing and immature bones or the mature skeleton. They can also cause other types of bony pathologic conditions such as metabolic diseases; for example, osteoporosis can be caused post-menopause because of the reduced amount of *oestrogen*, which causes an increase in bone resorption.

Pituitary gland

The anterior lobe of the pituitary gland produces growth hormone, which controls the rate of growth of the epiphyseal cartilage.

Gigantism: This occurs if hypersecretion takes place during childhood, resulting in excessive growth and thickened widened bones.

Acromegaly (Fig. 4.25) : This occurs if hypersecretion takes place during adulthood. It results in enlarged and thickened bones (especially the hands and mandible), widened joint spaces, and thickened soft tissue (e.g. the heel pad). Enlargement of the pituitary fossa is seen in the skull if the hypersecretion is caused by an *adenoma* (benign tumour of a gland).

Restricted growth: This occurs if hyposecretion takes place during childhood, resulting in delayed and lack of bone growth and, therefore, an individual of short stature. If it occurs in adulthood, it causes reduced skeletal muscle and cardiac function and increased body fat.

It should be noted that the more common form of restricted growth is *achondroplasia*, a genetic condition leading to impaired bone growth, particularly of the epiphyseal growth plates of long bones. Growth hormone does not affect this form of restricted growth.

Thyroid gland

The thyroid gland in the neck produces two thyroid hormones, *thyroxine* and *triiodothyronine*, which strongly affect metabolism in all tissues. Specifically, in the skeleton, they help ensure normal bone turnover and influence bone growth. Iodine in the diet is essential for the production of these hormones. An underactive thyroid, *hypothyroidism*, in babies and young children can cause significant delays in skeletal development and mental retardation.

The thyroid also produces a third hormone, *calcitonin*, which is associated with calcium and phosphate levels in bone and blood. It increases the amount of calcium in the bone (by inhibiting osteoclasts breaking it down) therefore reducing levels in the blood.

Fig. 4.25 Acromegaly; lateral skull. Enlarged pituitary fossa (sella turcica – arrow) caused by a pituitary adenoma. Note enlarged maxillary sinuses resulting from the acromegaly (arrowhead). (From STATdx © Elsevier 2022)

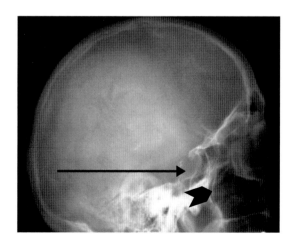

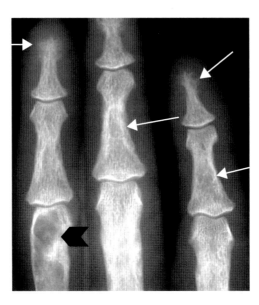

Fig. 4.26 Hyperparathyroidism; hand. Cortical bone resorption of the phalangeal tufts and shafts (arrows). Brown's tumour also seen as a lytic lesion (arrowhead). (From STATdx © Elsevier 2022)

Parathyroid glands

The paired parathyroid glands, which are attached to the thyroid, produce a hormone called *parathyroid hormone* (PTH), which works in opposition to calcitonin in calcium and phosphate homeostasis and storage. It increases the calcium level in the blood (and therefore reduces it in bones) by stimulating osteoclasts to break down bone.

Hyperparathyroidism (Figs. 4.26, 4.27, 4.28): increased secretion of PTH increases the rate at which calcium and phosphate are absorbed back in the blood from bone. It is most commonly caused by either a parathyroid adenoma or secondary to chronic kidney disease (called *renal osteodystrophy*).

Radiologically, the effects on the skeleton include osteopaenia, benign-appearing lytic lesions (Brown's tumours), and bone resorption in sub-periosteal and subchondral areas of bones (Fig. 4.26). In the spine, it may also cause a striped appearance in the vertebral bodies, sometimes called the 'rugger-jersey' sign (Fig. 4.27). The increased calcium levels in the blood may be deposited as soft tissue and vascular calcifications (Fig. 4.28).

Adrenal glands

The paired adrenal (suprarenal) glands produce two main types of hormones: *epinephrine* and *norepinephrine* (both involved in fight-or-flight response) and steroids, including *cortisol* and *androgens* (male sex hormones).

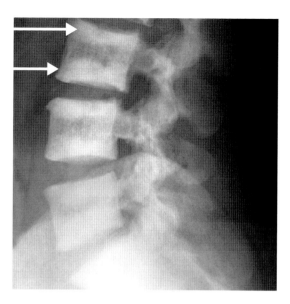

Fig. 4.27 Hyperparathyroidism secondary to renal disease; lumbar spine. 'Rugger-jersey' sign, seen as horizontal sclerotic bands in vertebral bodies (arrows). (From STATdx © Elsevier 2022)

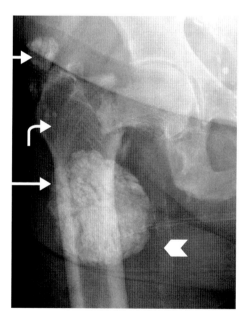

Fig. 4.28 Hyperparathyroidism; right hip. Soft tissue (arrows) and vascular (arrowhead) calcifications. Note the fractured neck of the femur with background osteopaenia causing a prominent trabecular pattern (curved arrow). (From STATdx © Elsevier 2022)

Increased secretion of the adrenal steroid hormones, such as in *Cushing's syndrome*, can affect calcium metabolism and is a cause of osteoporosis (as is overuse of steroids generally).

Infections

Infectious organisms such as bacteria and fungi can be introduced into bones and cause infection (*osteomyelitis*). Infection within a joint is known as *septic arthritis*.

Osteomyelitis (Figs. 4.29, 4.30, 4.31)

Bone infection most commonly comes from a *Staphylococcus* infection but sometimes from other organisms such as *tuberculosis*. It can be rapidly destructive and difficult to treat, leading to chronic infections and abscesses.

Fig. 4.29 Acute osteomyelitis; right forearm. There are ill-defined lytic areas throughout the radius (arrow) with periosteal reaction (arrowheads) along the bone. (From STATdx © Elsevier 2022)

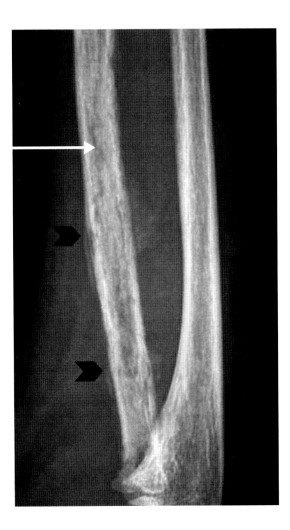

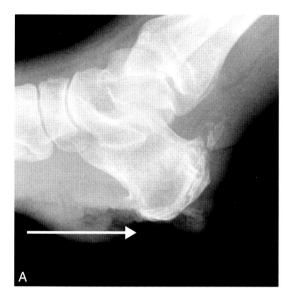
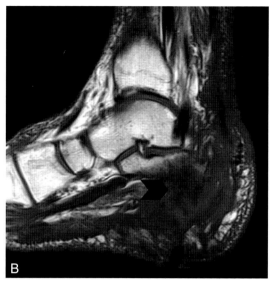

Fig. 4.30 Acute osteomyelitis. Lateral calcaneum radiograph (A) shows soft tissue ulcer only (arrow) with no bone destruction. The sagittal T1W MRI (B) shows marked signal loss in the calcaneum (arrowhead) compared to the other bones. (From STATdx © Elsevier 2022)

Causes

Haematogenous spread (from the blood) is most common, particularly in children where vessels enter close to the epiphyseal plate. Also, may be contiguous spread from open fractures, wounds, adjacent soft tissue infections (e.g. ulcers), and surgical interventions such as joint replacements (*prostheses*).

Radiological signs

The *acute* signs (Fig. 4.29) may not appear on radiographs for at least two weeks; the earliest sign is that the periosteum becomes elevated (*periosteal reaction*) followed by ill-defined bone destruction and lytic lesions, soft tissue swelling and loss of normal fat planes. MRI is much more sensitive (Fig. 4.30). The *sub-acute/chronic* sign is a well defined lytic lesion called *Brodie's abscess* (Fig. 4.31). If it persists despite treatment, this may become surrounded by a thick layer of dense sclerotic bone.

Arthritis

Arthritis (or arthropathy) refers to any pathologic condition affecting a joint. It may be because of any of the other causes of skeletal pathologic conditions, such as trauma, infection, or inflammation. The term arthritis (meaning joint inflammation) is sometimes a misnomer as not all pathologies affecting joints are inflammatory in nature.

Fig. 4.31 Brodie's abscess. Right knee radiograph (A) demonstrates well defined lytic lesion in the medial metaphysis (arrow). MRI (B) confirms that this crosses the epiphyseal plate (arrowhead). (From STATdx © Elsevier 2022)

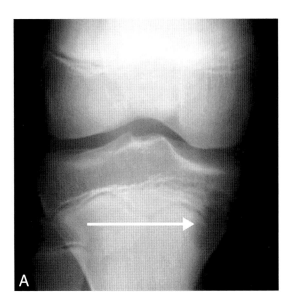

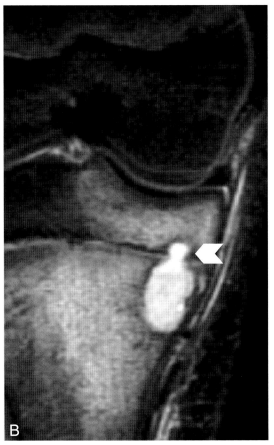

Numerous types of arthritis can be placed on a spectrum, from those that only produce bone and no bone destruction (e.g. osteoarthritis) to those that are purely erosive but form no new bone (e.g. rheumatoid arthritis). Other forms lie somewhere in between as a combination of bone formation and bone destruction.

Radiologically, the cardinal sign of arthritis is joint space narrowing caused by thinning of articular cartilage. Diagnosis is normally a combination of clinical history and laboratory testing, with radiological imaging often used to confirm and assess disease severity and progression.

Osteoarthritis (OA) (Figs. 4.32, 4.33)

It is also known as *degenerative joint disease* and is caused by degeneration and thinning of the articular hyaline cartilage. The underlying articular bone becomes thickened and sclerotic and forms *osteophytes* (spurs) around the joint margins. The most common sites are weight-bearing joints, including; hips, knees, hands and spine though it can affect any joint depending on the cause.

Causes

Primary OA: The causes are considered to be normal 'wear and tear' on weight-bearing joints, and the incidence increases with age.
Secondary OA: It can affect any joint but because of an underlying cause, such as obesity, previous trauma (such as an intra-articular fracture), and other underlying bone or joint pathologic conditions.

Radiological signs

The signs include a classic triad of *joint space narrowing*, *osteophyte formation*, and *subchondral sclerosis* of bone articular surfaces. Other features may include

Fig. 4.32 Osteoarthritis; left knee. Classic triad of osteophyte formation (arrows), joint space narrowing (curved arrow), and subchondral sclerosis (arrowhead). Interestingly the lateral joint is affected. More commonly, the medial compartment is affected first (although not in this case). (From STATdx © Elsevier 2022)

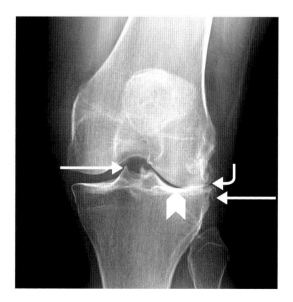

Fig. 4.33 Osteoarthritis; fingers. Osteophytes (arrows) and joint space narrowing of the distal interphalangeal joints. (From STATdx © Elsevier 2022)

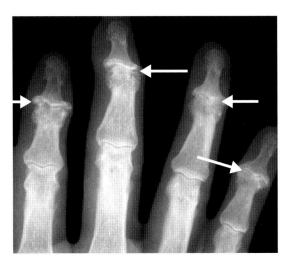

cysts that form in bone deep to the articular surface. Radiography remains a mainstay imaging modality.

Rheumatoid arthritis (Figs. 4.34, 4.35)

An autoimmune disease affecting many systems of the body and causing chronic inflammation, especially of joints. Causes destruction of articular hyaline cartilage and bone erosions, leading to deformities, particularly in the hands. It more commonly presents in females than males and typically first appears in the third to fifth decades.

Fig. 4.34 Rheumatoid arthritis; hand. Advanced erosive change and deformities at the metacarpophalangeal joints (arrows). Smaller erosions can be seen in the interphalangeal joints. Soft tissue joint swelling. (From STATdx © Elsevier 2022)

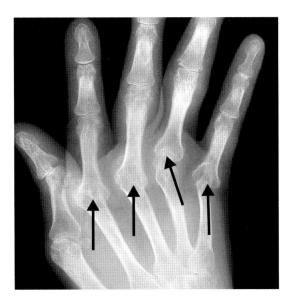

Fig. 4.35 Rheumatoid arthritis; colour Doppler ultrasound wrist. Synovial thickening and hyperaemia (increased blood flow shown by the colour) associated with tenosynovitis in a patient with rheumatoid arthritis. Radiographs were normal. (From STATdx © Elsevier 2022)

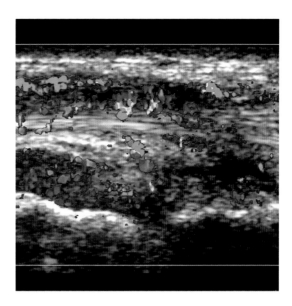

Causes

The causes are not well understood but considered to be genetic and hereditary. Infections and smoking are also thought to be potential contributing factors.

Radiological signs

They are usually symmetrical and include osteopaenia, joint space narrowing, bone erosions, soft tissue swelling, deformities and subluxations of the fingers and toes (Fig. 4.34). *Synovitis* (inflammation and thickening of the synovial membrane) is seen on ultrasound and MRI, which can often pick up signs earlier than radiographs (Fig. 4.35).

Gout (Fig. 4.36)

A metabolic disease caused by the deposition of sodium urate crystals in soft tissue and joints because of raised uric acid levels (hyperuricemia) in the blood. Most commonly presents in older males, often in the metatarsophalangeal joint of the hallux (big toe). Acute attacks of very painful, swollen, red joints (similar to septic arthritis).

Causes

Gout has been previously associated with very rich diets leading to high levels of uric acid. The causes may be idiopathic or associated with chronic diseases (e.g. of the kidney).

Radiological signs

The signs include large 'punched-out' erosions away from the articular surface. Dense, soft tissue opacities (called *tophi*) caused by deposits in soft tissue. Joint spaces and bone density are usually normal.

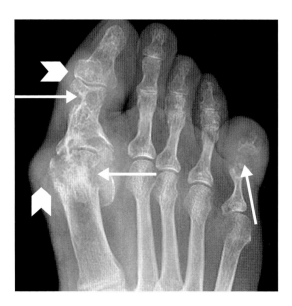

Fig. 4.36 Gout; right foot. Multiple large erosions (arrows). Soft tissue swelling and opacities (arrowheads) called *tophi* (From STATdx © Elsevier 2022)

UPPER LIMB

5

CHAPTER CONTENTS

Humerus	63	Phalanges	79
Radius	68	Elbow Joint	83
Ulna	71	Wrist Joint	91
Hand	77	First Carpometacarpal Joint	97
Carpal bones	77	Metacarpophalangeal and	
Metacarpal bones	78	Interphalangeal Joints	99

HUMERUS (FIGS. 5.1, 5.2)

Type
Long bone.

Position
The largest bone in the upper limb. Connects the upper limbs to the shoulder girdle.

Articulations
Head of the humerus with the glenoid cavity of the scapula to form the shoulder (*glenohumeral*) joint.
Trochlea of the humerus with the trochlear notch of the ulna and the *capitulum* of the humerus with the head of the radius; form the elbow joint.

Main parts
Features of the proximal end of the humerus
Head of the humerus – rounded; covered with articular hyaline cartilage.
Lesser tuberosity (tubercle) – anteriorly, the tendon of the subscapularis muscle is attached.
Greater tuberosity (tubercle) – posterolaterally; the supraspinatus tendon is attached to the superior aspect, infraspinatus tendon to the middle and the teres minor tendon to the infero- posterior aspect.
Intertubercular sulcus (bicipital groove) – between the tuberosities. Contains the tendon of the long head of the biceps.
Anatomical neck – adjoining the head, distal to the articular surface and proximal to tuberosities. Location of the epiphyseal growth plate.
Surgical neck – imaginary horizontal line across the proximal shaft, distal to tuberosities. Common fracture site (hence the name).

Features of the shaft (diaphysis) of the humerus
Triangular in cross-section – Medial border, Lateral border, Anterior border

Fig. 5.1 Right humerus
(anterior aspect).

A – Lesser tuberosity
(tubercle)
B – Greater tuberosity
(tubercle)
C – Intertubercular sulcus
(bicipital groove)
D – Deltoid tuberosity
E – Lateral border
F – Lateral supracondylar
ridge
G – Lateral epicondyle
H – Radial fossa
I – Capitulum
J – Trochlea
K – Medial epicondyle
L – Coronoid fossa
M – Medial supracondylar
ridge
N – Surgical neck
O – Anatomical neck
P – Head of the humerus.

Fig. 5.2 Right humerus
(posterior aspect).

1 – Head of the humerus
2 – Anatomical neck
3 – Surgical neck
4 – Medial border
5 – Medial supracondylar
ridge
6 – Olecranon fossa
7 – Medial epicondyle
8 – Groove for the ulnar
nerve
9 – Trochlea (note the
larger medial lip)
10 – Lateral epicondyle
11 – Lateral supracondylar
ridge
12 – Spiral groove
13 – Greater tuberosity
(tubercle).

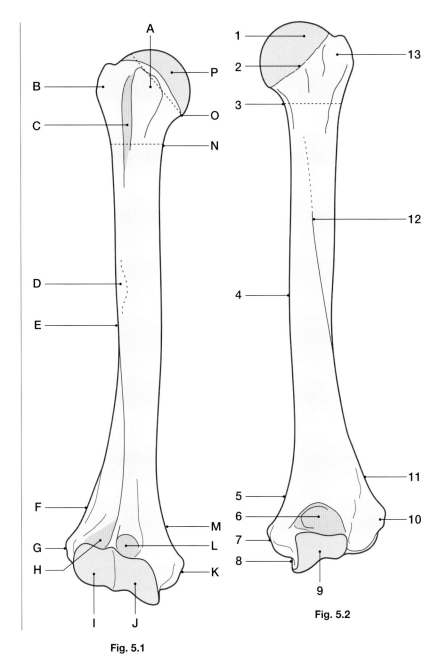

Fig. 5.1

Fig. 5.2

Posterior surface, Antero-lateral surface, Antero-medial surface – in the middle of which is the nutrient foramen.

Deltoid tuberosity – for the attachment of the deltoid muscle, located on the anterolateral surface.

Spiral groove – for the radial nerve.

Features of the distal end of the humerus

Lateral supracondylar ridge – distal end of the lateral border above the lateral epicondyle.

Medial supracondylar ridge – distal end of the medial border above the medial epicondyle.

Lateral epicondyle – superior to the capitulum.

Medial epicondyle – superior to the trochlea.

Capitulum – (lateral condyle) rounded; articulates with the head of the radius.

Trochlea – (medial condyle) pulley-shaped; articulates with the trochlear notch of the ulna. Has a larger medial lip which forms the 'carrying angle' (see elbow joint).

Groove for the ulnar nerve – posterior-medial aspect, medial to the trochlea.

Olecranon fossa – posteriorly, receives the olecranon process of the ulna when the elbow joint is extended.

Coronoid fossa – anteriorly, receives the coronoid process of the ulna when the elbow joint is fully flexed. Smaller than the olecranon fossa.

Radial fossa – anteriorly receives the head of the radius when the elbow joint is flexed.

Ossification (Figs. 5.5, 5.25)

Primary centre

Shaft (diaphysis) – appears in the eighth week of intrauterine life.

Secondary centres

Proximal end – three centres:
  humeral head – age six months;
  greater tuberosity – age one to two;
  lesser tuberosity – age four to five.
Fuse together to form a single epiphysis – age six;
Fuse with shaft – age 18–20.

Distal end – four centres:
  capitulum – age one;
  medial epicondyle – age four to six;
  trochlea – age nine to ten;
  lateral epicondyle – age 12.
Lateral epicondyle, trochlea and capitulum fuse together at puberty. Fuse with the shaft – age 14–16.
Medial epicondyle fuses with the shaft–age 20.

Radiographic appearances of the humerus (Figs. 5.3, 5.4)

Fig. 5.3 Right humerus: anteroposterior projection. (From Lampignano, Bontrager's Textbook of Radiographic Positioning and Related Anatomy, 10e, Elsevier)

A – Anatomical neck
B – Head of the humerus
C – Surgical neck
D – Shaft of the humerus (cortex)
E – Medullary cavity
F – Olecranon fossa
G – Olecranon (of the ulna)
H – Medial epicondyle
I – Trochlea
J – Radial head
K - Capitulum
L – Lateral epicondyle
M – Deltoid tuberosity
N – Lesser tuberosity
O – Greater tuberosity.

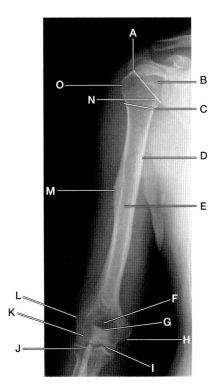

Fig. 5.4 Right humerus: lateral projection. (From Lampignano, Bontrager's Textbook of Radiographic Positioning and Related Anatomy, 10e, Elsevier)

1 – Lesser tuberosity
2 – Intertubercular sulcus (Bicipital groove)
3 – Capitulum
4 – Radius
5 – Olecranon process (of the ulna)
6 – Olecranon fossa
7 – Shaft of the humerus
8 – Head of the humerus.

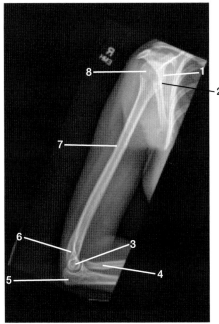

Fig. 5.5 Ossification centres of the (left) proximal humerus. (From STATdx © Elsevier).

A – Humeral head (age six months)
B – Greater tuberosity (age one to two years).
Not demonstrated - Lesser tuberosity (age four to five years)
Note the shape of the normal appearing epiphyseal growth plate (dotted line).

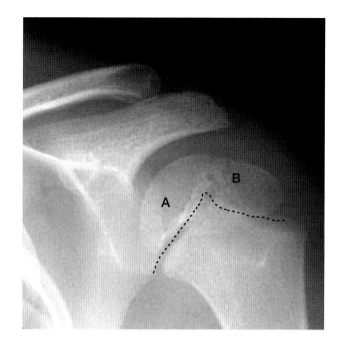

FRACTURES

Surgical neck

Cause – fall on an outstretched hand (FOOSH). Common in older people.
Example of treatment– often conservative (sling). May require ORIF or joint replacement (arthroplasty) in more complex, comminuted fractures.

Shaft

Usually the middle third; spiral, oblique or comminuted, dependent on the cause.
Cause – fall on the outstretched hand or direct blow (older persons) or high velocity injuries
Example of treatment–often conservative (sling) or immobilisation (cast). May require ORIF in complex/ displaced fractures.

Supracondylar (Fig. 5.6)

The distal bone fragment is displaced posteriorly with a significant risk of damage to the brachial artery and nerves. A common injury in younger children. They can be extremely subtle if minimally displaced.
Cause – fall on an outstretched hand with the elbow flexed.
Example of treatment– Limb immobilised in a cast with the elbow flexed. Reduction under anaesthesia with Kirschner (K) wire fixation may be required in displaced fractures.

Fig. 5.6 Minimally displaced supracondylar fracture; lateral left elbow projection. Elevated fat pads (arrows) indicate joint effusion. An anterior humeral line (dashed line) should normally pass through the capitulum (C), which it does not here. There is a very subtle fracture line evident (arrowhead). (From STATdx © Elsevier 2022)

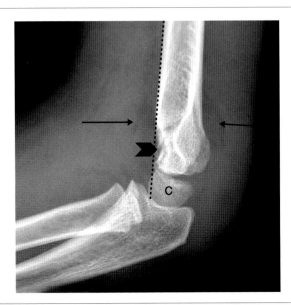

 INSIGHT

Age has a significant impact on the pattern of injury seen. A fall on an outstretched hand (FOOSH) in older people will more likely cause a surgical neck of humerus fracture, whereas young children are more likely to experience a supracondylar fracture. Different injuries occur in the forearm and wrist in other age groups.

RADIUS (FIGS. 5.7, 5.8)

Type	Long bone.
Position	Lateral bone of the forearm.
Articulations	*Head of the radius* with the radial notch of the ulna to form the superior radioulnar joint and with the capitulum of the humerus to form the lateral part of the elbow joint. *Distal end of the radius* with the head of the ulna to form the inferior radioulnar joint and with the scaphoid and lunate to form part of the wrist joint.
Main parts	**Features of the proximal end of the radius** *Head* – rounded, with a concave surface. *Neck* – narrow portion, inferior to the head. *Radial tuberosity* – medial aspect, inferior to the neck; provides attachment for the tendon of the biceps brachii muscle.

Fig. 5.7 Right radius (anterior aspect).

A – Head of the radius
B – Neck of radius
C – Radial tuberosity
D – Oblique line
E – Lateral border
F – Interosseous border
G – Distal end of radius
H – Radial styloid process

Right ulna (anterior aspect).
I – Ulnar styloid process
J – Medial border
K – Interosseous border
L – Ulnar tuberosity
M – Radial notch
N – Coronoid process
O – Trochlear notch
P – Olecranon process.

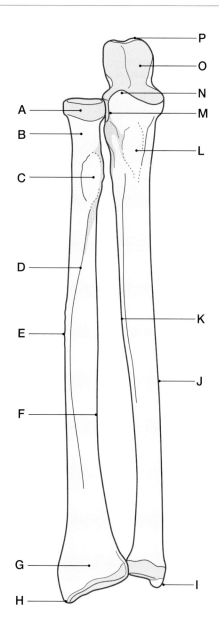

Fig. 5.8 Right radius (posterior aspect).

1 – Head of the radius
2 – Neck of radius
3 – Radial tuberosity
4 – Lateral border
5 – Interosseous border
6 – Radial styloid process
7 – Ulnar notch

Right ulna (posterior aspect).
8 – Ulnar styloid process
9 – Head of the ulna
10 – Interosseous border
11 – Medial border
12 – Olecranon process.

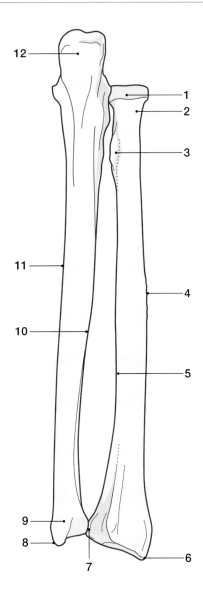

Features of the shaft of the radius

Anterior border, Posterior border
Interosseous border – attached to the lateral aspect of the ulna by an interosseous membrane to form the middle radioulnar joint (a fibrous syndesmotic joint).
Anterior surface – the location of the nutrient foramen.
Posterior surface, Lateral surface

Features of the distal end of radius

Ulnar notch – located on the medial aspect; articulates with the head of the ulna to form the inferior radioulnar joint.
Radial styloid process – a prominent process on the lateral aspect that can easily be palpated.
Lister's tubercle – palpable process on the dorsal aspect
Distal surface – two fossae, separated by a ridge, for articulation with the scaphoid and lunate.

Ossification (Figs. 5.25, 5.31)

Primary centre

Shaft (diaphysis) – eighth week of intrauterine life.

Secondary centres

Two centres:
>Distal end of the radius appears at age one;
>Head of the radius appears at age four to five.

Head of the radius fuses with the shaft at 14–17 years.
Distal end of the radius fuses with the shaft at 17–19 years.

ULNA (FIGS. 5.7, 5.8)

Type   Long bone.

Position   Medial bone of the forearm.

Articulations   *Radial notch* with the head of the radius to form the superior radioulnar joint.
Trochlear notch with the trochlea of the humerus to form the medial part of the elbow joint.
Head of the ulna with the ulnar notch of the radius to form the inferior radioulnar joint. The head of the ulna is covered with an articular disc of fibrocartilage and therefore does not directly take part in the formation of the wrist joint.

Main parts

Features of the proximal end of the ulna

Olecranon process – posterosuperior projection. It can easily be palpated on the posterior aspect of the elbow joint; it gives attachment to the triceps tendon.
Coronoid process – small anterior projection.
Ulnar tuberosity – situated on the anterior surface of the coronoid process; rough surface, provides attachment to the tendon of the brachialis muscle.
Radial notch – depression on the lateral aspect of the coronoid process; articulates with the head of the radius.
Trochlear notch – concave area between the coronoid and olecranon processes; articulates with the trochlea of the humerus.

Features of the shaft of the ulna

Anterior border. Posterior border
Interosseous border – attached to the medial aspect of the radius by an interosseous membrane to form the middle radioulnar joint (a fibrous syndesmotic joint).
Anterior surface – the location of the nutrient foramen.
Medial surface, Posterior surface

Features of the distal end of the ulna

Head – small and rounded.
Ulnar styloid process – small prominent process which can be palpated on the medial aspect of the wrist.

 INSIGHT

The heads of the radius and ulna are at opposite ends of the forearm; the head of the radius is part of the elbow joint, the head of the ulna is part of the wrist.

Ossification (Figs. 5.25, 5.31)

Primary centre
Shaft (diaphysis) – eighth week of intrauterine life.

Secondary centres
Two centres:
    Distal end of ulna appears age five to six;
    Olecranon appears age nine to 11.
Olecranon fuses with the shaft age 14–16.
Distal end fuses with the shaft age 17–18.

Radiographic appearances of the radius and ulna (Figs. 5.9, 5.10)

Fig. 5.9 Left forearm: anteroposterior projection. (From STATdx © Elsevier 2022)

A – Olecranon process
B – Trochlea
C – Coronoid process
D – Shaft of the ulna
E – Head of the ulna
F – Lunate
G – Scaphoid
H – Radial styloid process
I – Inferior radioulnar joint
J – Shaft of the radius
K – Radial tuberosity
L – Neck of the radius
M – Head of the radius
N – Capitulum
O – Shaft of the humerus.

Fig. 5.10 Left forearm: lateral projection. (From STATdx © Elsevier 2022)

1 – Epicondyles of the humerus (superimposed)
2 – Trochlea and capitulum (superimposed)
3 – Head of the radius
4 – Neck of the radius
5 – Radial tuberosity
6 – Shaft of the radius
7 – Lunate
8 – Scaphoid
9 – Ulnar styloid process
10 – Shaft of the ulna
11 – Coronoid process
12 – Trochlear notch
13 – Olecranon process.

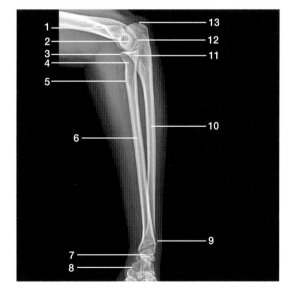

FRACTURES

Radial head

A common injury, particularly in young adults. Often very subtle and undisplaced; suspect with a history of trauma and evidence of joint effusion even in the absence of a visible fracture.
Cause – fall onto an outstretched hand, causes axial compression.
Example of treatment – often conservative with a sling.

Olecranon process

Usually occurs in adults. If complete, the fracture can be markedly displaced because of the pull of the triceps muscle.
Cause– fall on the olecranon process (tip of the elbow).
Example of treatment – cast, elbow flexed to 90°. Open reduction internal fixation with wires.

Plastic Bowing / Torus (Buckle) fracture / Greenstick fracture (Fig. 5.11)

Range of injuries that occur in children, typically aged five to 12 years. Bones tend to bend (plastic bowing), buckle (Torus fracture) or splinter (Greenstick fracture) rather than 'snap' because of their relative elasticity compared to mature bones.
Cause – fall onto an outstretched hand or other traumatic injuries.
Example of treatment – cast, elbow to wrist.

Fig. 5.11 Immature skeleton; right forearm. Plastic bowing of the radius without fracture (arrow). Incomplete 'greenstick' fracture of the ulna (arrowhead). (From STATdx © Elsevier 2022)

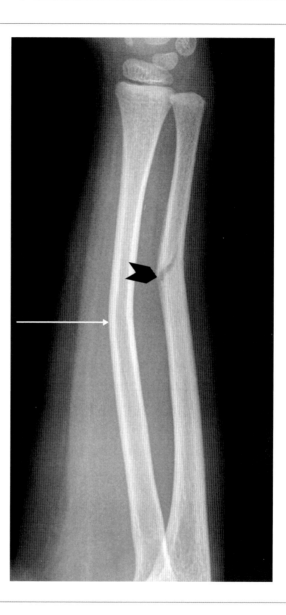

 INSIGHT

Due to the circular (ring) arrangement of the radius and ulna, a fracture of the shaft of one of the bones is usually associated with dislocation or fracture-dislocation of the other bone. Similar principles apply to other bony rings, such as in the pelvis, lower leg, and mandible. It is always important to consider more than one injury (satisfaction of search) and ensure adjacent joints are adequately assessed and imaged as necessary.

Monteggia fracture-dislocation (Fig. 5.12)

Fracture of the proximal third of the ulna with dislocation of the radial head.
Cause – fall on the hand with forced pronation (internal rotation) of the forearm.
Example of treatment – reduction of radial head dislocation, internal fixation of ulna fracture.

Fig. 5.12 Monteggia fracture-dislocation; left elbow/forearm. Displaced fracture of the proximal ulna (arrow). The radiocapitellar (dotted) line should always normally connect the radial head (R) and the capitulum (C), which it does not here, indicating dislocation of the radial head. (From STATdx © Elsevier 2022)

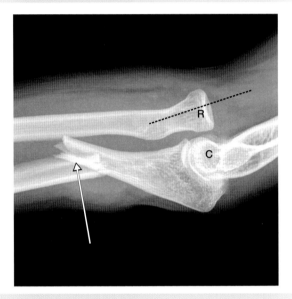

Galeazzi fracture-dislocation (Fig. 5.13)

Fracture of the distal third of the radius with dislocation of the head of the ulna at the inferior radioulnar joint. Less common than the Monteggia pattern of injury, the injuries seen are effectively the opposite.
Cause – fall on the hand with a rotational force.
Examples of treatment – reduction of ulna head dislocation, internal fixation of ulna fracture.

For fractures of the distal end of the radius and ulna, see the wrist joint.

Fig. 5.13 Galeazzi fracture-dislocation; left wrist/forearm. Displaced fracture of the mid radius (arrowhead). There is posterior dislocation of the head of the ulna from the inferior radioulnar joint (arrow). (From STATdx © Elsevier 2022)

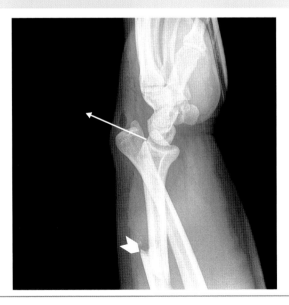

HAND (FIG. 5.14)

Carpal bones (Figs. 5.14–5.16)

Type   Short bones.

Position   Two rows (distal and proximal row) situated between the radius and the
                         bases of the metacarpals. They form a concave arch anteriorly (*carpal tunnel*)
                         containing structures including the median nerve and flexor tendons of the
                         fingers.

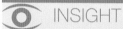 INSIGHT

To remember the position of the carpal bones, various mnemonics can be learned such as, as viewed on a
right wrist radiograph (Fig. 5.15);

5- Touch (TRAPEZIUM)	6- The (TRAPEZOID)	7- Cold (CAPITATE)	8- Hand (HAMATE)
1- Seldom (SCAPHOID)	2- Let (LUNATE)	3- The (TRIQUETRUM)	4- Patient (PISIFORM)

Articulations   *Scaphoid* with the radius, lunate, capitate, trapezium, trapezoid.
                        Lunate with the radius, scaphoid, capitate, triquetrum.
                        Triquetrum with the hamate, pisiform, lunate.
                        Pisiform with the triquetrum.
                        Hamate with the fourth and fifth metacarpals, capitate, triquetrum.
                        Capitate with the second, third and fourth metacarpals, hamate, lunate,
                        scaphoid, trapezoid.
                        Trapezoid with the second metacarpal, trapezium, scaphoid, capitate.
                        Trapezium with the scaphoid and trapezoid (the STT joint) and the first and
                        second metacarpals.

Main parts/features
Scaphoid – proximal and distal poles separated by the narrower waist.
Scaphoid tubercle on the anterior (volar) aspect of the distal pole.
Lunate – moon/crescent-shaped.
Triquetrum – three sides.

Pisiform – pea-shaped. Actually a sesamoid bone in the flexor carpi ulnaris tendon and not part of the wrist joint.

Hamate – wedge-shaped body and hook of the hamate (Hamulus) on the anterior surface.

Capitate – largest carpal bone, has proximal and distal poles separated by the waist.

Trapezoid – irregular, four-sided. Smaller than the trapezium.

Trapezium – four-sided. Concaved saddle-shaped distal surface for the thumb.

Ossification (Fig. 5.31)

Primary centres

Typically appear at the following ages though the date they ossify is subject to considerable variation.

Capitate – second month	*Scaphoid* – fourth to fifth year
Hamate – third month	*Trapezium* – fourth to fifth year
Triquetral – third year	*Trapezoid* – fourth to fifth year
Lunate – fourth year	*Pisiform* – ninth to 12th year

Metacarpal bones (Fig. 5.14)

Type

Miniature long bones.

Position

Distal to the carpal bones, proximal to the digits. Form the main part of the hand.

Articulations

First (thumb/pollex) metacarpal with the proximal phalanx of the thumb and the trapezium.

Second (index) metacarpal with the proximal phalanx of the index finger, the trapezium, trapezoid and capitate.

Third (middle) metacarpal with the proximal phalanx of the middle finger and the capitate.

Fourth (ring) metacarpal with the proximal phalanx of the ring finger, the capitate and hamate.

Fifth (little) metacarpal with the proximal phalanx of the little finger and the hamate.

The bases of the second–fifth metacarpals also articulate with the adjacent one(s).

Main parts

Head – distal, rounded; articulates with the corresponding proximal phalanx.

Neck – narrower part between the head and shaft.

Shaft – anterior border is concave along the length.

Base – proximal, expanded; articulates with the appropriate carpal bones.

Ossification (Fig. 5.31)

Primary centre

Shaft – ninth week of intrauterine life.

Secondary centres

One only per metacarpal:
> Base of the first metacarpal appears at age two to three.
> Head of the second–fifth metacarpals appears at age two.

Secondary centre unites with the shaft age 15–19.

 INSIGHT

Accessory ossification centres (pseudoepiphyses), which are normal variants, may also be seen in some individuals (Fig. 5.31) at the opposite end of the normal secondary centre. They can be confused for a fracture.

Phalanges (Fig. 5.14)

Type   Miniature long bones.

Position   Distal to the metacarpals, forming the fingers/thumb.

Articulations   *Five proximal phalanges* with the corresponding metacarpals proximally, distally with the corresponding middle phalanges except for the thumb with its distal phalanx (does not have a middle phalanx).
Four middle phalanges of the fingers (not thumb) with the corresponding proximal and distal phalanges.
Five distal phalanges with the corresponding finger middle phalanges or the proximal phalanx of the thumb.

Main parts   *Head* – distal, expanded. Middle and proximal phalanges have a bicondylar (rounded) articular surface with central depression. The distal phalangeal heads are even more expanded to form a phalangeal *'tuft'* to support the soft tissue of the fingertips.
Shaft – anterior border is concave along the length.
Base – proximal, expanded. Middle and distal phalanges have a biconcave articular surface with a central median ridge. Base of the proximal phalanx is concave.

Ossification (Fig. 5.31)

Primary centre
Shaft – eighth–twelfth week of intrauterine life.

Secondary centre

> One centre per phalanx: base of phalanges appears at age two to three years.
> Base unites with the shaft at age 15–18.

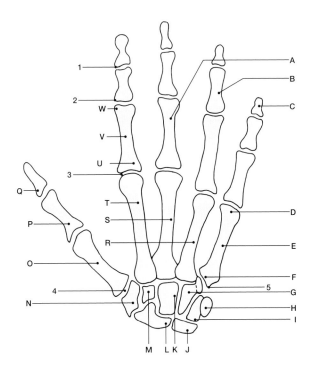

Fig. 5.14 Right hand, dorsal (posterior) aspect.

A – Shaft of proximal phalanx of the middle finger
B – Shaft of middle phalanx of the ring finger
C – Distal (terminal) phalanx of the little finger
D – Head of the fifth (little) metacarpal
E – Shaft of the fifth (little) metacarpal
F – Base of the fifth (little) metacarpal
G – Hamate
H – Pisiform
I – Triquetrum
J – Lunate
K – Capitate
L – Scaphoid
M – Trapezoid
N – Trapezium
O – Shaft of the first metacarpal
P – Base of the proximal phalanx of the thumb

Q – Base of the distal phalanx of the thumb
R – Shaft of the fourth (ring) metacarpal
S – Shaft of the third (middle) metacarpal
T – Shaft of the second (index) metacarpal
U – Base of the proximal phalanx of the index finger
V – Shaft of the proximal phalanx of the index finger
W – Head of the proximal phalanx of the index finger
1 – Distal interphalangeal joint of the index finger (synovial hinge joint)
2 – Proximal interphalangeal joint of the index finger (synovial hinge joint)
3 – Second metacarpophalangeal joint (synovial ellipsoid joint)
4 – First carpometacarpal joint (synovial saddle joint)
5 – Fifth carpometacarpal joint (synovial plane joint)

Radiographic appearances of the hand and wrist (Figs. 5.15–5.17)

Fig. 5.15 Right wrist: dorsi-palmar projection. (From STATdx © Elsevier 2022)

A – Scaphoid
B – Lunate
C – Triquetrum
D – Pisiform (hidden by triquetrum)
E – Trapezium
F – Trapezoid
G – Capitate
H – Hamate (hook of)
I – Radial styloid process
J – Radiocarpal (wrist) joint
K – Inferior (distal) radioulnar joint
L – Ulnar styloid process
M – Fifth (little) metacarpal
N – Third (middle) carpometacarpal joint
O – First (thumb) metacarpal.

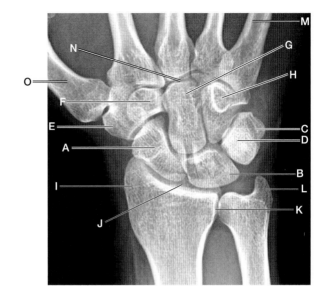

Fig. 5.16 Right wrist: lateral projection. (From STATdx © Elsevier 2022)

1 – Thumb metacarpal
2 – Trapezium
3 – Trapezoid
4 – Scaphoid
5 – Pisiform
6 – Lunate
7 – Radius
8 – Ulna
9 – Radiocarpal (wrist) joint
10 – Triquetrum
11 – Capitate
12 – Hamate
13 – Second to fifth metacarpals.

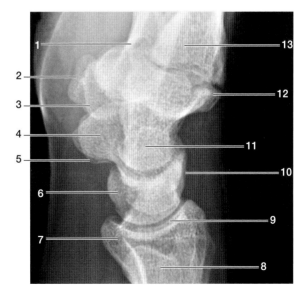

Fig. 5.17 Right hand: dorsi-palmar projection. (From STATdx © Elsevier 2022)

A – Distal interphalangeal joint (index finger)
B – Proximal interphalangeal joint (index finger)
C – Metacarpophalangeal joint (index finger)
D – Interphalangeal joint of the thumb
E – Proximal phalanx (thumb)
F – Sesamoid bones
G – Base of the second (index) metacarpal
H – Trapezoid
I – Trapezium
J – Capitate
K – Scaphoid
L – Distal radius
M – Distal ulna
N – Lunate
O – Pisiform (partly obscured by the triquetrum)
P – Triquetrum
Q – Hamate
R – shaft of the fifth (little) metacarpal
S – neck of the fifth (little) metacarpal
T – head of the fourth (ring) metacarpal
U – proximal phalanx
V – middle phalanx
W – distal phalanx
X – distal phalangeal (terminal) tuft.

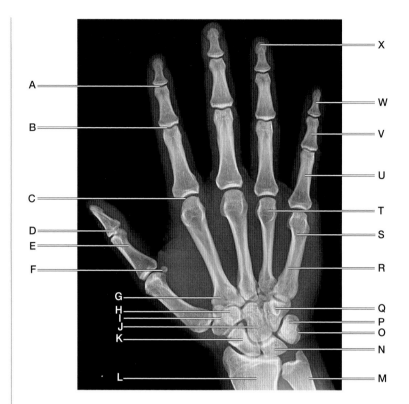

FRACTURES

Metacarpals (Fig. 5.18)

Typically occur at the base, shaft or neck.
Cause – because of a direct blow, for example, a punching injury (commonly of the neck of the fifth metacarpal)
Example of treatment – cast/splint, if minimal displacement. Reduction with K-wires if displaced.

Phalanges

Wide range; may be open, crush, oblique or avulsion dependent on mechanism.
Cause – may be to a direct blow (e.g. a hammer) or hyperextension/flexion (often because of a sports injury).
Example of treatment – splint/strapping with early rehabilitation to reduce loss of function.

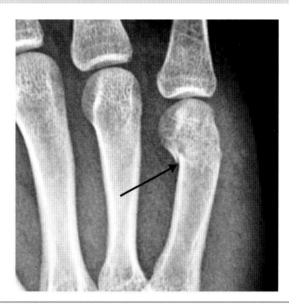

Fig. 5.18 Fracture of the neck of the fifth metacarpal. Commonly known as a 'boxer' fracture caused by a punching injury. This example is minimally displaced with only minor disruption of the cortex (arrow). (From STATdx © Elsevier 2022)

ELBOW JOINT (FIGS. 5.19–5.21)

Type

Two articulations make up the elbow joint proper. The humero-radial and humero-ulnar articulations form a synovial hinge joint to allow the elbow to flex and extend. A third articulation, the superior radioulnar joint, is a synovial pivot joint that allows pronation and supination of the forearm.

Bony articular surfaces

The *trochlea* of the humerus articulates with the *trochlear notch* of the ulna. The *capitulum* of the humerus articulates with the *head* of the radius. The *head of the radius* and *radial notch* of the ulna. The articular surfaces are covered with articular hyaline cartilage.

Fig. 5.19 Left elbow joint
(coronal section).

A – Humerus
B – Trochlea
C – Articular hyaline
cartilage
D – Synovial fluid
E – Synovial membrane
F – Ulna
G – Radius
H – Superior radioulnar joint
I – Head of the radius
J – Annular ligament
K – Fibrous capsule
L – Capitulum.

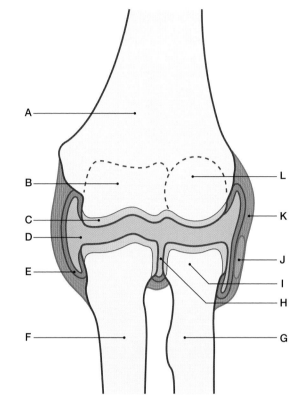

Fig. 5.20 Elbow joint
(sagittal section).

A – Humerus
B – Olecranon fossa
C – Posterior fat pad
D – Synovial membrane
E – Articular hyaline
cartilage of the trochlea
notch
F – Olecranon process of
the ulna
G – Radius
H – Annular ligament
I – Synovial fluid
J – Coronoid fossa
K – Anterior fat pad
L – Fibrous capsule.

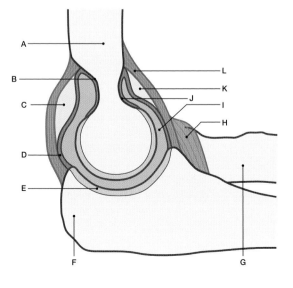

Fig. 5.21 Left elbow joint;
lateral aspect (A).

A – Radius
B – Ulna
C – Fibrous capsule
D – Radial collateral
    ligament
E – Humerus
F – Annular ligament.

Left elbow joint; medial
aspect (B).
1 – Humerus
2 – Ulnar collateral ligament
3 – Ulna
4 – Radius
5 – Annular ligament
6 – Fibrous capsule

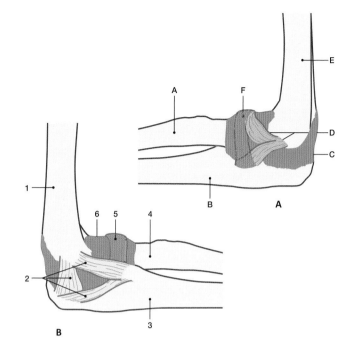

Fibrous capsule

Attached to the humerus at the level of the epicondyles, incorporating the coronoid and olecranon processes of the ulna and the neck of the radius and blending with the annular ligament of the superior radioulnar joint.

Synovial membrane

Lines the fibrous capsule and the coronoid, radial and olecranon fossae and is continuous with the superior radioulnar joint. The synovial membrane secretes synovial fluid, which lubricates the joint.

Intracapsular structures

Fat pads – anterior and posterior; situated between the synovial membrane and the fibrous capsule in the radial, coronoid and olecranon fossae.

 INSIGHT

The anterior and posterior fat pads in the elbow normally lie within the coronoid and olecranon fossae. Increased fluid in the joint (*effusion*), such as this may be caused by blood, inflammation, or infection, may displace these fat pads causing the 'sail sign.' This is an indicator of underlying joint effusion and, in trauma, is suspicious for fracture (Fig. 5.6).

Supporting ligaments

Ulnar collateral ligament – on the medial aspect of the joint, attached to the medial epicondyle of the humerus and the coronoid and olecranon processes of the ulna.

Radial collateral ligament – on the lateral aspect of the joint, attached to the lateral epicondyle of the humerus and the annular ligament.

Annular ligament – surrounds the head of the radius and is attached to the radial notch of the ulna, holds the radial head securely but allows it to rotate around its own axis.

Movements

Flexion by the biceps brachii, brachialis and brachioradialis muscles.
Extension by the triceps brachii and anconeus muscles.
Pronation/supination of the forearm at the superior radioulnar joint by the supinator and pronator teres and pronator quadratus muscles.

Blood supply

Brachial, ulnar, and radial arteries forming an anastamosis (union of different vessels).

Nerve supply

Musculo-cutaneous, radial and median nerves.

Carrying angle

The angle between the long axes of the humerus and ulna. The forearm is angled more laterally than the humerus (*valgus* angle). Greater in females than males, with the average angle being 163°.

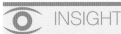 INSIGHT

The carrying angle is larger in females than males because females have a wider pelvis than males. The angle gets its name because it allows people to carry items with their arms straight without the forearm catching on the hips.

Imaging appearances of the elbow joint (Figs. 5.22–5.25)

Fig. 5.22 Left elbow joint: anteroposterior projection. (From Bruce, Merrill's Atlas of Radiographic Positioning; Procedures: Volume One, 14e, Elsevier)

A – Olecranon and coronoid fossae
B – Medial epicondyle
C – Olecranon
D – Trochlea
E – Coronoid process
F – Ulna
G – Shaft of radius
H – Radial tuberosity
I – Neck of the radius
J – Head of the radius
K – Capitulum
L – Lateral epicondyle
M – Radial fossa
N – Shaft of the humerus.

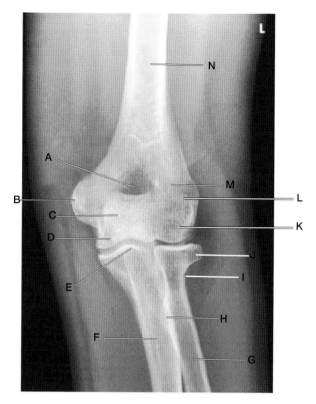

Fig. 5.23 Left elbow joint: lateral projection. (From STATdx © Elsevier 2022)

1 – Shaft of the humerus
2 - Anterior fat pad
3 – Coronoid fossa
4 - Head of the radius
5 - Neck of the radius
6 – Shaft of the ulna
7 – Coronoid process
8 – Olecranon process
9 – Trochlea notch
10 – Trochlea and capitulum (superimposed)
11 – Olecranon fossa (posterior fat pad hidden)
12 – Supracondylar ridge

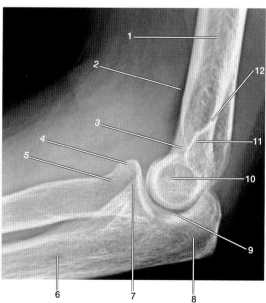

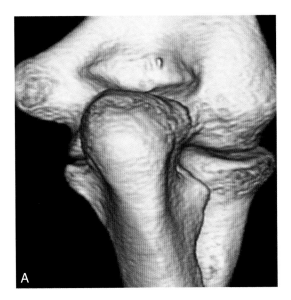
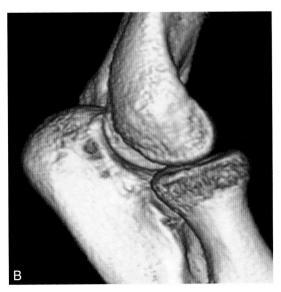

Fig. 5.24 Right elbow. CT 3D reformat images of the posterior (A) and lateral (B) aspects. (From STATdx © Elsevier 2022)

Fig. 5.25 Elbow ossification centres. The mnemonic CRITOL is a useful tool to remember the typical order in which they appear (From STATdx © Elsevier 2022)

C – Capitulum (age one)
R – Radial Head (age four to five)
I – Medial (internal) epicondyle (age four to six)
T – Trochlea (age nine to ten)
O – Olecranon (nine to 11 years)
L – Lateral epicondyle (12 years).

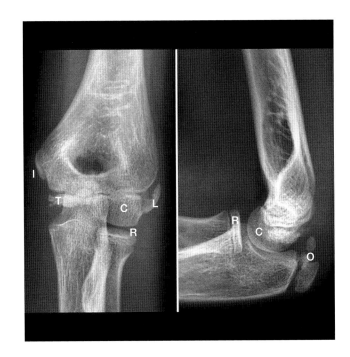

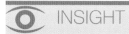 INSIGHT

The mnemonic CRITOL is a useful tool to remember the typical order in which the ossification centres of the elbow appear (Fig. 5.25). It is also helpful in identifying trauma in paediatrics if they appear out of order.

TRAUMA

Elbow dislocation (Fig. 5.26)

Cause – heavy fall on an outstretched hand. The radius and ulna displaced posteriorly or posterolaterally. Often associated with fractures and damage to the brachial artery or one of the nerves.
Example of treatment– reduction under anaesthesia.

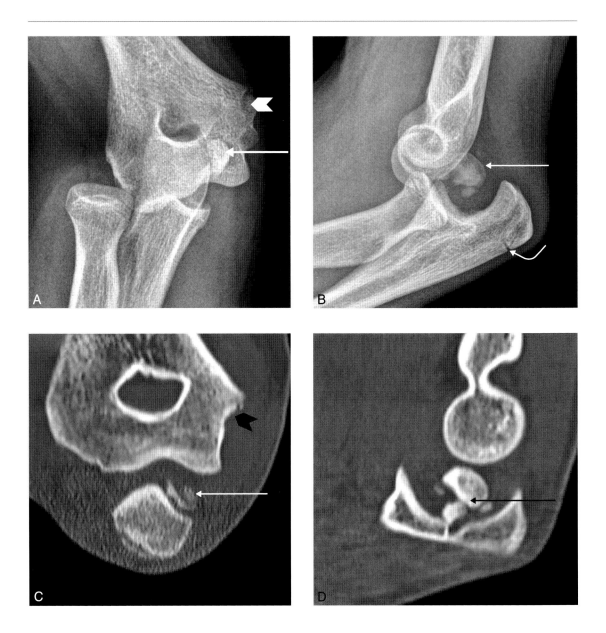

Fig. 5.26 Right elbow dislocation; antero-posterior (A) and lateral (B) radiographs. Coronal (C) and sagittal (D) CT images. Bone fragment (arrow) with associated donor site (arrowhead) represent an avulsion fracture of the medial epicondyle. Note the unfused normal olecranon ossification centre (curved arrow). (From STATdx © Elsevier 2022)

WRIST JOINT (FIGS. 5.27, 5.28)

The wrist as a unit comprises four separate joint cavities; the radiocarpal (wrist) joint joining the distal radius and ulna with the carpals, the inferior radioulnar joint, the intercarpal/carpometacarpal joints and the first (thumb) carpometacarpal joint.

Type

The wrist (radiocarpal) joint is a synovial ellipsoid joint. Intercarpal joints between individual carpals are a mixture of synovial plane and saddle joints. The inferior radioulnar joint is a synovial pivot joint.

Bony articular surfaces

The distal end of the radius with the scaphoid and lunate at its two corresponding fossae. *Articular disc* of the inferior radioulnar joint and distal ulna with the lunate and triquetrum. The articular surfaces are covered with articular hyaline cartilage.

Fibrous capsule

Of the radiocarpal joint; attached to the distal end of the radius and ulna, the margins of the articular disc and the proximal aspects of the scaphoid, lunate and triquetrum.

Fig. 5.27 Right wrist joint: dorsal aspect (dorsi-palmar projection).

A – Fibrous capsule
B – Synovial membrane
C – Articular hyaline cartilage
D – Distal radius
E – Inferior radioulnar joint
F – Head of the ulna
G – Articular disc (triangular fibrocartilage)
H – Synovial fluid
I – Triquetrum
J – Lunate
K – Scaphoid.

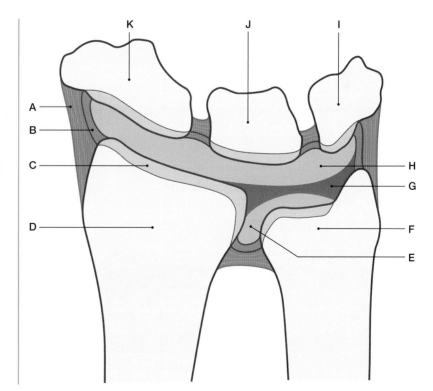

Fig. 5.28 Left wrist joint: palmar (anterior) aspect.

1 – Base of the first (thumb) metacarpal
2 – Trapezium
3 – Radial collateral ligament
4 – Palmar radiocarpal ligament
5 – Distal end of the radius
6 – Head of the ulna
7 – Palmar ulnocarpal ligament
8 – Ulnar collateral ligament
9 – Pisiform
10 – Hamate
11 – Capitate
12 – Trapezoid.

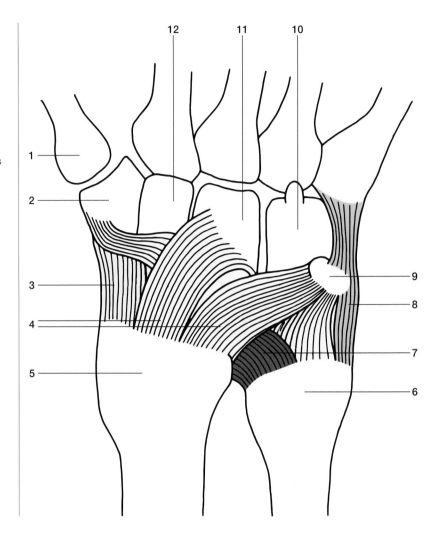

Synovial membrane

Lines the fibrous capsule, separating each of the four separate joint compartments. It covers the parts of the bones not covered with articular hyaline cartilage and secretes synovial fluid, which lubricates the joint.

Supporting ligaments

Can be divided into *intrinsic* ligaments connecting individual carpal bones (e.g., the scapholunate ligament) and *extrinsic*, connecting the radius, ulna, and metacarpals to the carpals, including:

Palmar (volar) radiocarpal ligament – from the radius to the scaphoid, lunate and triquetral on the anterior aspect of the joint. Forms a V-shape with:

Palmar (volar) ulnocarpal ligament – from the ulnar styloid process to the lunate and triquetrum on the anterior aspect of the wrist.

Dorsal radiocarpal ligament – from the radius to the scaphoid, lunate and triquetral on the posterior aspect of the wrist.
Ulnar collateral ligament – on the medial aspect of the wrist, attached to the ulnar styloid process and the triquetral and pisiform.
Radial collateral ligament – on the lateral aspect of the wrist, attached to the radial styloid process and the scaphoid.
Dorsal and palmar (volar) radioulnar ligaments – connecting the distal radius and ulna at the inferior radioulnar joint on their posterior and anterior surfaces, respectively.

Intracapsular structures
Articular disc – situated at the distal end of the ulna and inferior radioulnar joint separating them from the carpals; thick fibrocartilage disc called the *triangular fibrocartilage complex*.

Movements
Flexion by the flexor carpi radialis and flexor carpi ulnaris muscles.
Extension by the extensor carpi radialis and the extensor carpi ulnaris muscles.
Abduction by the flexor and extensor carpi radialis muscles, restricted by larger radial styloid.
Adduction by the flexor and extensor carpi ulnaris.

Blood supply
Radial and ulnar arteries.

Nerve supply
Ulnar, median and radial nerves.

Imaging appearances of the wrist joint (Figs. 5.15, 5.16, 5.29–5.31)

Fig. 5.29 Right wrist; coronal T1W MRI. (From STATdx © Elsevier 2022)

A – First (thumb) metacarpal
B – First carpometacarpal joint
C – Trapezium
D – Trapezoid
E – Extensor pollicis brevis and abductor pollicis tendons
F – Scaphoid
G – Radial styloid
H – Lunate
I – Inferior radioulnar joint
J – Ulnar styloid process
K – Triangular fibrocartilage (articular disc)
L – Triquetrum
M – Extensor carpi ulnaris tendon
N – Hamate
O – Fifth (little) metacarpal
P – Capitate
Q – Second (index) carpometacarpal joint.

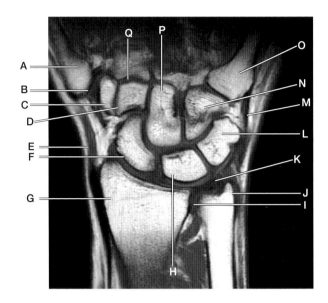

Fig. 5.30 Right wrist, distal carpals; axial T1W MRI. (From STATdx © Elsevier 2022)

1 – Body of the hamate
2 – Hook of the hamate
3 – Carpal tunnel (containing flexor tendons and median nerve)
4 – Trapezium
5 – Intercarpal (trapezo-trapezoid) joint
6 – Trapezoid
7 – Capitate
8 – Extensor tendons.

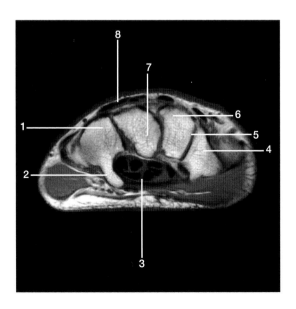

Fig. 5.31 Wrist ossification centres (left wrist). (From STATdx © Elsevier 2022)

A – Proximal phalanx epiphysis (age two to three years)
B – Fifth (little) metacarpal epiphysis (age two)
C – Hamate (three months)
D – Triquetrum (age three years)
E – Lunate (age four)
F – Distal ulnar epiphysis
G – Distal radius epiphysis
H – Scaphoid (age four to five years)
I – Trapezium (four to five years)
J – First (thumb) metacarpal epiphysis (age two to three years)
K – Accessory epiphysis second metacarpal (normal variant).

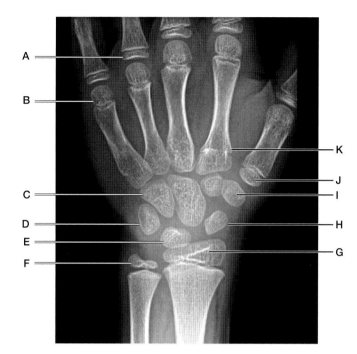

FRACTURES

Colles' fracture (Fig. 5.32)

Transverse fracture of the distal radius with posterior (dorsal) displacement of the distal fragment. The ulnar styloid process is also often fractured.
Cause – fall on a dorsiflexed outstretched hand. Most commonly seen in middle age, particularly females with osteopaenia.
Example of treatment – manipulation to reduce fracture, below elbow cast.

Scaphoid fracture (Fig. 5.33)

Most common carpal bone fracture. The patient typically presents with tenderness overlying the scaphoid in the *anatomical snuffbox*; a triangular depression at the base of the thumb formed between the extensor pollicis longus and abductor pollicis longus tendons.

Often not demonstrated radiographically until 10–14 days following injury, unless displaced. Most commonly a transverse fracture through the waist. Osteonecrosis of the proximal pole is a significant possible complication.
Cause – fall on a dorsiflexed outstretched hand. Most commonly seen in young adults.
Example of treatment – cast if undisplaced. Surgical intervention is indicated in displaced fractures or with complications such as delayed/non-union or osteonecrosis.

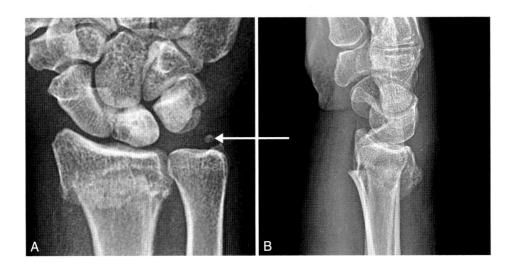

Fig. 5.32 Colles fracture right wrist; dorsi-palmar and lateral projections. Note the commonly associated ulna styloid fracture (arrow). (From STATdx © Elsevier 2022)

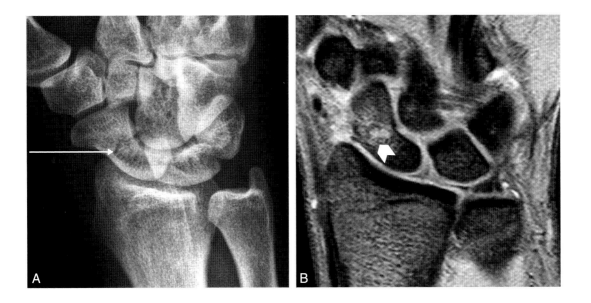

Fig. 5.33 Scaphoid fracture right wrist; DP oblique radiograph (A) and coronal T1W MRI image (B). The minimally displaced fracture (arrow) is obscured by high signal marrow oedema on MRI (arrowhead). (From STATdx © Elsevier 2022)

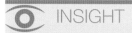 INSIGHT

If radiographs of the scaphoid are taken, and a fracture is not demonstrated, but pain or clinical suspicion persists, alternative imaging techniques such as MRI may be required to demonstrate the fracture.

FIRST CARPOMETACARPAL JOINT (FIG. 5.28)

Type

Synovial saddle joint to allow extensive mobility. Other carpometacarpal (CMC) joints (second to fifth) and inter-metacarpal joints are synovial planar joints with minimal movement.

Bony articular surfaces
The concave base of the first metacarpal with the convex, superior surface of the trapezium. The articular surfaces are covered with articular hyaline cartilage.

Fibrous capsule
Attached to the periphery of the base of the first metacarpal and the rough edge around the articular surface of the trapezium. The capsule is thickened dorsally and laterally.

Synovial membrane
Lines the fibrous capsule and is separated from the other carpometacarpal joints. It covers the parts of the bone not covered with articular hyaline cartilage and secretes synovial fluid, which lubricates the joint.

Supporting ligaments
Stabilised by a number of ligaments, including the:
Anterior oblique ligament – an oblique band from the palmar tubercle of the trapezium to the ulnar aspect of the base of the first metacarpal.
Dorsoradial ligament – from the lateral surface of the trapezium to the radial side of the base of the first metacarpal.
Posterior oblique ligament – an oblique band from the dorsal surface of the trapezium to the ulnar aspect of the base of the first metacarpal.

Movements
Flexion by the flexor pollicis brevis, opponens pollicis and flexor pollicis longus muscles.
Extension by the abductor pollicis longus, extensor pollicis brevis and extensor pollicis longus.
Abduction by the abductor pollicis brevis and the abductor pollicis longus.
Adduction by the adductor pollicis.
Axial rotation, a combination of the above movements.

Flexion is associated with medial rotation, and in full extension, the joint is slightly adducted.

Blood supply
Radial artery.

Nerve supply
Median and radial nerves.

FRACTURES

Bennett's fracture-dislocation

Oblique intra-articular fracture extending into the first carpometacarpal joint. The fracture fragment is held in place by the anterior oblique ligament whilst traction of the abductor pollicis longus tendon causes the rest of the thumb metacarpal to dislocate or sublux proximally and laterally. A similar injury, the Rolando fracture, displays a comminuted (rather than oblique) fracture (Fig. 5.34).

Cause – axial force on flexed metacarpal, such as a punching injury with a clenched fist.

Example of treatment – often requires open reduction internal fixation as is an unstable fracture.

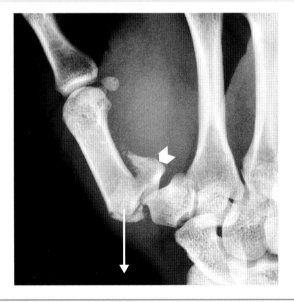

Fig. 5.34 Rolando fracture; right thumb. Volar fracture fragment (arrowhead) remains articulating with the trapezium whilst there is proximal and lateral displacement of the rest of the metacarpal (arrow). (From STATdx © Elsevier 2022)

METACARPOPHALANGEAL AND INTERPHALANGEAL JOINTS

Type

The metacarpophalangeal joints (MTPJs) are synovial ellipsoid joints whilst the interphalangeal joints (IPJs) are synovial hinge joints.

Bony articular surfaces
The concave base of the proximal phalanx articulates with the rounded head of the adjacent metacarpal in the metacarpophalangeal joints.

The head of each proximal and middle phalanx has a bicondylar (rounded) articular surface with central depression to accommodate the adjacent articular surface of the bases of the distal/middle phalanges, which have a biconcave surface with a central median ridge.

Fibrous capsule
Attach the neck of the metacarpal/phalanx to the base of the adjacent more distal phalanx. The thickened anterior (palmar) aspect of the capsule of the interphalangeal joints, called the *volar plate*, helps prevent hyperextension of the joint.

Synovial membrane
Lines the fibrous capsule, covers the parts of the bone not covered with articular hyaline cartilage and secretes synovial fluid, which lubricates the joint.

Supporting ligaments
Lateral and medial collateral ligaments – radial and ulna sides of the joint to stabilise abduction/adduction.
Palmar ligament – on the anterior part of joints to prevent hyperextension. Blends with the volar plate of the capsule to insert at the base of the phalanx.
Transverse metacarpal ligaments – connect the palmar ligaments of each metacarpal head to that adjacent to it (except the thumb).
Extensor hoods – extend over the dorsal aspect of the metacarpophalangeal joint to hold the tendons that extend the fingers in place and aid fine movement.

Movements
Movements of the hand and fingers are extremely complex and formed by a combination of extrinsic muscles in the forearm for strength and grip and the intrinsic muscles of the hand, which control finer, more delicate movements of the fingers. The predominate movements by the extrinsic muscles are:
Flexion – by the flexor digitorum (or pollicis in the thumb) muscles to each digit.
Extension – by the extensor digitorum (or pollicis) muscles to each digit.

Blood supply

Radial artery – thumb and lateral aspect of the index finger.
Ulnar artery – medial aspect of index finger and middle, ring, and little fingers.

Nerve supply

Radial, median, and ulnar nerves.

TRAUMA

Dislocation (Fig. 5.35)

Typically of the interphalangeal joints, more commonly the proximal joint. Important to rule out associated bony fracture, especially subtle volar plate avulsion at the base of the phalanx (Fig. 5.36).
Cause – hyperextension injury such as in basketball or netball.
Example of treatment – reduction and 'buddy' strapping to the adjacent finger. Rehabilitation essential.

Fig. 5.35 Distal interphalangeal joint dislocation; little finger lateral projection. This is a posterior (dorsal) dislocation as the distal phalanx is displaced posteriorly (arrow). (From STATdx © Elsevier 2022)

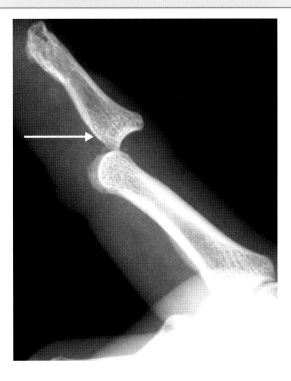

Fig. 5.36 Volar plate avulsion fracture; right middle finger. Small avulsion fracture (arrow) from the base of the middle phalanx. Note the lucent donor site (arrowhead). (From STATdx © Elsevier 2022)

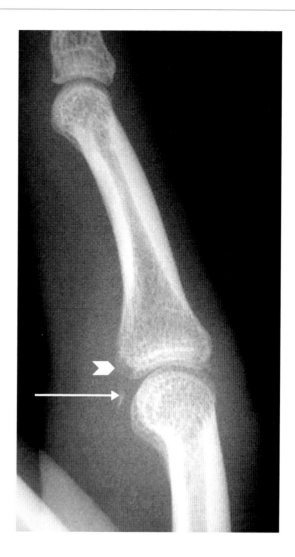

Mallet finger

Avulsion fracture (or extensor tendon rupture) at the base of the dorsal aspect of the distal phalanx (opposite surface to volar plate avulsion). Presents with flexion at the distal interphalangeal joint, the *mallet deformity*, which the patient cannot extend.

Cause – forced flexion of an extended finger, such as a blow on the end of a digit when trying to catch a ball.

Example of treatment – splint to maintain reduction. Surgical fixation *is* often difficult *because of* small fracture fragments.

CHAPTER CONTENTS

Clavicle	102	Trauma	116
Fractures	104	Pathology	121
Scapula	105	Acromioclavicular (AC) Joint	122
Fractures	110	Trauma	123
Shoulder Joint	112	Sternoclavicular (SC) Joint	124

The shoulder (or pectoral) girdle, consisting of the scapula and clavicle bones, is the attachment between the upper limb at the glenohumeral (shoulder) joint and the thorax through the sternoclavicular joint and muscular attachments. The two bones are connected at the acromioclavicular joint.

CLAVICLE (FIGS. 6.1, 6.2)

Type	Long bone, no medullary cavity.
Position	Runs horizontally from the base of the neck to the shoulder and is subcutaneous throughout. Informally referred to as the collar bone.
Articulations	The medial *sternal end* of the clavicle with the clavicular notch of the manubrium sterni to form the sternoclavicular joint. The lateral *acromial end* of the clavicle with the acromion process of the scapula to form the acromioclavicular joint.
Main parts	*Shaft* – 'S' shaped. Convex anteriorly on medial end, concave anteriorly on lateral end. *Sternal end* – medial; expanded, quadrangular. *Acromial end* – lateral; slightly expanded, flattened on end. *Facet for the first costal cartilage* – on the inferior aspect of the sternal end. *Costal tuberosity* – inferior surface of the sternal end, attachment for the costoclavicular ligament. *Conoid tubercle* – on the posteroinferior aspect of the acromial end, attachment for the conoid ligament. *Trapezoid line* – ridge extending laterally from the conoid tubercle; coracoclavicular ligament attached.

Fig. 6.1 Right clavicle (superior aspect).

A – Shaft
B – Posterior border
C – Acromial end
D – Anterior border
E – Sternal end

Fig. 6.2 Right clavicle (inferior aspect).

1 – Facet for the acromion
2 – Trapezoid line
3 – Conoid tubercle
4 – Posterior border
5 – Facet for the sternum
6 – Facet for the first costal cartilage
7 – Anterior border

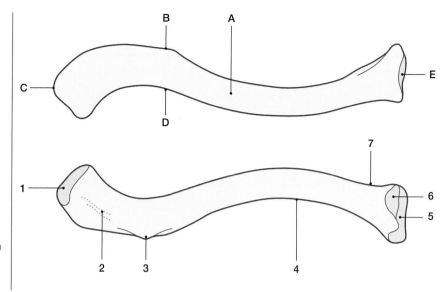

Ossification

Intramembranous rather than a hyaline cartilage model. It is the first bone to ossify but one of the last to fuse.

Primary centres
Two centres in the shaft – appears in the fifth week of intrauterine life. Then they fuse to form one centre at age 45 days.

Secondary centres
One centre – sternal end appears at age 18–20 years. Sternal end fuses with the shaft at age 18–25 years.

Radiographic appearances of the clavicle (Fig. 6.3)

Fig. 6.3 Left clavicle: anteroposterior (A) and inferosuperior (axial) (B) projection. (From Lampignano, Bontrager's Textbook of Radiographic Positioning and Related Anatomy, 10e, Elsevier)

A – Sternal end
B – Shaft
C – Acromial end
D – Acromioclavicular joint (ACJ)
E – Acromion
F – Sternoclavicular joint (SCJ)
G – Conoid tubercle

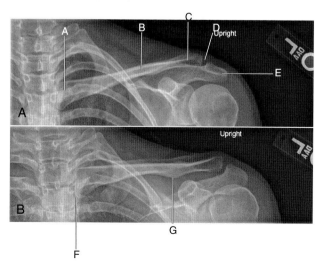

FRACTURES (FIGS. 6.4, 6.5)

A common fracture, particularly in children. Most occur in the middle third, where the bone changes direction between the two curves. Non-union, or mal-union, may occur in more displaced fractures and cause a residual deformity.

Cause – fall on the outstretched hand, force transmitted through upper limb to the trunk

Example of treatment – often treated conservatively with a sling but severely displaced may require surgical fixation.

Fig. 6.4 Left clavicle fracture. Transverse fracture of the mid clavicle with inferior displacement of the lateral part. (From STATdx © Elsevier 2022)

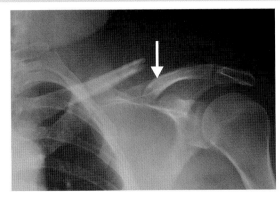

Fig. 6.5 Right clavicle fracture. The fracture is occult on the anteroposterior radiograph (A) because of overlying bony structures. Axial CT image (B) demonstrates a greenstick fracture (arrow) in this paediatric case. (From Guillaume Bierry, Skeletal Trauma, 1e, Elsevier)

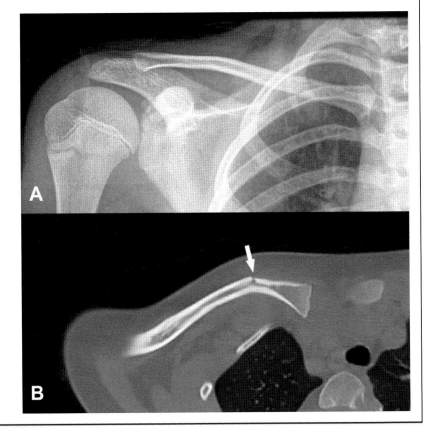

INSIGHT

Where there is a change in direction or orientation within a bone, this is a natural weak point and a commonplace for fracture or injury.

SCAPULA (FIGS. 6.6, 6.7)

Type

Flat bone. Complex, roughly triangular-shaped bone with several projections.

Position

Posterior bone of the shoulder girdle, lying on the posterolateral aspect of the bony thorax extending from the second to seventh ribs. Known informally as the shoulder blade.

Articulations

Acromion process of the scapula with the acromial end of the clavicle to form the acromioclavicular joint.
Glenoid cavity of the scapula with the head of the humerus to form the glenohumeral (shoulder) joint.
The anterior costal aspect articulates with the thoracic cage via the *scapulothoracic joint*. Not a true joint, the scapula is held against the ribs by muscles that allow a range of movements.

Main parts

Posterior aspect
Body – triangular in shape.
Spine – prominent narrow ridge on posterior surface dividing the superior third from the inferior two-thirds; forms attachment for the trapezius and deltoid muscles.
Supraspinous fossa – depression superior to the spine for the supraspinatus muscle.
Infraspinous fossa – depression inferior to the spine for the infraspinatus muscle.
Acromion process – broadened lateral aspect of the spine. Palpable as the tip of the shoulder. On its medial border, there is an articular facet for the clavicle.
Superior angle – at the junction between the superior and medial borders.
Inferior angle – at the junction between the medial and lateral borders; most inferior part
Medial (vertebral) border – palpable for most of its length.
Lateral (axillary) border – teres minor muscle is attached below the infraglenoid tubercle.
Spinoglenoid notch – at the junction of the spine and the neck.
Acromial angle – junction of the acromion and spine, posteriorly.

Lateral aspect
Head of the scapula – at the lateral angle, formed at the junction of the superior and lateral borders.

Fig. 6.6 Left scapula: costal (anterior) aspect.

A – Scapular notch
B – Superior border
C – Superior angle
D – Subscapular fossa
E – Medial border
F – Inferior angle
G – Lateral border
H – Neck
I – Infraglenoid tubercle
J – Glenoid cavity (fossa)
K – Head
L – Coracoid process
M – Acromion process
N – Articular facet for the clavicle

Fig. 6.7 Left scapula: dorsal (posterior) aspect.

1 – Acromion process
2 – Acromial angle
3 – Supraglenoid tubercle
4 – Spinoglenoid notch
5 – Glenoid cavity (fossa)
6 – Infraglenoid tubercle
7 – Lateral border
8 – Inferior angle
9 – Medial border
10 – Infraspinous fossa
11 – Spine
12 – Supraspinous fossa
13 – Superior angle
14 – Superior border
15 – Scapular notch
16 – Coracoid process

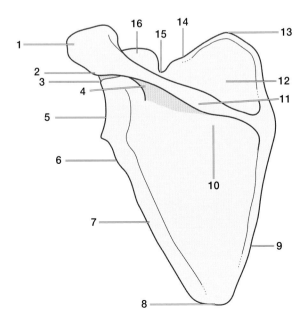

Glenoid cavity (fossa) – 'pear-shaped' depression for the head of the humerus to form the glenohumeral joint on the lateral aspect of the head of the scapula.
Supraglenoid tubercle – superior aspect of the glenoid cavity, tendon of the long head of the biceps brachii attached.
Infraglenoid tubercle – inferior to the glenoid cavity; provides attachment for the tendon of the long head of the triceps brachii muscle.

Anterior aspect
Subscapular fossa – large depression for the subscapularis muscle.
Superior border – lateral to the superior angle.
Scapular notch – lateral end of the superior border.
Coracoid process – long 'finger-like' expanded portion, lateral to the scapular notch; provides attachment for the coracoclavicular ligament and short head of the biceps brachii and coracobrachialis muscle tendons.

Ossification (Fig. 6.11)

Primary centre
Body and spine first appear near the glenoid cavity – eighth week of intrauterine life.

Secondary centres
Seven centres, though the number and ages at which they appear vary:
coracoid process (two centres) – age 12–18 months, fuses age 15 years
glenoid – age 10–11 years, fuses age 16–18 years
inferior angle – puberty, age 14-20 years
acromion process (two centres) – puberty, age 14–20 years
medial border – puberty, age 14–20 years
Unless otherwise stated, fuse with body, age 20–25 years

Radiographic appearances of the scapula (Figs. 6.8–6.11)

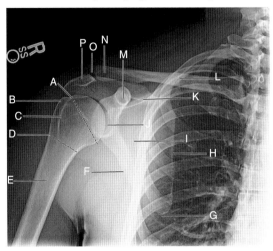

Fig. 6.8 Shoulder joint and scapula: anteroposterior projection. Note the normal overlap between the head of the humerus and glenoid cavity. (From Lampignano, Bontrager's Textbook of Radiographic Positioning and Related Anatomy, 10e, Elsevier)

A – Anatomical neck of the humerus
B – Greater tuberosity
C – Lesser tuberosity
D – Surgical neck of the humerus
E – Shaft of the humerus
F – Lateral border
G – Inferior angle
H – Medial border
I – Body
J – Glenoid fossa
K – Spine
L – Superior angle
M – Coracoid process
N – Acromial end of the clavicle
O – Acromioclavicular joint
P – Acromion process

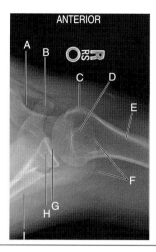

Fig. 6.9 Right shoulder joint and scapula: superoinferior axial projection. (From Lampignano, Bontrager's Textbook of Radiographic Positioning and Related Anatomy, 10e, Elsevier)

A – Clavicle
B – Coracoid process
C – Lesser tuberosity

D – Head of the humerus
E – Shaft of the humerus
F – Acromion process

G – Glenoid cavity (fossa)
H – Head of the scapula
I – Spine of the scapula

Fig. 6.10 Right shoulder joint and scapula: lateral scapula/Y-projection. (From Lampignano, Bontrager's Textbook of Radiographic Positioning and Related Anatomy, 10e, Elsevier)

A – Acromion process
B – Spine of the scapula
C – Head of the humerus
D – Body
E – Inferior angle
F – Ribs
G – Glenoid cavity (at the junction of Y)
H – Coracoid process
I – Superior angle
J – Acromial end of the clavicle

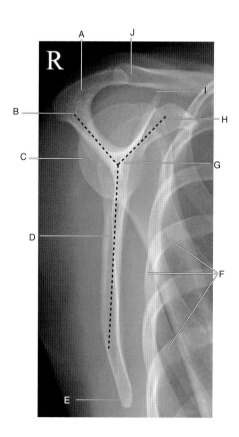

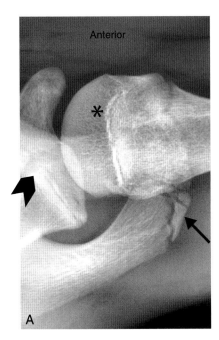
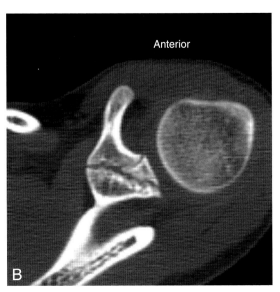

Fig. 6.11 Selected scapula ossification centres . Axial right shoulder projection (A) demonstrates the acromial (arrow) and glenoid (arrowhead) ossification centres and that of the humeral head (*). Axial CT (B) shows the unfused ossification centres of the coracoid and glenoid. (From STATdx © Elsevier 2022)

FRACTURES

Body and neck (Fig. 6.12)

Fractures to the body or neck usually result from high energy trauma such as road traffic collisions. Due to the mechanism of injury, there is a need to consider other injuries such as head and lung trauma and other fractures. Often intra-articular, computed tomography (CT) 3D reformat images are used to assess complex fractures

Cause – direct blow. Usually a high velocity injury.

Example of treatment – conservative, sling, for comfort, unless complex when surgical intervention may be required, such as when associated with a clavicle fracture ("floating shoulder" Fig. 6.12)

Acromion and coracoid process

Usually avulsion fractures or high energy injuries. May be confused with unfused ossification centres.

Cause – direct trauma or avulsion fractures during sports.

Example of treatment – conservative, sling, for comfort.

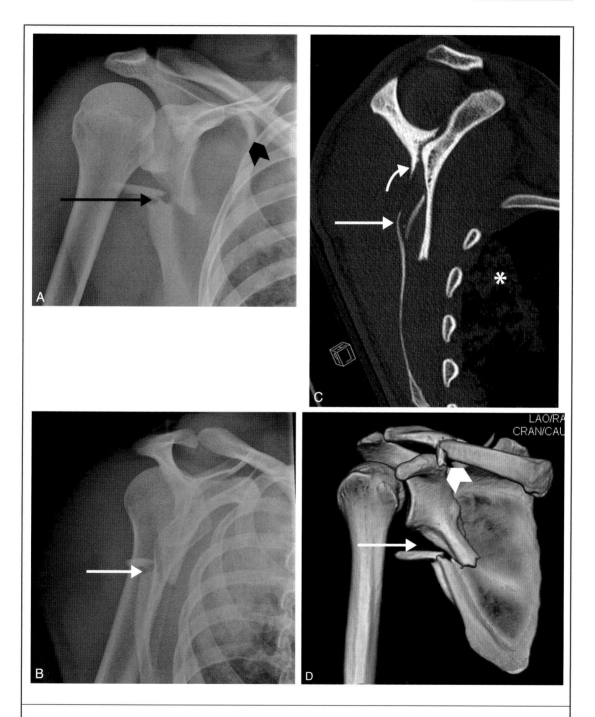

Fig. 6.12 Scapula fracture "floating shoulder." Right anteroposterior (A) and lateral (B) projections show a comminuted fracture of the body (arrow) with associated fracture of the clavicle (arrowhead). Sagittal CT (C) and 3D CT (D) reformat demonstrate the extent of the scapula fracture (arrow), clavicle fracture (arrowhead), and fracture of the acromion (curved arrow). There is also an underlying lung contusion (*). Open reduction and internal fixation were indicated in this case (E). (From STATdx © Elsevier 2022)

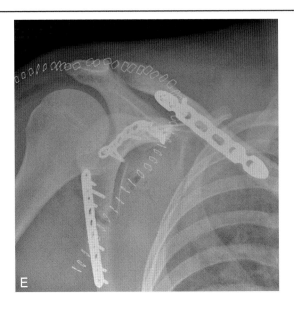

Fig. 6.12 (*Cont.*)

SHOULDER JOINT (FIGS. 6.13, 6.14)

More precisely, the glenohumeral joint (GHJ).

Fig. 6.13 Right shoulder joint (coronal section).

A – Fibrous capsule
B – Synovial membrane
C – Synovial membrane
D – Long head of the
    biceps tendon
E – Surgical neck of the
    humerus
F – Fibrous capsule
    (axillary recess)
G – Synovial membrane
H – Glenoid labrum
I – Glenoid cavity of the
    scapula
J – Articular hyaline
    cartilage
K – Synovial fluid
L – Glenoid labrum
M – Supraglenoid tubercle

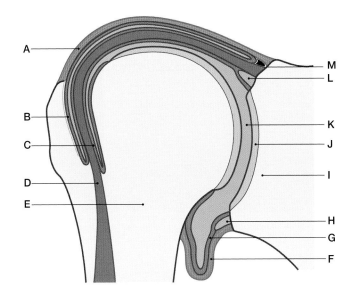

Fig. 6.14 Right shoulder joint (anterior aspect).

1 – Coracoacromial
      ligament
2 – Coracohumeral
      ligament
3 – Transverse humeral
      ligament
4 – Long head of biceps
      tendon
5 – Fibrous capsule
      (axillary recess)
6 – Inferior glenohumeral
      ligament
7 – Middle glenohumeral
      ligament
8 – Superior
      glenohumeral
      ligament

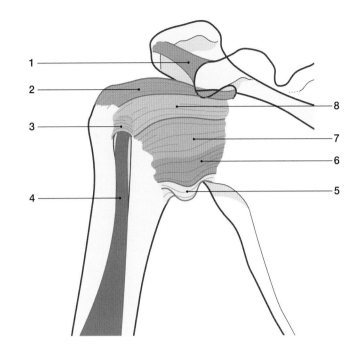

Type

Synovial ball and socket joint. The most freely moveable synovial joint.

Bony articular surfaces
Head of the humerus with the glenoid cavity of the scapula. The articular surfaces are covered with articular hyaline cartilage.

Fibrous capsule
Forms a cylindrical sleeve that is attached medially to the rim of the glenoid and laterally to the anatomical neck of the humerus. The capsule is loose inferiorly to allow movement with several expanded recesses (anterior, posterior, axillary).

Synovial membrane
Lines the fibrous capsule, encloses the tendon of the long head of biceps and is medially reflected over the glenoid labrum. The membrane secretes synovial fluid, which lubricates the joint. In addition, there are several associated bursae, including:
Subscapular bursa – lies between the joint and the subscapularis muscle anteriorly.
Subacromial bursa – lies between the shoulder joint, superficial to the supraspinatus muscle, and the acromion process.

Strengthening ligaments

Glenohumeral ligaments (superior, middle and inferior) – from the anterior glenoid of the scapula to the lesser tuberosity and the anatomical neck of the humerus.

Coracohumeral ligament – from the coracoid process of the scapula to the greater tuberosity of the humerus.

Transverse humeral ligament – between the lesser and greater tuberosities of the humerus; maintains the tendon of the long head of biceps within the intertubercular sulcus (bicipital groove).

Tendons

The muscles increase joint stability and hold the humerus in the glenoid without reducing mobility. Their tendons blend with and reinforce the joint capsule and form the '*rotator cuff*':

Supraspinatus tendon attached to the superior aspect of the greater tuberosity of the humerus.

Infraspinatus tendon attached to the middle of the greater tuberosity of the humerus.

Teres minor attached to the infero-posterior aspect of the greater tuberosity of the humerus.

Subscapularis tendon attached to the anterior aspect of the lesser tuberosity of the humerus.

Intracapsular structures

Glenoid labrum – fibrocartilaginous rim around the glenoid cavity to deepen the socket.

Tendon of the long head of biceps brachii – proximal attachment at the supraglenoid tubercle, then passing inferiorly through the joint capsule and bicipital groove to where it becomes the muscle. Surrounded by a synovial tendon sheath to reduce friction within the groove.

Movements

Flexion by the pectoralis major and the anterior fibres of the deltoid muscles.

Extension by the posterior fibres of the deltoid and teres major, assisted by the latissimus dorsi.

Abduction by the deltoid, assisted by the supraspinatus (up to about 15 degrees).

Adduction by the pectoralis major and latissimus dorsi, assisted by the teres major.

Medial rotation by the pectoralis major, anterior fibres of the deltoid, teres major and subscapularis.

Lateral rotation by the posterior fibres of the deltoid, infraspinatus and teres minor.

Circumduction – a combination of the above movements.

Blood supply

Branches of the axillary and subclavian arteries.

Nerve supply

Suprascapular, axillary and lateral pectoral nerves.

Imaging appearances of the shoulder joint (Figs. 6.8–6.10, 6.15, 6.16)

Fig. 6.15 Right shoulder; Oblique coronal T1W MRI arthrogram arthrogram. (From STATdx © Elsevier 2022)

A – Acromion
B – Supraspinatous tendon
C – Greater tuberosity
D – Cortex of the humerus
E – Remnant of the epiphyseal growth plate
F – Axillary joint recess (pouch)
G – Inferior glenoid labrum
H – Articular cartilage of glenoid cavity
I – Superior glenoid labrum

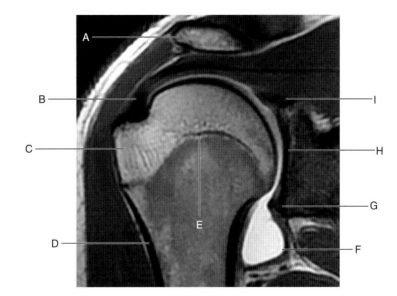

Fig. 6.16 Right shoulder; Axial T1W MR arthrogram. (From STATdx © Elsevier 2022)

1 – Long head of the biceps tendon
2 – Greater tuberosity
3 – Infraspinatous tendon
4 – Posterior joint recess
5 – Posterior glenoid labrum
6 – Glenoid
7 – Articular hyaline cartilage
8 – Anterior glenoid labrum
9 – Anterior joint recess
10 – Subscapularis tendon
11 – Lesser tuberosity

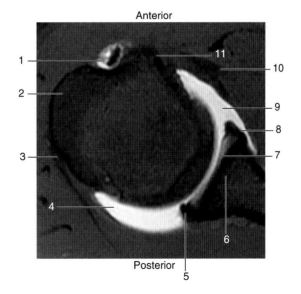

TRAUMA

 INSIGHT

As with all joint or intra-articular trauma, a combination of bony and soft tissue injuries must be considered.

Anterior dislocation (Figs. 6.17, 6.18)

The shoulder (glenohumeral) joint is the most commonly dislocated joint in the body, of which 95% are anterior dislocations. The humeral head displaces anteriorly, medially, and inferiorly, often lying inferior to the coracoid.

Associated with other injuries when the humeral head strikes the glenoid, such as an impaction fracture of the greater tuberosity (Hill-Sachs fracture) or fracture of the bone or fibrocartilage labrum of the glenoid (Bankart lesion).

Cause – fall on an outstretched hand or direct blow.

Example of treatment – reduction under anaesthetic. Sling for support. May require surgical intervention for recurrent dislocations and instability.

Fig. 6.17 Anterior dislocation right shoulder; anteroposterior (A) and axial (B) projections. The humeral head (arrow) has displaced anteriorly, inferiorly, and medially from the glenoid (arrowhead), now positioned inferior to the coracoid process (*). (From STATdx © Elsevier 2022)

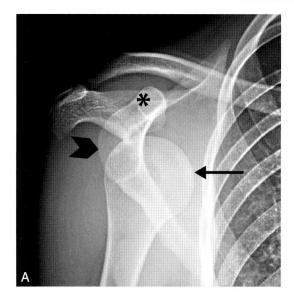

Fig. 6.17—Con't

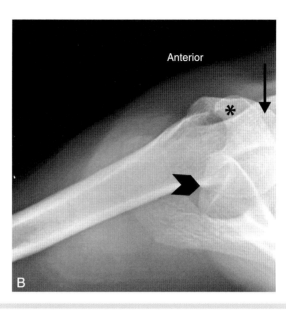

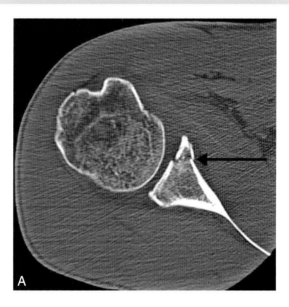

Fig. 6.18 Anterior dislocation right shoulder; post-reduction. Axial (A) and 3D CT reformat (B) imaging demonstrated a Bankart fracture of the glenoid (arrow) and small Hill-Sachs impaction fracture of the greater tuberosity (arrowhead). (From STATdx © Elsevier 2022)

Fig. 6.18—Cont'd

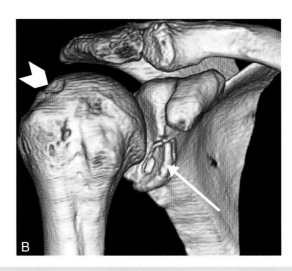

Posterior dislocation (Fig. 6.19)

Much less common than anterior. Usually dislocates directly posteriorly with fixed internal rotation ("lightbulb sign"). Also associated with impaction fractures of the humeral head or glenoid abnormality.
Cause – most commonly during an epileptic seizure or electric shock. Direct blow to the anterior shoulder.
Example of treatment – reduction under anaesthetic. Sling for support. May require surgical intervention for
   recurrent dislocations and instability.

Fig. 6.19 Posterior dislocation right shoulder; anteroposterior (A) and axial (B) projections. The humeral head (arrow) is interiorly rotated, producing the classic 'lightbulb' sign, and is perched on the posterior aspect of the glenoid (arrowhead). Note the widened glenohumeral joint space (*). (From STATdx © Elsevier 2022)

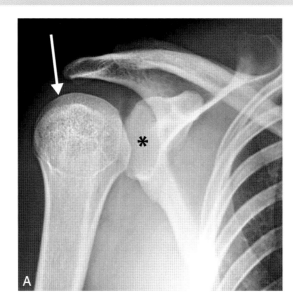

Fig. 6.19—Cont'd

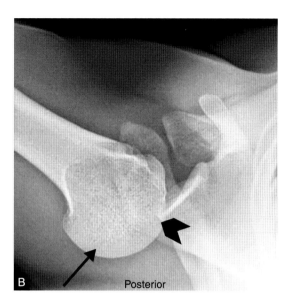

B   Posterior

Glenoid labrum tears

May occur instead of, or as well as, bony or other soft tissue injury. Several variants include superior labrum anteroposterior and anteroinferior (Bankart lesion) tears. Best imaged using MRI arthrogram.

Cause – various but include overhead arm movements, fall on an outstretched hand, and associated with glenohumeral joint dislocations.

Example of treatment – often conservative, but surgery may be indicated in more severe tears.

Rotator cuff tears (Fig. 6.20)

May be partial, full or complete thickness depending on how much of the tendon is affected. Incidence increases with age. Supraspinatus most commonly affected. Imaged using ultrasound or MRI.

Cause – acute; because of a fall or lifting a heavy object, or chronic; because of underlying diseases such as tendinopathy (tendon degeneration) or impingement.

Example of treatment – dependent on severity; analgesia, physiotherapy, or surgical repair.

Fig. 6.20 Full thickness tear of the supraspinatus tendon. Longitudinal (A) and transverse (B) ultrasound images demonstrate a gap (arrow) in the normal tendon fibres of the tendon, proximal to the greater tuberosity (*). Note that the overlying bursa (arrowhead) is depressed, partly filling the gap. (From STATdx © Elsevier 2022)

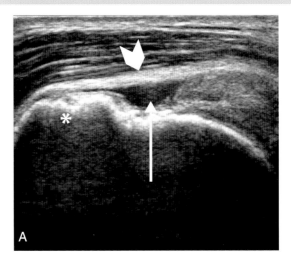

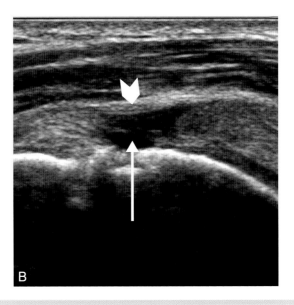

PATHOLOGY

Calcific tendinopathy (Fig. 6.21)

Calcification (same mineral *hydroxyapatite* as found in bone) within tendons and bursae. Most common in the rotator cuff (particularly supraspinatus) but can affect any tendon in the body. Well visualised on radiographs and ultrasound.

Causes – idiopathic (unknown), may be associated with metabolic causes.

Treatment – usually self-limiting (resolves without treatment), but options such as shock wave therapy can accelerate the resolution of symptoms.

Fig. 6.21 Calcific tendinopathy of the supraspinatous. Anteroposterior right shoulder projection (A), and longitudinal ultrasound of the supraspinatous tendon (B) demonstrate a large calcified opacity (arrow). Note that this causes shadowing (*) of the ultrasound beam deep to the calcification. (From STATdx © Elsevier 2022)

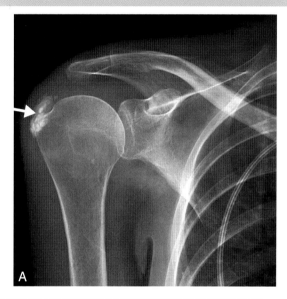

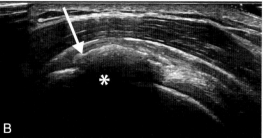

ACROMIOCLAVICULAR (AC) JOINT (FIG. 6.22)

Type   Synovial plane joint.

Bony articular surfaces
Acromial end of the clavicle with the medial aspect of the acromion process of the scapula. Unlike most synovial joints, articular surfaces are covered with fibrocartilage rather than hyaline cartilage.

Fibrous capsule
Attached to the lateral end of the clavicle and the medial aspect of the acromion process of the scapula.

Synovial membrane
Lines the fibrous capsule and is reflected over the lateral aspect of the articular disc. The membrane secretes synovial fluid, which lubricates the joint.

Supporting ligaments
Acromioclavicular ligament – from the superior aspect of the acromion process to the superior aspect of the clavicle.
Coracoacromial ligament – from the coracoid process of the scapula to the acromion surface of the scapula.
Coracoclavicular ligaments – from the coracoid process of the scapula to the conoid tubercle (conoid ligament) and the trapezoid line of the clavicle (trapezoid ligament).

Intracapsular structure
Articular disc – fibrocartilage; in the superior aspect of the joint, wider superiorly. Sometimes absent.

Fig. 6.22 Right acromioclavicular joint (coronal section).

A – Fibrous capsule
B – Articular disc
C – Fibrocartilage
D – Acromion process of the scapula
E – Synovial fluid
F – Synovial membrane
G – Fibrous capsule
H – Fibrocartilage
I – Acromial end of the clavicle

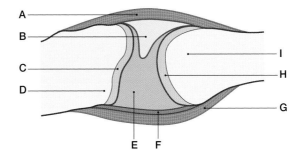

Movements
Gliding.

Blood supply
Suprascapular artery – branch of the subclavian artery.
Thoracoacromial artery – branch of the axillary artery.

Nerve supply
Suprascapular and lateral pectoral nerves.

Radiographic appearances of the acromioclavicular joint (Figs. 6.3, 6.8)

TRAUMA

Subluxation and dislocation (Figs. 6.23, 6.24)
Range from a mild ligament sprain to complete dislocation with rupture of the acromioclavicular and coracoclavicular ligaments. Demonstrated as widening of acromioclavicular joint (>6 mm) and coracoclavicular distance, and loss of alignment of the inferior surface of the acromion and clavicle.
Cause – fall on the point of the shoulder.
Example of treatment – conservative, sling worn for support.

Fig. 6.23 Right acromioclavicular joint subluxation. There is a loss of alignment of the acromion and clavicle (dotted line), but the coracoclavicular distance (arrow) is normal, suggesting these ligaments are intact. (From STATdx © Elsevier 2022)

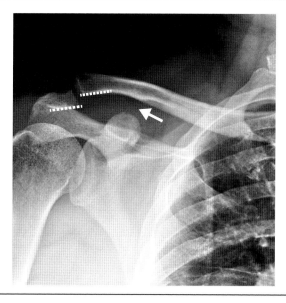

Fig. 6.24 Right acromioclavicular joint dislocation. There is marked superior displacement of the clavicle in relation to the acromion (dotted lines). Widening of the coracoclavicular distance (arrow) suggests ligament rupture. (From STATdx © Elsevier 2022)

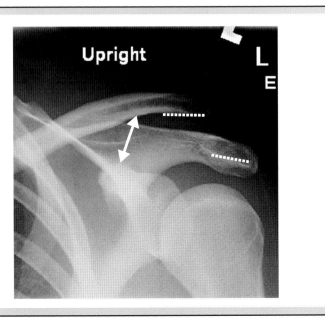

STERNOCLAVICULAR (SC) JOINT (FIG. 6.25)

Type   Synovial saddle joint, permits a wide range of movement.

Bony articular surfaces
The sternal end of the clavicle with the clavicular notch of the manubrium sterni and first costal cartilage. The articular surfaces are covered with fibrocartilage.

Fig. 6.25 Right sternoclavicular joint (coronal section).

A – Sternal end of the clavicle
B – Fibrocartilage
C – Synovial fluid
D – Articular disc
E – Fibrous capsule
F – Synovial fluid
G – Fibrocartilage
H – Clavicular notch of manubrium sterni
I – Synovial membrane
J – Fibrous capsule

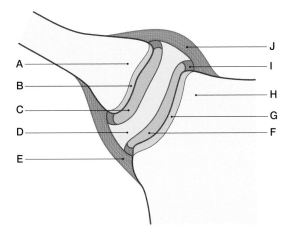

Fibrous capsule

Attached to the sternal end of the clavicle and the lateral aspect of the manubrium sterni. The capsule thins superiorly and inferiorly.

Synovial membrane

Lines the fibrous capsule and is reflected over the articular disc. The membrane secretes synovial fluid, which lubricates the joint.

Strengthening ligaments

Anterior and posterior sternoclavicular ligaments – between the manubrium sterni and sternal end of the clavicle.
Interclavicular ligament – unites the sternal ends of the left and right clavicles.
Costoclavicular ligament – between the anterior costal cartilage of the first rib to costal tuberosity on the inferior clavicle.

Intracapsular structure

Articular disc – fibrocartilage, divides the joint into two distinct parts.

Movements

Elevation.
Depression.
Anterior movement in a gliding horizontal direction.
Posterior movement in a gliding horizontal direction.
Circumduction.

Blood supply

Internal mammary arteries and *suprascapular arteries*, which are branches of the subclavian artery.

Nerve supply

Anterior supraclavicular nerve.

Imaging appearances of the sternoclavicular joint (Fig. 6.26)

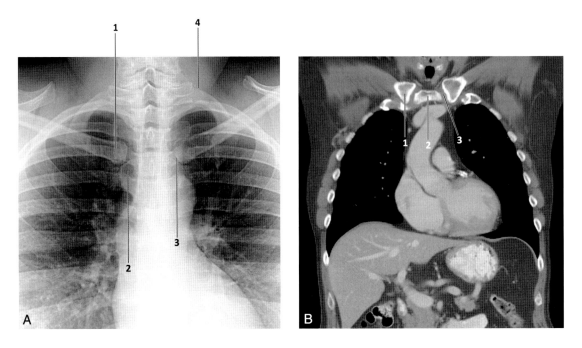

Fig. 6.26 Imaging appearances of the sternoclavicular joints; cropped posteroanterior chest projection (A) and coronal CT (B). (From STATdx © Elsevier 2022)

1 – Sternal end of right clavicle
2 – Manubrium sterni
3 – Left sternoclavicular joint
4 – Left first rib

LOWER LIMB

7

CHAPTER CONTENTS

Femur	127	Knee Joint	164
Patella	136	Proximal Tibiofibular Joint	178
Tibia	140	Distal Tibiofibular Joint	178
Fibula	144	Ankle Joint	179
Foot	150	Intertarsal Joints	188
Tarsal bones	151	Tarsometatarsal Joints	190
Metatarsal bones	155	Metatarsophalangeal and	
Phalanges	156	Interphalangeal Joints	192

FEMUR (FIGS. 7.1, 7.2)

Type

Long bone. Longest, heaviest, and strongest bone in the body.

Position

Forming the thigh between the hip and knee joints. Angles medially (varus) from the hip to the knee joints, more so in females because the pelvis is broader.

Articulations

Head of the femur with the acetabulum of the hip bone to form the hip joint (see Chapter 8).

Femoral condyles with the tibial plateaus of the tibial condyles and the *patellar articular surface* of the femur with the posterior aspect of the patella to form the knee joint.

Main parts

Features of the proximal end of the femur

Head of the femur – rounded, forming two-thirds of a sphere.

Fovea – depression in the head of the femur for the ligament of the head of the femur.

Neck – narrow portion about 5 cm long joining the head to the shaft; lies at an average angle of approximately 125 degrees (it is more acute in males than females).

Fig. 7.1 Right femur (anterior aspect).

A – Fovea
B – Head of the femur
C – Neck of the femur
D – Greater trochanter
E – Intertrochanteric line
F – Shaft
G – Lateral border
H – Lateral epicondyle
I – Lateral condyle
J – Patellar articular surface
K – Medial condyle
L – Medial epicondyle
M – Adductor tubercle
N – Medial border
O – Lesser trochanter

Fig. 7.2 Right femur (posterior aspect).

1 – Fovea
2 – Head of the femur
3 – Lesser trochanter
4 – Spiral line
5 – Linea aspera
6 – Medial supracondylar line
7 – Adductor tubercle
8 – Medial condyle
9 – Intercondylar notch
10 – Lateral condyle
11 – Lateral supracondylar line
12 – Gluteal tuberosity
13 – Intertrochanteric crest
14 – Greater trochanter
15 – Trochanteric fossa

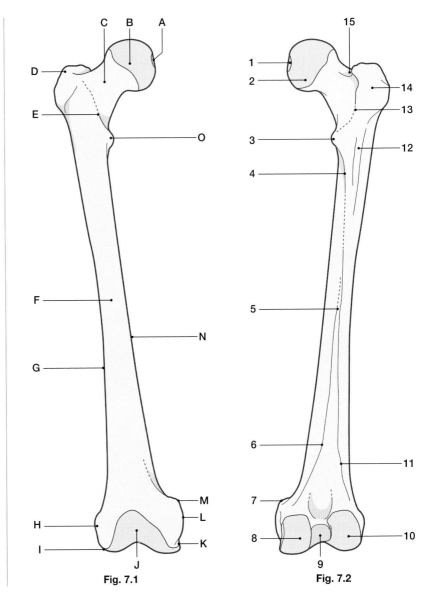

Fig. 7.1

Fig. 7.2

Greater trochanter – lies more superiorly on the lateral aspect at the junction of the shaft with the neck; provides insertion for the gluteus, piriformis, obturator, and gemellus muscles.
Lesser trochanter – more inferiorly on the medial aspect of the junction between the neck and the shaft; provides insertion of the iliopsoas muscle.
Intertrochanteric line – the anterior line between the trochanters; marks part of the junction between the neck and shaft.
Intertrochanteric crest – posterior crest, between the trochanters; marks part of the junction between the neck and the shaft.

Trochanteric fossa – depression inferior to the medial aspect of the greater trochanter.

Features of the shaft (diaphysis) of the femur
Spiral line – posterior aspect, continuous with the intertrochanteric line.
Gluteal tuberosity – lateral surface of the proximal end of the shaft, insertion for the gluteus maximus muscle.
Linea aspera – sharp ridge forming the posterior border below the junction of the spiral line and gluteal tuberosity. Insertion for adductor muscles.
Medial and lateral borders
Anterior, medial, and lateral surfaces – is roughly triangular in cross-section. Nutrient foramina on the medial surface.

Features of the distal end of the femur
Medial and lateral condyles – articular surfaces with the tibia; fused together anteriorly, separated by the intercondylar notch posteriorly.
Medial epicondyle – most prominent point of the medial condyle; provides attachment for the tibial (medial) collateral ligament.
Lateral epicondyle – most prominent point of the lateral condyle; provides attachment for the fibular (lateral) collateral ligament.
Intercondylar notch/fossa – between the condyles, inferiorly and posteriorly.
Patellar articular surface – anterior aspect of the distal end of the femur, joining the condyles.
Adductor tubercle – superior to the medial epicondyle; provides attachment for the adductor magnus muscle.
Medial supracondylar line – from the adductor tubercle to the linea aspera.
Lateral supracondylar line – from the lateral epicondyle to the linea aspera.
Popliteal surface – flattened triangular area between the supracondylar lines.
Popliteal sulcus – groove on the lateral condyle for the popliteus tendon

Ossification (Fig. 7.3)

Primary centre
Shaft – appears in the seventh week of intrauterine life.

Secondary centres
Four centres:
    Distal epiphysis – appears just before birth;
    Head – appears at six months old;
    Greater trochanter – appears at age four;
    Lesser trochanter – appears at age 12.
Fuse with shaft at age 16–18.

Fig. 7.3 Ossification centres of the (left) femur and patella. (From STATdx © Elsevier 2022)

A – Shaft (*in utero*)
B – Distal epiphysis (just before birth)
C – Femoral head (age six months)
D – Greater trochanter (age four years)
E – Lesser trochanter (age 12 years)
F – Patella (age three to six years)

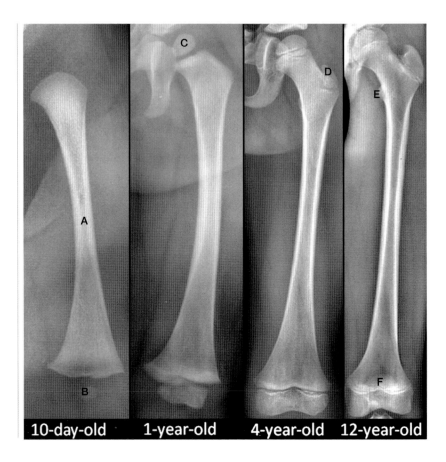

Radiographic appearances of the femur (Figs. 7.4–7.7)

Fig. 7.4 Left femur, proximal; anteroposterior projection. (From STATdx © Elsevier 2022)

A – Fovea
B – Head of the femur
C – Lesser trochanter
D – Shaft
E – Intertrochanteric crest
F – Greater trochanter
G – Neck
H – Acetabulum

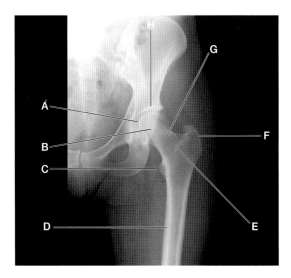

Fig. 7.5 Left femur, proximal; lateral projection. (From STATdx © Elsevier 2022)

1 – Head
2 – Lesser trochanter
3 – Shaft
4 – Greater trochanter
5 – Acetabulum

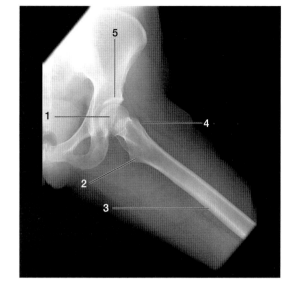

Fig. 7.6 Left femur, distal; anteroposterior projection. Note the medial angulation from the hip to the knee. (From STATdx © Elsevier 2022)

A – Cortex of shaft
B – Medial supracondylar line
C – Adductor tubercle
D – Medial condyle
E – Lateral condyle
F – Patella
G – Lateral supracondylar line
H – Linea aspera

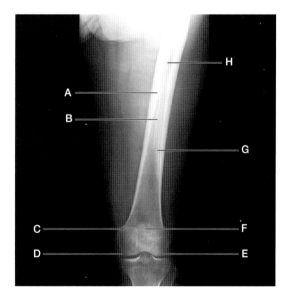

Fig. 7.7 Left femur, distal; lateral projection. (From STATdx © Elsevier 2022)

1 – Linea aspera
2 – Medial femoral condyle
3 – Patella
4 – Lateral femoral condyle

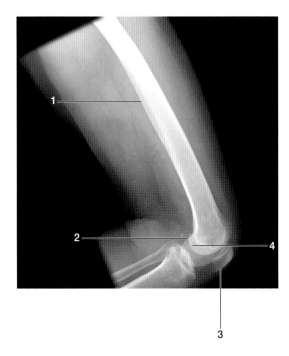

FRACTURES

 INSIGHT

Proximal femoral fractures can be divided into whether they are within or outside the hip joint capsule. This heavily influences management mainly because of the location of the blood supply to the head, which passes through the neck.

There are three main types depending on their location: the neck of the femur, inter-trochanteric, or sub-trochanteric.

They are common in older females (in particular), associated with osteoporosis, and can occur even with simple falls.

Neck of the femur (Figs. 7.8, 7.9)

Intracapsular. Involves the neck between the head and intertrochanteric line. Osteonecrosis of the head is relatively common as blood vessels are often damaged. Can be very subtle or occult on radiographs, so further imaging (computed tomography (CT) or magnetic resonance imaging (MRI)) is required if still clinically suspected.

Cause – typically because of a fall. Stress fractures may occur.

Example of treatment – reduction under anaesthetic; hemiarthroplasty to replace the femoral head, internal fixation (screws) if undisplaced.

Fig. 7.8 Neck of a right femur fracture; anteroposterior and lateral projections. There is medial (varus) and posterior angulation at the fracture site (arrows) in the middle of the neck. (From STATdx © Elsevier 2022)

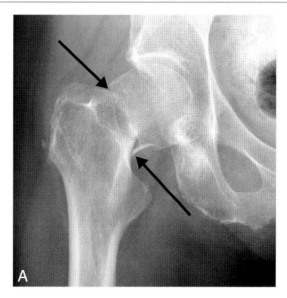

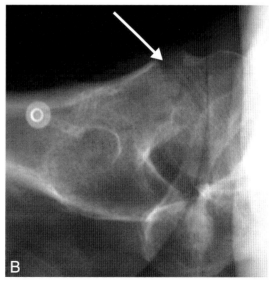

Fig. 7.9 Subtle neck of a right femur fracture. Subtle sclerosis (arrow) is the only sign of fracture on the anteroposterior projection (A). The coronal T2W MR image (B) demonstrates a linear fracture (arrow) with extensive surrounding marrow oedema (arrowhead). (From STATdx © Elsevier 2022)

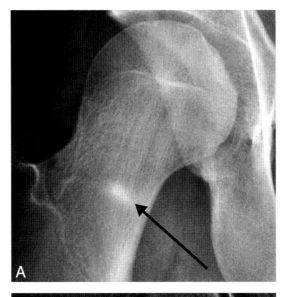

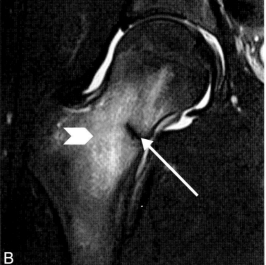

Intertrochanteric fracture (Fig. 7.10)

Extracapsular. Occur between and involving the greater and lesser trochanters. Osteonecrosis is uncommon as it occurs distal to the blood vessels supplying the head.
Cause – because of a fall.
Example of treatment – reduction under anaesthetic; internal fixation, dynamic hip screw.

Fig. 7.10 Intertrochanteric fracture right femur; anteroposterior (A) and lateral (B) projections. The fracture (arrow) extends from the greater trochanter to the lesser trochanter (arrowhead). There is medial (varus) and posterior angulation at the fracture site. (From STATdx © Elsevier 2022)

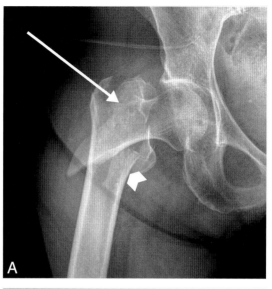

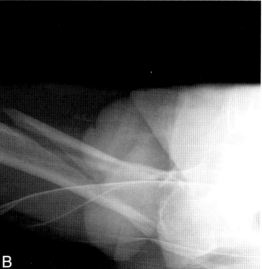

Sub-trochanteric/shaft of the femur (Fig. 7.11)

Extracapsular. Fracture patterns variable. It may be associated with neurovascular injury if displaced or comminuted.

Cause – because of high energy trauma, e.g., a road traffic collision; or because of an underlying pathologic condition, e.g., osteoporosis, tumour.

Example of treatment – internal fixation using an intramedullary nail.

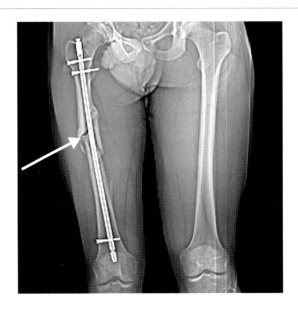

Fig. 7.11 Right femur midshaft fracture; anteroposterior CT topogram. This comminuted fracture (arrow) has been treated with an intramedullary nail. (From STATdx © Elsevier 2022)

PATELLA (FIGS. 7.12, 7.13)

Type	Sesamoid bone, the largest in the skeletal system. Triangular in shape.
Position	Anterior to the distal end of the femur within the quadriceps femoris tendon. Increases the efficiency of the quadriceps femoris muscle and protects the knee joint.
Articulation	Two *facets* of the patella with the femoral condyles form the patellofemoral part of the knee joint.
Main parts	*Base* – superior aspect, attached to the quadriceps femoris muscle by the quadriceps tendon. *Apex* – inferior aspect, attached by the patellar tendon to the tibial tuberosity. *Facet for the lateral condyle of the femur* – large, on the posterolateral aspect. *Facet for the medial condyle of the femur* – small, on the posteromedial aspect.

Ossification (Fig. 7.3)

Primary centre

Appears at age three to six. Ossification is complete at puberty.

A normal variant of a bipartite (Fig. 7.14) or tripartite patella may be seen in some people caused by additional unfused secondary ossification centres. Not to be confused with a fracture.

Fig. 7.12 Left patella
(anterior aspect).

A – Base
B – Apex

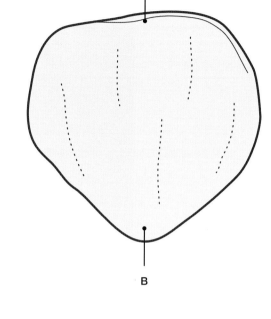

Fig. 7.13 Left patella
(posterior aspect).

1 – Facet for lateral condyle
of the femur
2 – Apex
3 – Facet for medial condyle
of the femur
4 – Base

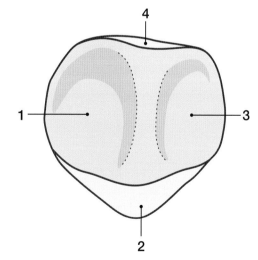

Fig. 7.14 Bipartite patella, right knee; anteroposterior projection. The superolateral position (arrow) is classic for this normal variant. It is round and smooth, unlike a fracture. (From STATdx © Elsevier 2022)

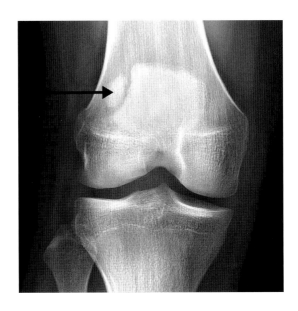

Imaging appearances of the patella (Figs. 7.15, 7.16)

Fig. 7.15 Right patella; axial (skyline) projection. (From STATdx © Elsevier 2022)

A – Lateral patellar facet
B – Lateral femoral condyle
C – Trochlea groove of the femur
D – Medial femoral condyle
E – Medial patellar facet

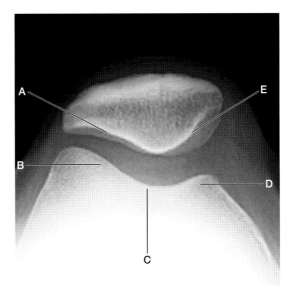

Fig. 7.16 Right knee: axial CT image. (From STATdx © Elsevier 2022)

A – Patella
B – Trochlea groove of the femur
C – Lateral femoral condyle
D – Intercondylar notch
E – Medial femoral condyle
F – Patellofemoral joint

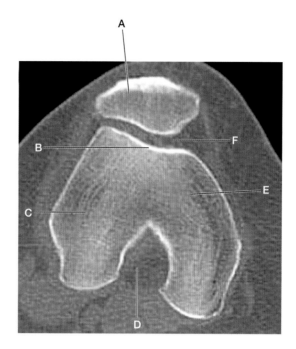

FRACTURES

Transverse (Fig. 7.17)

Orientation of the fracture line and traction of the quadriceps tendon may cause marked displacement.
Cause – sudden, violent contraction of the quadriceps femoris muscle.
Examples of treatment – internal surgical fixation.

Longitudinal

Often minimally displaced and very subtle on radiographs.
Cause – direct blow.
Example of treatment – immobilisation, cast.

Comminuted

Also known as 'stellate,' fracture lines radiate like the points on a star.
Cause – direct blow.
Example of treatment – internal surgical fixation or excision of the patella (patellectomy).

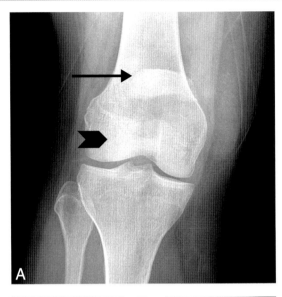

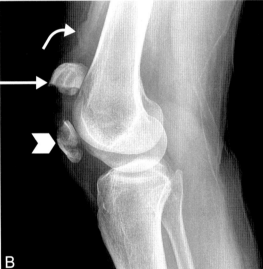

Fig. 7.17 Transverse right patella fracture: anteroposterior (A) and lateral (B) projections. Note the displacement of the proximal part (arrow) compared to the distal part (arrowhead) and how the quadriceps tendon has retracted (curved arrow). (From STATdx © Elsevier 2022)

TIBIA (FIGS. 7.18, 7.19)

Type	Long bone. Larger, weight-bearing bone of lower limb.
Position	Medial bone of the lower limb.
Articulations	*Tibial plateaus* (articular surface of the *Tibial condyles)* with the femoral condyles to form the knee joint.

Fig. 7.18 Left tibia (anterior aspect).

A – Fibular facet
B – Lateral condyle
C – Tubercles of the intercondylar eminence (tibial spines)
D – Medial condyle
E – Tibial tuberosity
F – Interosseous border
G – Anterior border
H – Medial surface
I – Medial malleolus
J – Fibular notch

Left fibula (anterior aspect).
K – Head of the fibula
L – Interosseous border
M – Lateral surface
N – Lateral malleolus

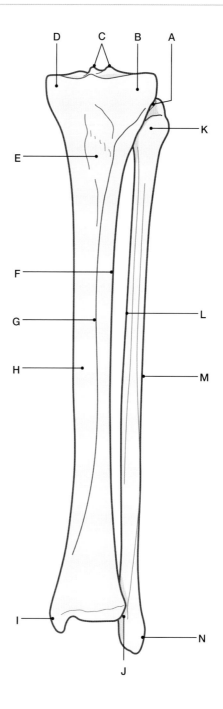

Fig. 7.19 Left tibia
(posterior aspect).

1 – Lateral condyle
2 – Tubercles of the
    intercondylar eminence
    (tibial spines)
3 – Medial condyle
4 – Soleal line
5 – Medial border
6 – Interosseous border
7 – Fibular notch
8 – Medial malleolus

Left fibula (posterior aspect).
9 – Head of the fibula
10 – Interosseous border
11 – Posterior border
12 – Lateral malleolus
13 – Malleolar fossa

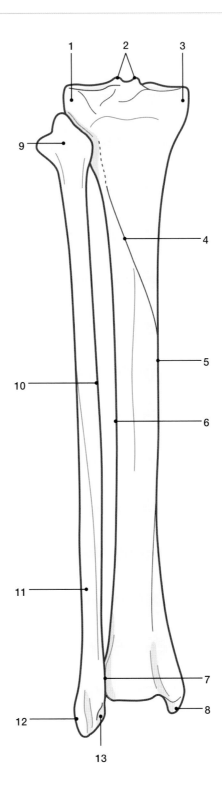

Articular facet on the lateral condyle of the proximal tibia with the head of the fibula to form the superior tibiofibular joint.

Distal end of tibia with the talus to form part of the ankle joint.

Fibular notch of the distal tibia with the distal end of the fibula to form the inferior tibiofibular joint.

Main parts

Features of the proximal end of the tibia

Medial condyle – medial part of the proximal end, larger of the two condyles.

Lateral condyle – lateral part of the proximal end.

Medial tibial plateau – concave articular surface of the medial condyle.

Lateral tibial plateau – flattened articular surface of the lateral condyle.

Tubercles of the intercondylar eminence (tibial spines) – on the superior aspect of the tibia between the articular surfaces. Attachment for cruciate ligaments.

Articular facet – on the posterolateral aspect of the lateral condyle for the head of the fibula.

Tibial tuberosity – anterior aspect; can be palpated 2.5 cm below the condyles; forms attachment for the patellar tendon.

Features of the shaft of the tibia

Soleal line – 'horseshoe-shaped' oblique line on the posterior aspect of the shaft, which receives the soleus muscle.

Medial surface, Lateral surface, Posterior surface – bone is triangular in cross-section. Nutrient foramen is situated on the posterior surface, inferior to the soleal line.

Anterior border – subcutaneous and easily palpated.

Medial border

Interosseous border – attached to the medial aspect of the fibula by an interosseous membrane to form the middle tibiofibular joint (a fibrous syndesmotic joint).

Features of the distal end of the tibia

Medial malleolus – palpable feature at the medial aspect of the ankle.

Posterior malleolus – expanded portion on the posterior aspect of the distal tibia.

Fibular notch – lateral aspect of the distal end, for the distal end of the fibula.

Inferior articular surface – Tibial '*plafond*' (French for ceiling); concave for articulation with the superior surface of the talus.

Ossification (Figs. 7.43, 7.56)

Primary centre

Shaft – seventh week intrauterine life.

Secondary centres

Two centres:

Proximal epiphysis – appears just before or after birth; fuses with the shaft at age 16–18.

Distal epiphysis – appears at age one. Fuses with the shaft at age 15–17. Often leaves a visible sclerotic remnant.

FIBULA (FIGS. 7.18, 7.19)

Type   Long bone. Narrowest of all long bones in relation to its length.

Position   Lateral bone of the lower leg. Non-weight-bearing, but an important muscle attachment site.

Articulations   *Head of the fibula* with the articular facet of the lateral condyle of the tibia to form the superior tibiofibular joint.
Distal end of the fibula with the fibular notch of the tibia to form the inferior tibiofibular joint.
Lateral malleolus of the fibula with the talus to form part of the ankle joint.

Main parts   ## Features of the proximal end of the fibula
Head – rounded aspect; can be palpated 2.5 cm inferior to the lateral aspect of the knee joint.
Styloid process – pointed superior part of the head.
Neck – narrow area inferior to the head.

Features of the shaft of fibula
Anterior border, Posterior border
Interosseous (medial) border – connected to the lateral aspect of the tibia by an interosseous membrane to form the middle tibiofibular joint (syndesmotic fibrous joint).
Nutrient foramen

Features of the distal end of the fibula
Lateral malleolus – lateral aspect of the distal end; bulbous, easily palpated at the ankle. Approximately 1 cm longer than the medial malleolus.
Articular facet – on the medial aspect of the lateral malleolus.
Malleolar fossa – depression on the posteromedial aspect of the distal end; provides attachment for part of the lateral ligaments at the ankle joint.

Ossification (Figs. 7.43, 7.56)

Primary centre
Shaft – eighth week of intrauterine life.

Secondary centres
Two centres:
Distal epiphysis (lateral malleolus) – appears at age one; fuses with the shaft at age 17–19.
Proximal epiphysis (head) – appears at age three to four; fuses with shaft at age 15–17.

Radiographic appearances of the tibia and fibula (Figs. 7.20, 7.21)

Fig. 7.20 Left tibia and fibula: anteroposterior projection.

A – Tubercles of intercondylar eminence (tibial spine)
B – Medial tibial condyle
C – Tibial tuberosity
D – Interosseous borders
E – Cortex of the tibia
F – Medullary cavity
G – Medial border
H – Medial malleolus
I – Talus
J – Lateral malleolus
K – Inferior tibiofibular joint
L – Shaft of the fibula
M – Neck of the fibula
N – Head of the fibula
O – Superior tibiofibular joint
P – Lateral tibial condyle
Q – Femur

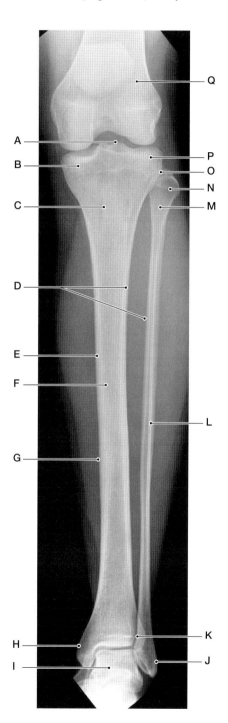

Fig. 7.21 Left tibia and fibula: lateral projection.

1 – Condyles of the femur
2 – Head of the fibula
(superimposed by tibia)
3 – Shaft of the fibula
4 – Calcaneus
5 – Talus
6 – Ankle joint
7 – Shaft of the tibia
8 – Anterior border
9 – Tibial tuberosity
10 – Knee joint
11 – Patella

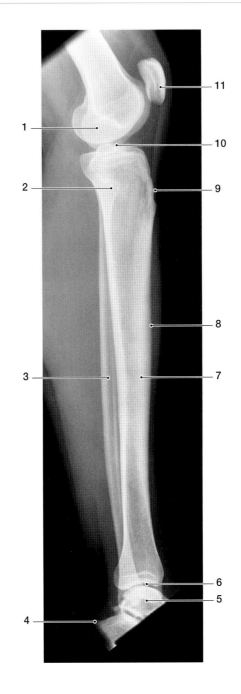

FRACTURES

Shaft of tibia and/or fibula (Fig. 7.22)

Range from simple to highly complex comminuted injuries. Transverse and comminuted fractures usually result from higher velocity injury than spiral fractures. Non-union is relatively common because of poor blood supply.

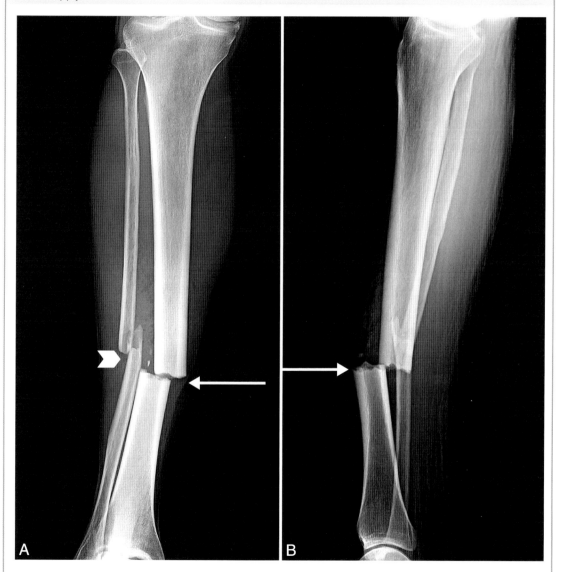

Fig. 7.22 Transverse fractures of the right tibia and fibula; anteroposterior (A) and lateral (B) projections. There is anterolateral displacement of the tibial fracture (arrow) and medial displacement of the fibular fracture (arrowhead). There is a relatively high risk of non-union of fractures in this area. (From STATdx © Elsevier 2022)

Cause – wide range including sports injuries and road traffic collisions.
Example of treatment – dependent on complexity; cast, tibial intramedullary nail, external fixation devices (e.g. Ilizarov frame).

Tibial condyles (plateaus) (Figs. 7.23, 7.24)

Most commonly (80%) are lateral tibial plateau as the most common mechanism is a lateral force on knee; e.g., car bumper striking a pedestrian, hence 'bumper' (or fender) fracture. May be very subtle (or occult) on radiographs. CT is useful to demonstrate the extent of injury and plan management.
Cause – abduction of the tibia on the femur caused by lateral force.
Example of treatment – reduction under anaesthetic and internal fixation.

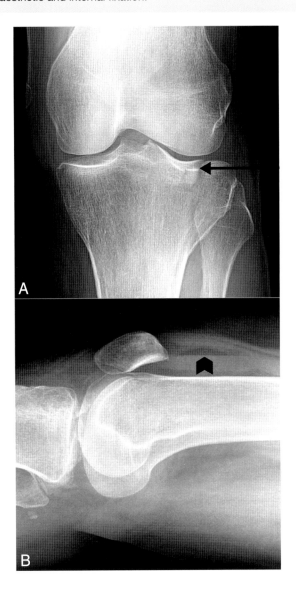

Fig. 7.23 Lateral tibial plateau fracture; anteroposterior (A) and lateral (B) projections left knee. Note the minimally displaced vertical fracture (arrow). Lipohaemarthrosis is also present, demonstrated by the horizontal line (arrowhead) in the suprapatellar bursa. (From STATdx © Elsevier 2022)

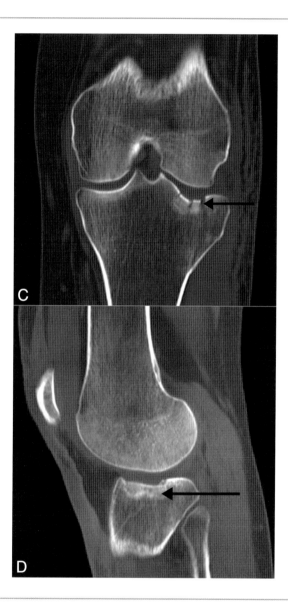

Fig. 7.24 Lateral tibial plateau fracture; coronal (C) and sagittal (D) CT images left knee. Same patient as Fig. 7.23. The CT demonstrates depression of the fracture fragment (arrow), which will need reducing surgically. (From STATdx © Elsevier 2022)

INSIGHT

Lipohaemarthosis (Fig. 7.23) is a useful indicator of an otherwise occult intraarticular fracture, such as of the tibial plateaus, femoral condyles, and patella. Blood and fatty bone marrow collect in the joint cavity and, because they do not mix, cause a horizontal line on imaging (but only if the leg is horizontal). If present, an intraarticular fracture is certain. However, its absence does not exclude a fracture.

FOOT (FIG. 7.25)

The bones of the foot can be divided into three regions:
Forefoot – metatarsals and phalanges.
Midfoot – cuneiforms, cuboid, and navicular bones.
Hindfoot – calcaneus and talus bones.

Fig. 7.25 Right foot (dorsal aspect).

A – Distal phalanx of the hallux
B – Proximal phalanx of the hallux
C – Shaft of the first metatarsal
D – Medial cuneiform
E – Intermediate cuneiform
F – Lateral cuneiform
G – Navicular
H – Head of the talus
I – Trochlea of the talus (talar dome)
J – Calcaneus
K – Cuboid
L – Base of the fifth metatarsal
M – Shaft of the fifth metatarsal
N – Head of the fifth metatarsal
O – Proximal phalanx of the fifth toe
P – Middle phalanx of the fourth toe
Q – Distal phalanx of the third toe
1 – Interphalangeal joint of the hallux (synovial hinge joint)
2 – First metatarsophalangeal joint (synovial ellipsoid joint)
3 – Fifth distal interphalangeal joint (synovial hinge joint)
4 – Second proximal interphalangeal joint (synovial hinge joint)

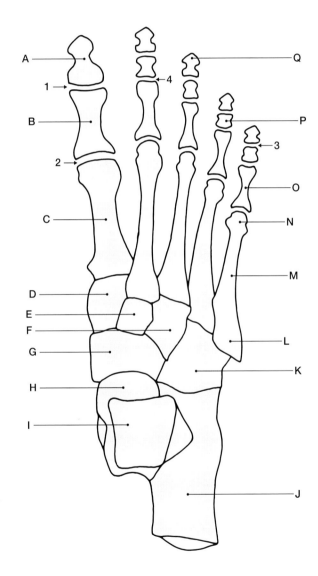

Tarsal bones

The *tarsus* (ankle) is comprised of seven tarsal bones which form the proximal part of the foot.

Type

Short bones.

Position

Three rows situated between the distal tibia proximally and the bases of the metatarsals distally.

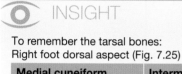
INSIGHT

To remember the tarsal bones:
Right foot dorsal aspect (Fig. 7.25)

Medial cuneiform	Intermediate cuneiform	Lateral cuneiform	Cuboid
Nearest the midline	The middle cuneiform	The cuneiform nearest the cuboid	Cube shaped
Navicular			
Boat-shaped			
Talus			**Calcaneus**
Forms the ankle joint (talus means ankle bone)			Largest tarsal bone

Articulations

Talus with the tibia, fibula, calcaneus, and navicular.
Calcaneus with the talus and cuboid.
Navicular with the talus, cuboid, medial cuneiform, intermediate cuneiform, and lateral cuneiform.
Cuboid with the calcaneus, navicular, lateral cuneiform, fourth metatarsal, and fifth metatarsal.
Lateral cuneiform with the navicular, cuboid, intermediate cuneiform, second, third and fourth metatarsals.
Intermediate cuneiform with the navicular, lateral cuneiform, medial cuneiform, and second metatarsal.
Medial cuneiform with the navicular, intermediate cuneiform, first and second metatarsals.

Individual bones

Proximal row
Talus (Fig. 7.26)
Shaped like a snail. Forms articulation between lower leg and foot at ankle joint.
Head – rounded distal end of the bone; articulates with the navicular.
Neck – narrowed section proximal to the head.

Fig. 7.26 Right talus (medial aspect).

A – Neck
B – Head
C – Articular surface of the head (for navicular)
D – Middle articular facet (on the inferior surface)
E – Sulcus tali
F – Body
G – Trochlea articular surface (talar dome)

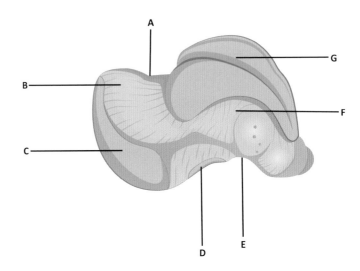

Body – cuboidal in shape.
Trochlear articular surface (Talar dome) – convex, superior upper aspect of the body. Covered in articular cartilage, forms the ankle joint with the tibia and fibula.
Inferior surface – carries the anterior, posterior and middle articular facets for articulation with the calcaneus to form the talocalcaneal (subtalar) joints.
Sulcus tali – deep groove on the inferior surface of the neck between the middle and posterior articular facets.

Calcaneus (Fig. 7.27)

Largest of the tarsal bones, situated inferiorly and slightly lateral to the talus. Divided into three parts; anterior process, body, and posterior (calcaneal) tuberosity.
Superior surface – has three facets (anterior, middle and posterior) for the talus to form the talocalcaneal (subtalar) joints.
Sulcus calcanei – lies between the middle and posterior facets on the superior surface. Forms a large gap, tarsal sinus, between the anterolateral parts of the calcaneum and talus.
Inferior (plantar) surface – slightly concave.
Posterior surface – large and convex; provides insertion for the Achilles tendon.
Calcaneal tuberosity – thickened inferior aspect of inferoposterior surface; weight-bearing portion; has a medial and lateral process on the inferior surface.
Medial surface – concave.
Sustentaculum tali – 'shelf-like' projection from the anterosuperior aspect of medial surface; supports the head of the talus.
Anterior surface – small; articulates with the cuboid.
Lateral surface – flattened except for the peroneal tubercle.

Fig. 7.27 Right calcaneum; superior aspect.

A – Anterior articular facet
B – Middle articular facet
C – Sulcus calcanei
D – Sustentaculum tali
E – Posterior articular facet
F – Posterior (calcaneal) tuberosity (insertion of Achilles tendon)
G – Peroneal tubercle
H – Body
I – Anterior process

Right calcaneum; inferior (plantar) surface.
1 – Calcaneal tubercle
2 – Lateral process of calcaneal tuberosity
3 – Posterior surface of calcaneal tuberosity
4 – Medial process of calcaneal tuberosity
5 – Sustentaculum tali
6 – Articular surface of anterior surface (for cuboid)

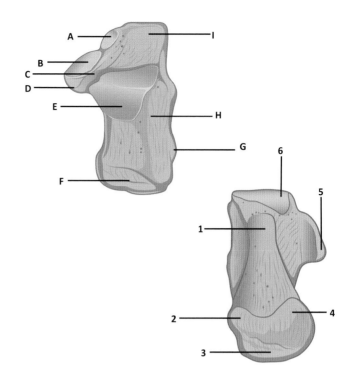

Radiographic appearances of the calcaneus and talus (Figs. 7.28, 7.29)

Intermediate row
Navicular
Roughly disc or 'boat'-shaped.
Proximal surface – concave; articulates with the head of the talus.
Distal surface – convex; three facets which articulate with the three cuneiform bones.
Inferior surface – tuberosity on the medial aspect for insertion of the tibialis posterior tendon.

Distal row
Cuneiform bones
'Wedge'-shaped bones. Medial, intermediate, and lateral.

Cuboid
Flattened, six-sided, 'cube'-shaped bone.
Lateral and inferior (plantar) surfaces – have a deep groove for the peroneus longus tendon.

Fig. 7.28 Right calcaneus: axial projection.

A – Medial surface
B – Sustentaculum tali
C – Middle talocalcaneal (subtalar) joint
D – Medial malleolus
E – Posterior talocalcaneal (subtalar) joint
F – Base of the fifth metatarsal
G – Lateral surface
H – Posterior surface

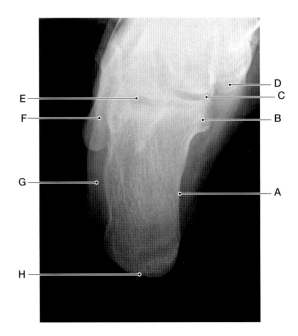

Fig. 7.29 Right calcaneus and talus: lateral projection. (From Lampignano, Bontrager's Textbook of Radiographic Positioning and Related Anatomy, 10e, Elsevier)

1 – Tibia
2 – Neck of the talus
3 – Head of the talus
4 – Navicular
5 – Intermediate cuneiform
6 – Base of the fifth metatarsal
7 – Cuboid
8 – Anterior process of the calcaneus
9 – Body of the calcaneus
10 – Calcaneal (posterior) tuberosity
11 – Posterior surface of calcaneus
12 – Middle talocalcaneal (subtalar joint)
13 – Posterior talocalcaneal (subtalar joint)
14 – Body of the talus
15 – Trochlea of the talus (talar dome)
16 – Fibula

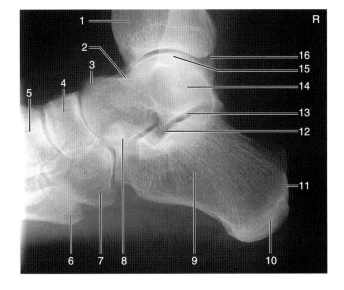

Ossification (Fig. 7.33)

Primary centres

One per tarsal bone

Calcaneus – third to fourth month of intrauterine life.
Talus – sixth month of intrauterine life.
Cuboid – ninth month of intrauterine life.
Lateral cuneiform – age one.
Medial cuneiform – age two.
Intermediate cuneiform – age three.
Navicular – age three.

Secondary centres

Calcaneus – Posterior aspect of the calcaneus appears at age six to eight. Fuses at puberty.
Talus – May have a secondary centre at the posterior aspect. If the centre does not fuse, it is called the *os trigonum*.

Metatarsal bones (Fig. 7.25)

Type	Miniature long bones.
Position	Distal to the tarsal bones. Numbered one to five from medial to lateral.
Articulations	The *head of the metatarsals* with the proximal phalanges to form the metatarsophalangeal joints.
	The *base of the metatarsals* with the tarsal bones to form the tarsometatarsal joints.
	First metatarsal with the proximal phalanx of the hallux (great toe) and the medial cuneiform.
	Second metatarsal with the proximal phalanx of the second toe and the medial, intermediate and lateral cuneiform bones.
	Third metatarsal with the proximal phalanx of the third toe and the lateral cuneiform.
	Fourth metatarsal with the proximal phalanx of the fourth toe, the lateral cuneiform and the cuboid.
	Fifth metatarsal with the proximal phalanx of the fifth toe and the cuboid.
	The *bases of the second – fifth metatarsals* with the adjacent metatarsal at the intermetatarsal joints.
Main parts	*Head* – distal, rounded; articulates with the corresponding proximal phalanx.
	Shaft – plantar aspect concave, dorsal aspect convex.
	Base – proximal, expanded; articulates with the appropriate tarsal bone(s).

First metatarsal

Short and thick. Two articular facets on the plantar aspect of the head for two sesamoid bones.

Second metatarsal

Longest.

Fifth metatarsal

Tuberosity – projects laterally from the base. Insertion of peroneus brevis tendon. Common site of an avulsion fracture.

Ossification (Fig. 7.33)

Primary centre

Shaft – ninth to tenth week of intrauterine life.

Secondary centre

One centre per bone only:

Base of the first metatarsal – appears at age three.
Heads of the second to fifth metatarsals – appear at age three to four.

Secondary centre unites with the shaft at age 17–20.

Phalanges (Fig. 7.25)

Type

Miniature long bones.

Position

Distal to the metatarsals, forming the toes; named one to five from medial to lateral. This first is also known as the hallux (great toe).

Articulations

The *base of the proximal phalanx* with the metatarsal to form the metatarsophalangeal joints.

With each other to form the interphalangeal joints; distal and proximal (except the first, which only has one joint).

Five proximal phalanges with the corresponding metatarsal; the first with the distal phalanx of the hallux, and the second to fifth with the corresponding middle phalanx.

Four middle phalanges with the corresponding proximal and distal phalanges.

Five distal phalanges with the corresponding second to fifth middle phalanges and the proximal phalanx of the hallux.

Main parts

Head – distal, expanded.
Shaft – plantar aspect is concave.
Base – proximal, expanded; articulates with either the phalanx or the metatarsal proximal to it.

Ossification (Fig. 7.33)

Primary centre
Shaft – ninth to 15th week of intrauterine life.

Secondary centre
One centre:
    Base of phalanges appears at age two to eight.
    Base unites with the shaft at age 18.

Arches of the foot
Support and distribute the weight of the body onto the bony and soft tissues of the foot. Provide leverage on walking; not rigid and absorb shock.

Medial longitudinal arch – formed by the calcaneus, talus, navicular, three cuneiform bones and first, second and third metatarsals; higher than the lateral longitudinal arch.

Lateral longitudinal arch – formed by the calcaneus, cuboid and the fourth and fifth metatarsals.

Radiographic appearances of the foot (Figs. 7.30–7.33)

Fig. 7.30 Right foot: dorsiplantar projection.

A – Head of the distal phalanx of the hallux
B – Base of the proximal phalanx of the hallux
C – Medial and lateral sesamoid bones
D – First tarsometatarsal joint
E – Medial cuneiform
F – Intermediate cuneiform
G – Navicular
H – Head of the talus
I – Medial malleolus of the tibia
J – Lateral malleolus of the fibula
K – Calcaneum
L – Cuboid
M – Base of the fifth metatarsal
N – Lateral cuneiform
O – Shaft of the fifth metatarsal
P – Head of the fifth metatarsal

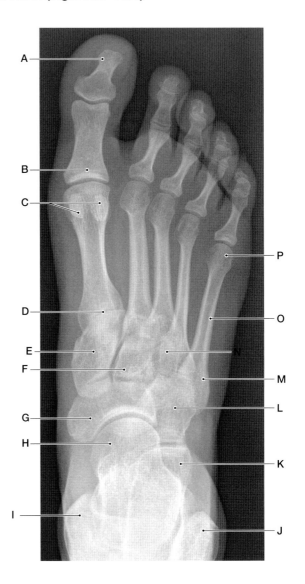

Fig. 7.31 Right foot: dorsiplantar oblique projection. (From Bruce, Merrill's Atlas of Radiographic Positioning & Procedures: Volume One, 14e, Elsevier)

1 – Distal phalanx of the hallux
2 – Medial and lateral sesamoid bones
3 – First metatarsal bone
4 – Medial cuneiform
5 – Intermediate cuneiform
6 – Navicular
7 – Head of the talus
8 – Neck of the talus
9 – Body of the talus
10 – Ankle joint
11 – Tibia
12 – Fibula
13 – Calcaneus
14 – Tarsal sinus
15 – Cuboid
16 – Base of the fifth metatarsal bone
17 – Lateral cuneiform
18 – Second intermetatarsal joint
19 – Fifth metatarsal bone

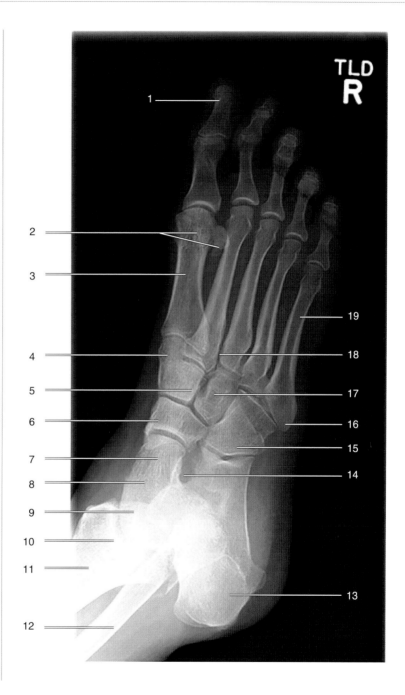

Fig. 7.32 Right foot: lateral projection. (From STATdx © Elsevier 2022)

A – Body of the calcaneus
B – Medial and lateral processes of the calcaneum
C – Anterior process of the calcaneum
D – Cuboid
E – Base of the fifth metatarsal
F – Sesamoid bones
G – Proximal phalanx of the hallux
H – Head of the first metatarsal
I – Cuneiform bones
J – Navicular
K – Head of the talus
L – Trochlea of the talus (talar dome)

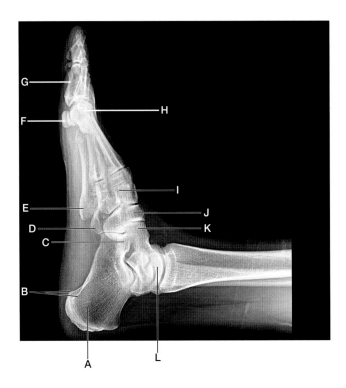

Fig. 7.33 Ossification centres of the foot. Lateral (A) and dorsiplantar (B) projections of the right foot of a two-year-old. Lateral calcaneus projection (C) of a 10-year-old. (From STATdx © Elsevier 2022)

A – Calcaneus (*in utero*)
B – Posterior calcaneal tuberosity (age six to eight years)
C – Talus (*in utero*)
D – Cuboid (*in utero*)
E – Lateral cuneiform (age one year)
F – Metatarsals
G – Epiphysis (base) of the first metatarsal (age three years)
H – Epiphysis (head) of the second to fifth metatarsals (age three to four years)
I – Phalanges (*in utero*)
J – Epiphysis (base) of phalanges (age two to eight years)
Note, the metatarsals and phalanges only have one epiphysis, either distal or proximal.

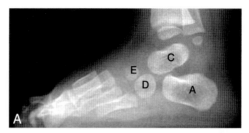

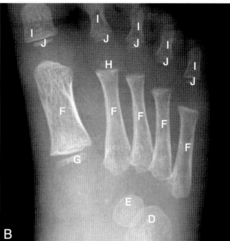

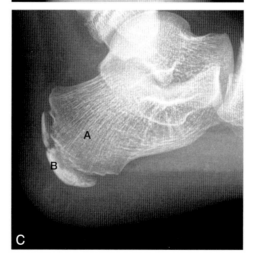

FRACTURES

Calcaneus (Figs. 7.34, 7.35)

Flattening of the shape of the calcaneus may be the only radiographic sign. Often complex and intraarticular. CT is used for a full evaluation and to plan management.

Cause – compression, because of a fall from a height. Often associated with vertebral compression fractures because of forces transmitted to the spine.

Example of treatment – conservative if undisplaced; open reduction internal fixation.

Metatarsals

Cause – direct blow, often because of a heavy object falling on the foot.

Example of treatment – cast.

Stress fractures (Fig. 3.1)

Most commonly of shafts of the metatarsals (March fracture) or calcaneus.

Cause – repetitive strain/injury; prolonged walking/running.

Example of treatment – conservative; remove cause.

Phalanges

Cause – crush injury; stubbing toe.

Example of treatment – conservative.

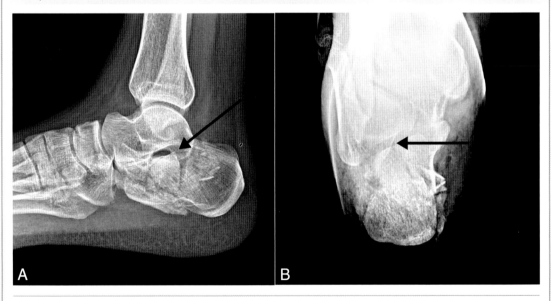

Fig. 7.34 Comminuted compression fracture right calcaneum; lateral (A) and axial (B) projections. Note the flattening of the shape of the calcaneum and intrarticular involvement of the posterior subtalar joint (arrow). (From STATdx © Elsevier 2022)

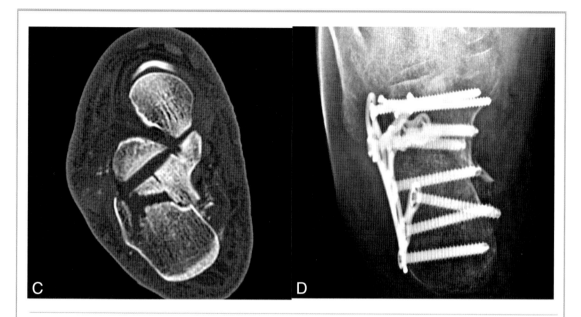

Fig. 7.35 Comminuted compression fracture right calcaneum; axial CT image (C) and post-ORIF axial projection (D). Same patient as Fig. 7.34. Note the reduced bone density caused by disuse in image D. (From STATdx © Elsevier 2022)

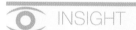 INSIGHT

A large number of normal variants, sesamoid bones and accessory ossification centres are seen around the foot, which can be mistaken for a fracture. They appear smooth, have a cortical edge, and are found at typical locations. It is useful to learn the most common ones.

PATHOLOGY

Hallux valgus

Lateral (valgus) deviation of the hallux at the first metatarsophalangeal joint. Causes a prominent lump at the joint on the medial aspect of the foot, also known as a 'bunion.'

Cause – wearing tight fitting shoes/high heels; family history.

Radiological sign – hallux angle greater than 10-15 degrees (Fig. 7.36)

Fig. 7.36 Normal assessment of the hallux valgus; dorsiplantar projection left foot. A normal hallux angle of 10-15 degrees at the metatarsophalangeal joint. More than this is indicative of hallux valgus. (From STATdx © Elsevier 2022)

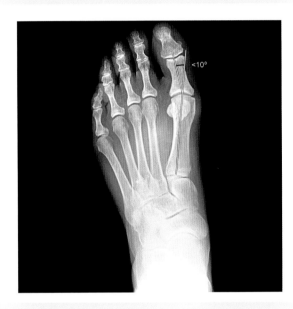

Diabetic foot complications

The foot is commonly involved in diabetes. More common manifestations include vascular (arterial) calcification, soft tissue ulcers and *osteomyelitis* (Fig. 4.30), osteopaenia and stress/insufficiency fractures (Fig. 3.1), and destructive forms of arthritis. Often people with diabetes perceive no foot pain or pain is masked by neuropathy of the nerves.

KNEE JOINT (FIGS. 7.37–7.40)

The largest and most complex joint. The joint is supported by a large number of soft tissue structures, both intra- and extracapsular, to increase its strength and stability.

Type

Synovial bicondylar joint.

Fig. 7.37 Right knee joint (coronal section).

A – Femur
B – Fibrous capsule
C – Articular hyaline cartilage
D – Popliteus tendon, enclosed in the synovial membrane
E – Synovial fluid
F – Synovial membrane
G – Tibia
H – Fibula
I – Articular hyaline cartilage
J – Medial meniscus
K – Synovial membrane
L – Anterior cruciate ligament
M – Posterior cruciate ligament
N – Fibrous capsule
O – Synovial membrane

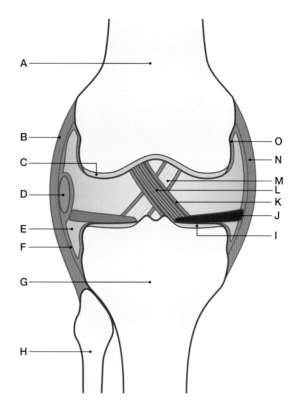

 INSIGHT

The knee joint is sometimes classified as a hinge joint; when the joint is flexed and extended, there is a slight amount of medial and lateral rotation to lock the joint on extension, making it a synovial bicondylar joint.

Bony articular surfaces

The femoral condyles with the articular surface of the tibial condyles; the tibial plateaus. Posterior aspect of the patella with the patellar articular surface of the femur. These three articulations are known as the medial and lateral (femorotibial) and patellofemoral compartments. The articular surfaces are covered with articular hyaline cartilage.

Fibrous capsule

Blends with the suprapatellar (quadriceps) tendon and the patellar tendon; elsewhere, it is attached to the margins of the femoral and tibial condyles and to the head of the fibula.

Synovial membrane

Lines part of the fibrous capsule and covers the intracapsular popliteus tendon. Anteriorly it forms the *suprapatellar bursa* and covers the anterior and lateral

Fig. 7.38 Right knee joint (anterior aspect). Patella reflected over the tibia.

1 – Fibular (lateral) collateral ligament
2 – Lateral meniscus
3 – Patellar tendon
4 – Quadriceps tendon (cut)
5 – Tibial (medial) collateral ligament
6 – Medial meniscus
7 – Anterior cruciate ligament
8 – Posterior cruciate ligament

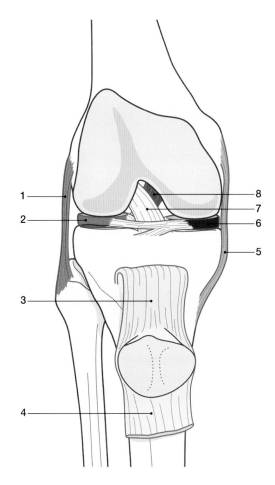

surfaces of the cruciate ligaments. The central posterior aspect of the joint has no synovial covering.

The membrane secretes synovial fluid, which lubricates the joint. There are several synovial bursae around the knee that reduce friction at key points, including:

Suprapatellar bursa – a sac containing synovial fluid situated above the patella between the distal end of the femur and the quadriceps. Direct communication with the synovial joint capsule. Commonly demonstrated site of fluid collection in joint effusion/haemarthrosis on imaging (Fig. 7.23).

Infrapatellar bursae – two extra-articular sacs (deep and superficial) containing synovial fluid. Situated inferior to the patella between the proximal tibia and the patellar tendon; one deep to the tendon, the other superficial to it.

Prepatellar bursa – an extra-articular sac containing synovial fluid, situated between the anterior surface of the patella and the skin.

Fig. 7.39 Left knee joint (sagittal section).

A – Quadriceps tendon
B – Suprapatellar bursa
C – Patella
D – Prepatellar bursa
E – Articular hyaline
cartilage
F – Infrapatellar (Hoffa's)
fat pad
G – Synovial membrane
H – Patellar tendon
I – Deep infrapatellar bursa
J – Tibia
K – Fibrous capsule
L – Posterior cruciate
ligament
M – Anterior cruciate
ligament
N – Femur

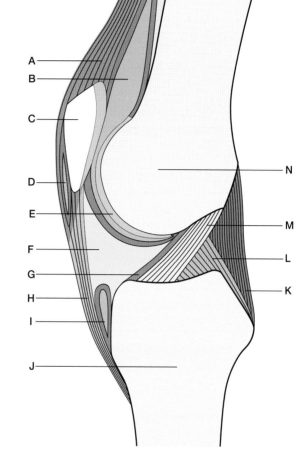

Fig. 7.40 Right tibia (superior aspect).

1 – Transverse ligament
2 – Anterior cruciate
ligament
3 – Medial meniscus
4 – Posterior cruciate
ligament
5 – Lateral meniscus

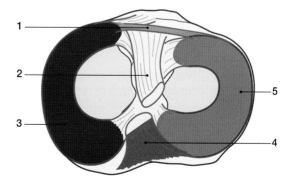

Supporting ligaments and tendons

Provide a lot of support and strength, these include:

Quadriceps tendon – attached to the superior aspect of the patella. The quadriceps muscles in the thigh are the main extensor of the knee.

Patellar tendon – attached to the inferior aspect of the patella and inserts into the tibial tuberosity. Sometimes referred to as the patella ligament (bone-to-bone), it is actually a continuation of the quadriceps tendon with the patella (a sesamoid bone) within it.

Popliteal tendon – inserts on the lateral surface of the lateral condyle and extends inferomedially as the popliteus muscle, which originates on the posterior tibia; rotates the tibia on the femur to unlock the knee and allow flexion.

Tibial (medial) collateral ligament – medial condyle of the tibia and the medial epicondyle of the femur. Prevents excess lateral angulation at knee.

Fibular (lateral) collateral ligament – lateral epicondyle of the femur to the head of the fibula. Prevents excess medial angulation at knee.

Oblique popliteal ligament – extension of the semimembranosus tendon on the posteromedial tibia, which then extends obliquely to the posterior surface of the lateral condyle of the femur. Blends with the fibrous capsule.

Arcuate popliteal ligament – Y-shaped ligament on the lateral aspect of the joint. Two parts, one extends from the head of the fibula to the lateral epicondyle of the femur, the other arching over the popliteus tendon to the posteromedial tibia.

Intracapsular structures

Anterior cruciate ligament (ACL) – anterior and medial part of the intercondylar area of the tibia to the medial surface of the lateral condyle of the femur. Prevents the tibia from moving anteriorly on the femur.

Posterior cruciate (PCL) – posterior and lateral part of the intercondylar area of the tibia to the lateral surface of the medial condyle of the femur. Prevents the tibia from moving posteriorly on the femur. Crosses (hence cruciate- 'cross') the ACL within the intercondylar area of the knee; in between the synovial membrane and outer fibrous capsule.

Medial semilunar cartilage (meniscus) – half-moon shaped fibrocartilage disc situated on the medial aspect of the proximal end of the tibia. The peripheral border is attached to the fibrous capsule.

Lateral semilunar cartilage (meniscus) – half-moon shaped fibrocartilage disc situated on the lateral aspect of the proximal end of the tibia. The menisci help increase the congruity between the tibia and femur.

Infrapatellar (Hoffa's) fat pad – situated inferior to the patella between the patellar tendon and the synovial membrane.

Movements

Flexion by the hamstring muscles aided by the gastrocnemius.

Extension by the quadriceps femoris muscles.

When the knee is in flexion, there is a minimal degree of:
> *Medial rotation* by the popliteus muscle.
> *Lateral rotation* by the biceps femoris of the hamstrings.

Blood supply

Branches of the femoral, popliteal and anterior tibial arteries, forming an anastomosis.

Nerve supply

Obturator, femoral, tibial and common peroneal nerves.

Fabella

Sesamoid bone found in the lateral head of the gastrocnemius muscle, where it passes over the lateral condyle of the femur. Smooth, round structure posterior to the knee joint on a lateral radiograph. Not always present, a normal variant.

Imaging appearances of the knee (Figs. 7.15, 7.16, 7.41–7.47)

Fig. 7.41 Right knee anteroposterior projection. (From Lampignano, Bontrager's Textbook of Radiographic Positioning and Related Anatomy, 10e, Elsevier)

A – Patella
B – Lateral femoral epicondyle
C – Popliteal sulcus (for popliteus tendon)
D – Lateral femoral condyle
E – Lateral tibial plateau
F – Lateral tibial condyle
G – Styloid process of the fibula
H – Head of the fibula
I – Tubercles of intercondylar eminences (tibial spines)
J – Medial tibial condyle
K – Medial tibial plateau
L – Medial femoral condyle
M – Medial femoral epicondyle
N – Adductor tubercle

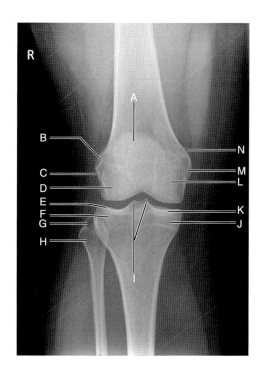

Fig. 7.42 Right knee: lateral projection. (From STATdx © Elsevier 2022)

1 – Femur
2 – Patella
3 – Patellar tendon
4 – Tibial plateaus (superimposed)
5 – Tibial tuberosity
6 – Tibia
7 – Neck of the fibula
8 – Proximal patellofemoral joint
9 – Tubercles of intercondylar eminences (tibial spines)
10 – Medial femoral condyle
11 – Lateral femoral condyle
12 – Adductor tubercle

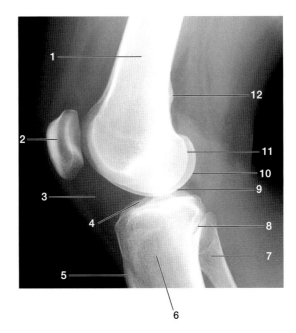

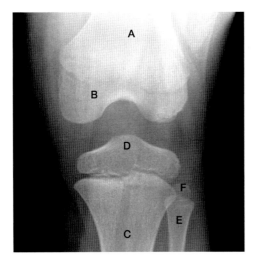

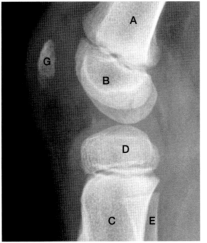

Fig. 7.43 Ossification centres around the (left) knee. These images are of a six-year-old. (From STATdx © Elsevier 2022)

A – Femoral shaft (*in utero*)
B – Distal femoral epiphysis (just before birth)
C – Tibial shaft (*in utero*)
D – Proximal tibial epiphysis (at birth)
E – Fibular shaft (*in utero*)
F – Proximal fibular epiphysis, head (age three to four years)
G – Patella (age three to six years)

Fig. 7.44 Right knee: Coronal T1W MRI images. (From STATdx © Elsevier 2022)

A – Lateral femoral condyle
B – Lateral meniscus
C – Lateral tibial condyle
D – Anterior cruciate ligament
E – Medial intercondylar eminence (spine)
F – Medial tibial condyle
G – Medial meniscus
H – Tibial (medial) collateral ligament
I – Posterior cruciate ligament
J – Medial femoral condyle
K – Intercondylar notch

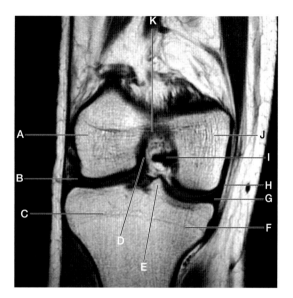

Fig. 7.45 Right knee: Sagittal T1W MRI images at the intercondylar notch (A) and lateral femoral condyle (B). (From STATdx © Elsevier 2022)

1 – Vastus medialis muscle (part of quadriceps)
2 – Infrapatellar (Hoffa's) fat pad
3 – Anterior cruciate ligament
4 – Proximal tibia
5 – Lateral gastrocnemius muscle
6 – Femur
7 – Quadriceps tendon
8 – Suprapatellar bursa
9 – Patella
10 – Articular hyaline cartilage
11 – Patellar tendon
12 – Anterior horn of the lateral meniscus
13 – Proximal tibiofibular joint
14 – Posterior horn of the lateral meniscus
15 – Lateral condyle of the femur
16 – Biceps femoris (hamstring) muscle

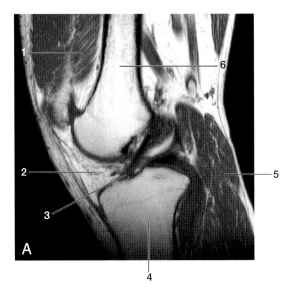

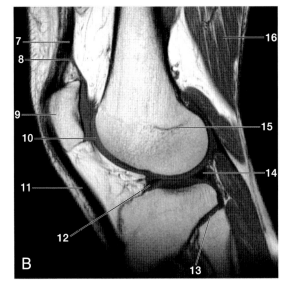

Fig. 7.46 Right knee: longitudinal (sagittal) panoramic ultrasound of the anterior (extensor) aspect. Note the shadowing (*) deep to the bone cortex caused by the strong reflection of the ultrasound beam. Structures deep to bone surfaces cannot be visualised on ultrasound. (From STATdx © Elsevier 2022)

A – Vastus medialis muscle (part of quadriceps)
B – Quadriceps tendon
C – Cortex of the patella
D – Patellar tendon
E – Infrapatellar (Hoffa's) fat pad
F – Cortex of the tibia
G – Suprapatellar bursa
H – Cortex of the femur

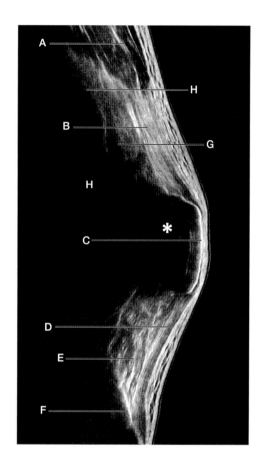

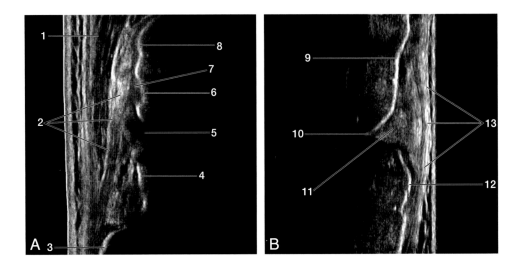

Fig. 7.47 Right knee: longitudinal (sagittal) ultrasound of the lateral (A) and medial (B) aspects of the joint. (From STATdx © Elsevier 2022)

1 – Biceps femoris (hamstring) muscle
2 – Fibular (lateral) collateral ligament
3 – Cortex of the fibular head
4 – Cortex of the lateral tibial condyle
5 – Knee joint space
6 – Popliteal sulcus (for popliteus tendon)
7 – Popliteus tendon

8 – Cortex of the lateral femoral condyle
9 – Cortex of the medial femoral condyle
10 – Knee joint space
11 – Lateral meniscus
12 – Cortex of the medial tibial condyle
13 – Tibial (medial) collateral ligament

PATHOLOGY

Osteoarthritis (also see Chapter 4, page 59) (Figs 4.32, 7.48)

One of the most common joints affected; usually of medial compartment because of greater weight-bearing forces. Severe disease treated with knee replacement (arthroplasty).

Osteochondritis dissecans (Fig. 7.49)

Chronic disorder that is most common in adolescent athletes, causing abnormality of the articular hyaline cartilage and subchondral bone. Also may be seen in the ankle, elbow and hip joints.
Cause – unknown but thought to be related to repetitive trauma; may be genetic.
Radiological signs – smooth bone fragments in the region of the femoral condyle with a defect in the underlying femoral condyle. MRI required for a full assessment.

Fig. 7.48 Advanced osteoarthritis: right knee. Classic triad of osteophytes (arrow), joint space narrowing (arrowhead), and subchondral sclerosis (curved arrow). Note how the medial joint space is significantly narrower than the lateral and patellofemoral joints. (From STATdx © Elsevier 2022)

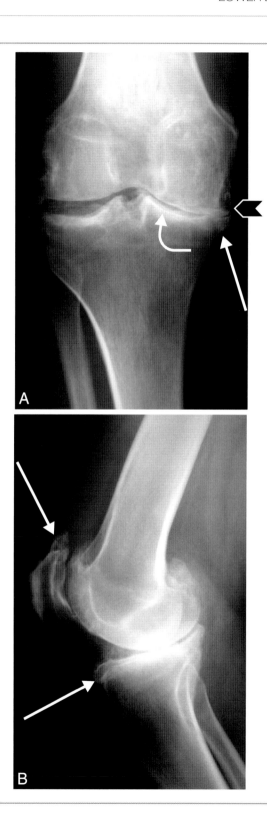

Fig. 7.49 Osteochondritis dissecans: right knee. Intercondylar notch ('tunnel') projection (A) and sagittal T2W MRI (B) demonstrate an osseous fragment (arrow) and underlying defect of the medial femoral condyle (arrowhead). Note the unfused epiphyseal plates in this immature skeleton. (From STATdx © Elsevier 2022)

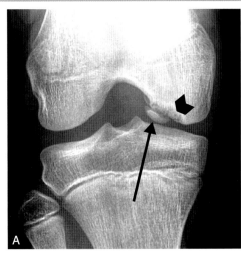

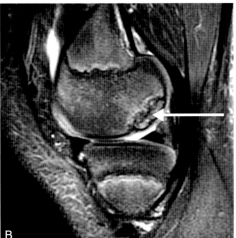

Osgood–Schlatter's disease (Fig. 7.50)

Non-inflammatory condition of the insertion of the patellar tendon at the tibial tuberosity in adolescents. Diagnosis is typically made clinically, and radiographs are not normally indicated.
Cause – repetitive microtrauma during ossification of the tibial tuberosity until skeletal maturity.
Radiological signs – fragmentation of the tibial tuberosity and adjacent soft tissue swelling.

ACL tears (Fig. 7.51)

Often associated with tears of the meniscus and collateral ligaments.
Cause – usually a twisting force with the foot planted on the floor; most commonly a sports injury.
Radiological signs – radiographs may show non-specific joint effusion but sometimes demonstrate associated small avulsion fractures. MRI is the imaging investigation of choice for all intraarticular soft tissue injuries.

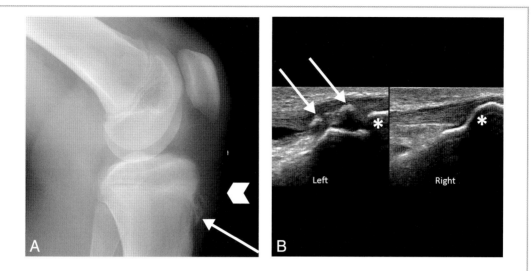

Fig. 7.50 Osgood–Schlatter Disease: left knee. Lateral radiograph (A) demonstrates fragmentation (arrow) of the tibial tuberosity and soft tissue swelling (arrowhead). Longitudinal (sagittal) ultrasound images (B) show the abnormal left knee compared to the normal right where the patellar tendon inserts on the tibial tuberosity (*). (From STATdx © Elsevier 2022)

Fig. 7.51 Complete tear of the ACL: right knee. T2W MRI shows no fibres of the proximal part of the ligament (arrow). Normal fibres are demonstrated of the distal part (arrowhead) at its insertion on the tibia. (From STATdx © Elsevier 2022)

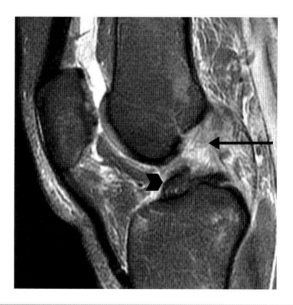

PROXIMAL TIBIOFIBULAR JOINT

Type   Synovial plane joint. Located on the posterolateral aspect of the tibia.

Bony articular surfaces

Lateral condyle of the tibia with the head of the fibula. Both surfaces are covered with articular hyaline cartilage.

Fibrous capsule
Attached to the margins of the articular facets on the tibia and fibula.

Synovial membrane
Lines the fibrous capsule and secretes synovial fluid, which lubricates the joint.

Supporting ligaments
Anterior ligament.

Movements
Gliding.

Blood supply
Branches of the anterior tibial artery.

Nerve supply
Common peroneal nerve.

Radiographic appearances of the proximal tibiofibular joint (Figs. 7.41, 7.42)

DISTAL TIBIOFIBULAR JOINT

Type   Fibrous syndesmosis.

Bony articular surfaces
Distal end of the fibula and the fibular notch of the tibia.

Strengthening ligaments
  Anterior tibiofibular ligament.
  Posterior tibiofibular ligament.
  Inferior transverse (intermalleolar) ligament.
  Interosseous ligament.

Movements
Minimal.

Blood supply

Branches of the peroneal artery; branches of the anterior and posterior tibial arteries.

Nerve supply

Deep peroneal, tibial and saphenous nerves.

Radiographic appearances of the inferior tibiofibular joint (Figs. 7.54, 7.55)

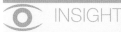 INSIGHT

The distal tibiofibular joint (syndesmosis) is integral to the stability and strength of the ankle joint, and it resists the fibula and tibia being pulled apart. Injury involving the syndesmosis ligaments is heavily associated with the stability of the injury. Because the ankle and lower leg are ring structures (see Chapter 5, page 75), widening of the syndesmosis without visible bone fracture is suspicious for a proximal fibula fracture (Fig. 7.60).

ANKLE JOINT (FIGS. 7.52, 7.53)

Type

Synovial saddle joint (not a synovial hinge joint because of the accessory movements in plantar flexion).

Fig. 7.52 Left ankle joint (coronal section).

A – Tibia
B – Medial malleolus
C – Fibrous capsule
D – Synovial membrane
E – Talus
F – Articular hyaline cartilage
G – Lateral malleolus
H – Synovial fluid
I – Synovial membrane
J – Distal tibiofibular joint (syndesmosis)
K – Fibula
L – Interosseous ligament of middle and inferior tibiofibular joint

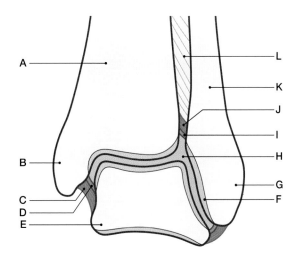

Fig. 7.53 Left ankle joint (lateral aspect).

A – Tibia
B – Anterior tibiofibular ligament
C – Talus
D – Anterior talofibular ligament
E – Talonavicular ligament
F – Navicular
G – Cervical ligament
H – Calcaneus
I – Calcaneofibular ligament
J – Posterior talofibular ligament
K – Posterior tibiofibular ligament
L – Fibula

Left ankle joint (medial aspect).
1 – Tibia
2 – Posterior tibiofibular ligament
3 – Deltoid ligament
4 – Calcaneus
5 – Navicular
6 – Talonavicular ligament

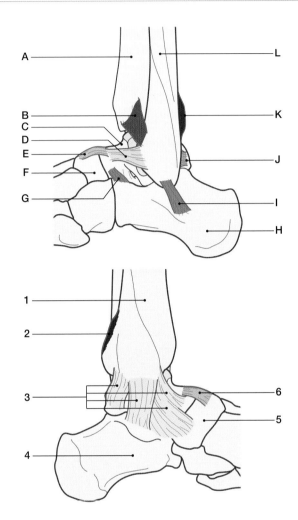

Bony articular surfaces

The distal end (plafond) and medial malleolus of the tibia and the medial aspect of the lateral malleolus of the fibula, with the talus. The articular surfaces are covered with articular hyaline cartilage.

 INSIGHT

The bone structure of the ankle joint between the tibia, fibula, and talus resembles a mortise-and-tenon joint used in woodwork; hence it is commonly referred to as the *mortise joint* on imaging. Its joint space should be consistent on all sides (Fig. 7.54).

Fig. 7.54 Right ankle joint: anteroposterior mortise projection. (From STATdx © Elsevier 2022)

A – Fibula
B – Distal tibiofibular joint (syndesmosis) space
C – Lateral malleolus
D – Calcaneus
E – First metatarsal
F – Navicular
G – Body of the talus
H – Ankle joint space
I – Medial malleolus
J – Remnant of the epiphyseal growth plate
K – Tibia

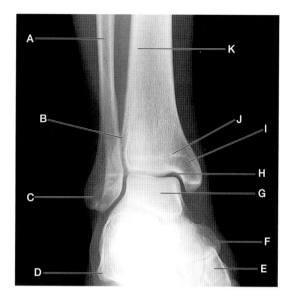

Fig. 7.55 Right ankle joint: lateral projection. (From STATdx © Elsevier 2022)

1 – Tibia
2 – Head of the talus
3 – Navicular
4 – Cuneiforms
5 – Base of the fifth metatarsal
6 – Cuboid
7 – Anterior process of the calcaneus
8 – Calcaneal tuberosity
9 – Posterior talocalcaneal (subtalar) joint
10 – Body of the talus
11 – Malleoli (superimposed)
12 – Fibula

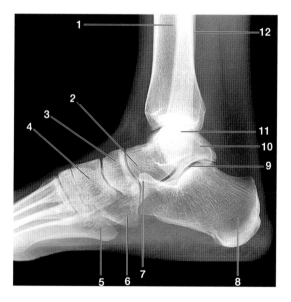

Fibrous capsule

Attached to the tibia and fibula above the malleoli, to the posterior and lateral surfaces of the talus, and anteriorly to the neck of the talus. The capsule is weak anteriorly and posteriorly but is strengthened laterally and medially by ligaments.

Synovial membrane

Lines the fibrous capsule and the parts of the bone not covered with articular hyaline cartilage. A small fold extends between the distal ends of the tibia and fibula. The synovial membrane secretes synovial fluid, which lubricates the joint.

Supporting ligaments

Medial collateral or deltoid – triangular in shape, apex attached to the medial malleolus, and inserts on the navicular, calcaneus and talus.
Lateral collateral – consists of three ligaments.
Anterior talofibular – attached to the lateral malleolus and the talus.
Posterior talofibular – attached to the malleolar fossa and the talus.
Calcaneofibular – attached to the lateral malleolus and the calcaneus.

Movements

Main movements

Dorsiflexion by the anterior tibialis muscle (pulls foot superiorly). Dorsiflexion effectively locks the ankle joint as the talus becomes 'wedged' between the malleoli.
Plantarflexion by the soleus and gastrocnemius muscles (points toes).

Accessory movements

Abduction ⎫	
Adduction ⎬	slight movement in plantar-flexion.
Rotation ⎭	

Blood supply

Branches of the anterior tibial and peroneal arteries.

Nerve supply

Posterior and lateral popliteal nerves.

Imaging appearances of the ankle joint (Figs. 7.54–7.58)

Fig. 7.56 Ossification centres around the (left) ankle. This image is of a nine-year-old. (From STATdx © Elsevier 2022)

A – Tibial shaft (*in utero*)
B – Distal tibial epiphysis (age one year)
C – Fibular shaft (*in utero*)
D – Distal fibular epiphysis (age one year)
E – Talus (*in utero*)

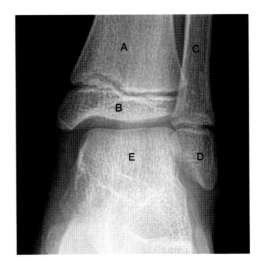

Fig. 7.57 Right ankle joint: Sagittal T1W MRI. (From STATdx © Elsevier 2022)

A – Anterior tibialis tendon
B – Tibia
C – Body of the talus
D – Head of the talus
E – Navicular
F – Origin of plantar fascia
G – Calcaneus
H – Posterior talocalcaneal (subtalar) joint
I – Achilles tendon
J – Ankle joint
K – Flexor hallucis longus muscle

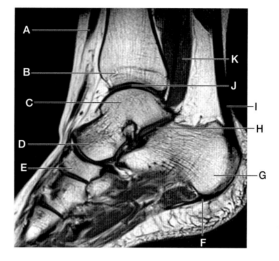

Fig. 7.58 Achilles tendon: longitudinal (sagittal) ultrasound. (From STATdx © Elsevier 2022)

A – Flexor hallucis longus muscle
B – Posterior malleolus of the tibia
C – Talar dome
D – Calcaneus
E – Insertion of the Achilles tendon
F – Achilles tendon
G – Soleus muscle

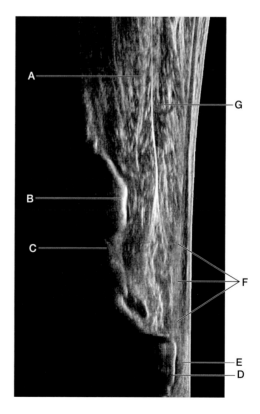

FRACTURES

 INSIGHT

Due to a combination of forces, ankle injuries are often a combination of more than one injury; bony fracture and ligamentous sprain.

Weber classification of fibular fractures (Fig. 7.59)

Corresponds to the location of fibula fractures in relation to the tibial plafond at the ankle joint. Correlates with fracture stability; the more proximal the fracture, the more unstable the injury. Weber A distal to the ankle joint; stable. Weber B at the level of the ankle joint; variable stability. Weber C proximal to the ankle joint; unstable. Need to consider other bone and soft tissue injuries too.

Cause – twisting forces; eversion or inversion of the ankle.

Treatment – dependent on stability; typically cast for stable, open reduction internal fixation for unstable.

Maissoneuve injury (Fig. 7.60)

A type of Weber C injury where the fracture occurs in the proximal fibula rather than around the ankle. Suspect when there is a widening of the medial ankle joint and/or tibiofibular syndesmosis and no visible fibular fracture. Further imaging of the lower leg is required. Unstable injury.

Cause – twisting; pronation and external rotation of the ankle

Treatment – internal fixation of tibiofibular syndesmosis injury and cast.

Pilon Fracture (Figs. 7.61, 7.62)

Intra articular tibial fracture involving the tibial plafond. Usually comminuted and often also involve the distal fibula and tibiofibular syndesmosis. CT is used for a full assessment of the fracture. Resultant osteoarthritis is common.

Cause – high energy, axial loading of the ankle pushing talus into tibial plafond (e.g., road traffic collision).

Example of treatment – surgical open reduction internal fixation.

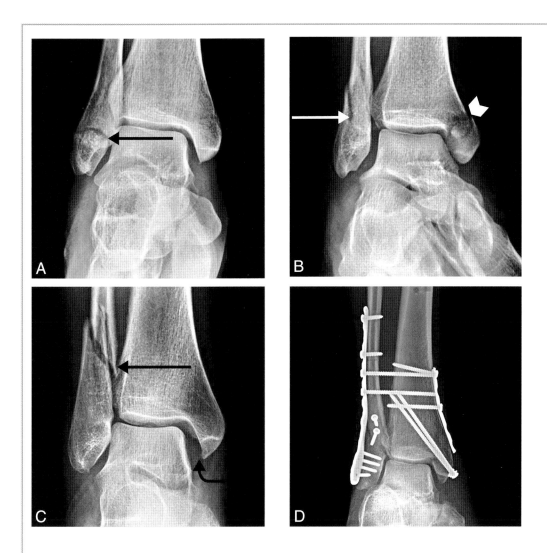

Fig. 7.59 Weber classification of ankle fractures; mortise projections right ankle. Fibular fractures (arrows) are demonstrated; Weber A; distal to the ankle joint (A). Weber B; at the level of the ankle joint (B) with an associated medial malleolus fracture (arrowhead). Weber C; proximal to the ankle joint (C). Note widening of the medial joint space (curved arrow) indicative of ligamentous injury. ORIF of a complex Weber B fracture (D). (From STATdx © Elsevier 2022)

Fig. 7.60 Maisonneuve injury; right leg. Ankle mortise (A) and anteroposterior knee (B) projections show widening of the tibiofibular syndesmosis (arrow) and medial ankle joint space (arrowhead). The injury extends in the interosseous membrane and exits as a proximal fibular fracture (curved arrow). (From STATdx © Elsevier 2022)

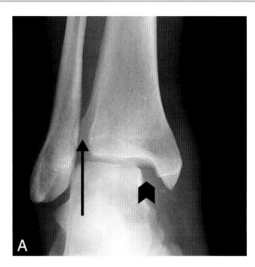

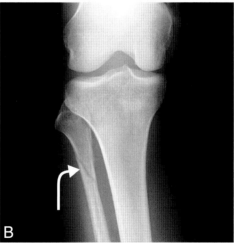

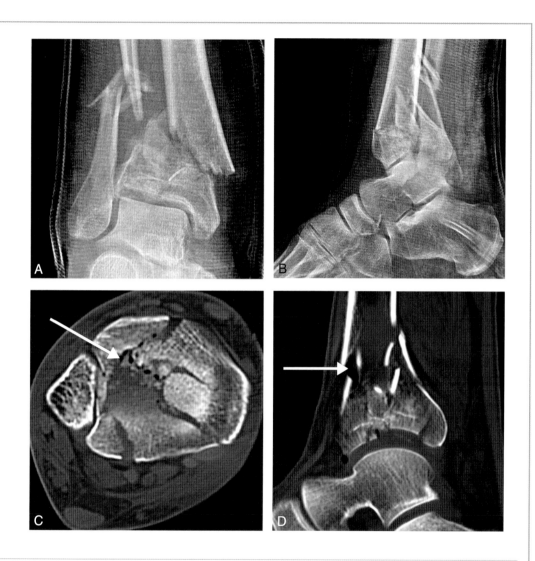

Fig. 7.61 Pilon fracture; right ankle. Mortise (A) and lateral (B) projections. Note the air (arrows) demonstrated in the axial (C) and sagittal (D) CT images; this was an open fracture. (From STATdx © Elsevier 2022)

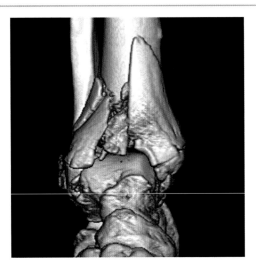

Fig. 7.62 Pilon fracture right ankle; 3D CT reconstruction. CT demonstrates excellent detail of complex fractures to help plan management. (From STATdx © Elsevier 2022)

INTERTARSAL JOINTS

Type

All synovial. The talocalcaneal (subtalar), naviculocuneiform, cuboideonavicular, and intercuneiform are all plane joints. The talocalcaneonavicular joint may be considered a form of the ball-and-socket joint. The calcaneocuboid joint is a modified saddle joint.

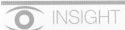 INSIGHT

The talonavicular and calcaneocuboid joints combined form the '*Chopart' joint*, separating the mid and hindfoot.

Bony articular surfaces

Subtalar joint – anterior, middle and anterior facets on the inferior surface of the talus with corresponding facets on the superior surface of the calcaneus.
Talonavicular joint – convex head of talus with the concave surface of the proximal navicular.
Talocalcaneonavicular joint – the convex head of the talus with a concavity formed by the concave posterior surface of the navicular, anterior surface of calcaneus, and plantar calcaneonavicular ligament.
Calcaneocuboid joint – facet on the anterior calcaneum with the facet on the posterior aspect of the cuboid.

Naviculocuneiform joints – three convex facets on the distal navicular with the concave facet on the corresponding medial, intermediate and lateral cuneiforms.

Intercuneiform joints – obliquely orientated; the lateral surface of the medial cuneiform with the medial surface of the intermediate cuneiform. Lateral surface of the intermediate cuneiform with the medial surface of lateral cuneiform.

Joint capsules

The three separate facets of the subtalar joint have two separate joint capsules; the posterior facets and the middle/anterior facets. Despite having three facets, the naviculocuneiform articulations have one single joint capsule. The remaining joints have a single joint capsule each.

Supporting ligaments

A strong and complex system of ligaments support the intertarsal joints and arches of the foot, including:

Interosseous talocalcaneal ligament – within the tarsal sinus.

Talonavicular ligament – superiorly between the neck of the talus and navicular.

Plantar calcaneonavicular (Spring) ligament – on the medial aspect of the foot between the sustentaculum tali of calcaneus and navicular. Maintains the medial arch of the foot.

Short plantar (calcaneocuboid) ligament – from calcaneal tuberosity to cuboid. Short, wide and strong, supports the lateral arch of the foot.

Bifurcate ligament – two parts from anterior process of calcaneum to the navicular and cuboid.

Movements

Each individual joint provides relatively minimal (mainly gliding) movement but combined allow inversion, eversion, pronation, and supination of the foot. Most movement is seen at the subtalar, talocalcaneonavicular, and calcaneocuboid joints.

Blood supply

Anterior and posterior tibial and peroneal arteries.

Nerve supply

Tibial, deep and superficial peroneal and sural nerves.

TARSOMETATARSAL JOINTS

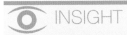

The tarsometatarsal joints combined form the *'Lisfranc' joint*, separating the mid and forefoot.

Type

Synovial plane joints.

Joint capsules

There are three separate joint capsules; the first metatarsophalangeal joint, the second to third metatarsophalangeal joints, and the fourth to fifth metatarsophalangeal joints.

Supporting ligaments

Lisfranc ligament – from the medial cuneiform to the base of the second metatarsal. Dorsal, plantar, and thicker interosseous bands. Stabilises the Lisfranc joint.

First tarsometatarsal ligaments – dorsal, plantar, and medial collateral; from the medial cuneiform to the base of the first metatarsal.

Second to fifth tarsometatarsal ligaments – dorsal and plantar; between the base of the second to fifth metatarsal with the corresponding tarsal bone.

Intermetatarsal ligaments – dorsal and plantar; between the bases of adjacent second to fifth metatarsals at the intermetatarsal joints.

Movements

Second to fifth tarsometatarsal joints have limited gliding movements. The first metatarsophalangeal joint allows some flexion, extension and rotation and assists in pronation and supination of the foot.

FRACTURES

Lisfranc (tarsometatarsal joint) fracture dislocation (Fig. 7.63)

Combination of fractures of the base of metatarsals and dislocation of the tarsometatarsal (Lisfranc) joints.
May be obvious or subtle; assess for normal alignment on radiographs, CT beneficial.
Cause – plantar flexion with rotation, often high velocity; road traffic collisions, sports injuries.
Treatment – open reduction internal fixation.

Fig. 7.63 Lisfranc fracture dislocation left foot; dorsiplantar projections. Note the loss of normal alignment of the tarsometatarsal and intermetatarsal joints. Radiographs often cannot fully assess the extent of the injury. (From STATdx © Elsevier 2022)

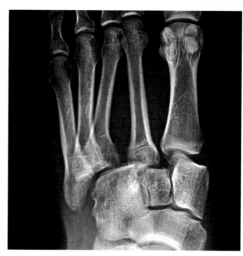

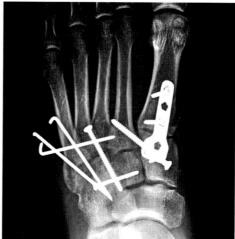

METATARSOPHALANGEAL AND INTERPHALANGEAL JOINTS (FIG. 7.25)

Type

The metatarsophalangeal joints are synovial ellipsoid joints whilst the interphalangeal joints are synovial hinge joints.

Bony articular surfaces

The concave base of the second to fifth proximal phalanx articulates with the rounded head of the adjacent metatarsal in the second to fifth metacarpophalangeal joints.

The head of the first metatarsal may be flat, convex or have a central prominence. Facets on the plantar surface for two sesamoid bones.

The head of each proximal and middle phalanx has a bi-condylar (rounded) articular surface with central depression to accommodate the adjacent articular surface of the bases of the distal/middle phalanges, which have a biconcave surface with a central median ridge.

Fibrous capsule

Attach the neck of the metatarsal/phalanx to the base of the adjacent more distal phalanx. The thickened fibrocartilaginous plantar aspect of the capsule, called the *plantar plate* (akin to the volar plate in the fingers), helps support the body weight and restrict dorsiflexion.

Synovial membrane

Lines the fibrous capsule, covers the parts of the bone not covered with articular hyaline cartilage and secretes synovial fluid, which lubricates the joint.

Supporting ligaments

Lateral and medial collateral ligaments – medial and lateral sides of the joint to stabilise abduction/adduction.

Intermetatarsal ligaments – between adjacent metatarsal heads.

Movements

Metatarsophalangeal joints allow flexion and extension with limited abduction, adduction, and rotation. Dorsiflexion is important in pushing off when walking.

Interphalangeal joints allow flexion and extension only.

Nerve supply

Plantar and dorsal digital nerves accompany blood vessels on medial and lateral aspects of the metatarsals and phalanges.

PELVIC GIRDLE

8

CHAPTER CONTENTS

Pelvis	194	Pathology	214
Hip bone	198	Sacroiliac joints (SIJs)	217
Fractures	203	Pathology	219
Hip joint	206	Symphysis pubis	220
Trauma	211	Pathology	220

The pelvic (hip) girdle is formed by the two hip bones, the sacrum and the coccyx (for notes on the sacrum and coccyx, see Chapter 10). It forms the connection between the axial skeleton and lower limb, supports the spine and protects the pelvic organs.

PELVIS (FIGS. 8.1, 8.2)

The pelvis is formed posteriorly by the sacrum and coccyx and laterally and anteriorly by the two hip bones. It is considered an osseous ring structure. Each half of the pelvis is known as a hemipelvis (left and right).

Greater (False) Pelvis

The superior portion of the pelvis is referred to as the greater pelvis. It is larger than the lesser (true) pelvis and lies superior to the *pelvic brim*; an oblique plane formed:
- Posteriorly – the sacral promontory
- Laterally – the arcuate line and iliopubic (iliopectineal) lines
- Anteriorly – the pubic tubercle, crest and the superior border of the symphysis pubis

The greater pelvis is considered part of the abdominal cavity.

Lesser (true) pelvis

The lesser pelvis lies inferior to the *pelvic brim* and contains the organs of the pelvis. It can be divided into three areas:

Fig. 8.1 Female pelvis (anterior aspect).

A – Iliac crest
B – Iliac fossa
C – Sacral promontory
D – Pelvic brim (dotted line)
E – Ischial spine
F – Acetabulum
G – Obturator foramen
H – Symphysis pubis
I – Pubic arch
J – Coccyx
K – Arcuate line
L – Sacrum
M – Anterior superior iliac spine
N – Sacroiliac joint

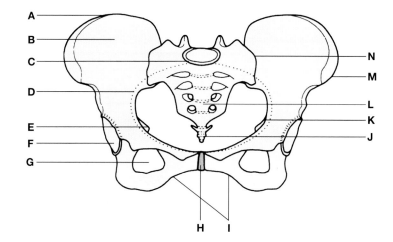

Fig. 8.2 Male pelvis (anterior aspect).

A – Sacrum
B – Pelvic brim (dotted line)
C – Ischial tuberosity
D – Pubic arch
E – Symphysis pubis
F – Arcuate line
G – Greater sciatic notch

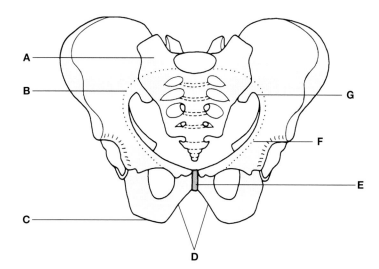

The pelvic inlet – bounded by the pelvic brim.
The pelvic outlet – formed by:
- the *pubic arch;* the rami of the ischium and pubis anteriorly.
- the sacrotuberous ligaments and the ischial tuberosities laterally.
- the apex of the sacrum posteriorly.

The pelvic cavity – The space between the inlet and the outlet; contains the rectum, bladder and parts of the reproductive system.

Imaging Appearances of the Pelvis (Figs. 8.3–8.5)

Fig. 8.3 Female pelvis: anteroposterior projection. (From Lampignano, Bontrager's Textbook of Radiographic Positioning and Related Anatomy, 10e, Elsevier)

A – Gas-filled bowel
B – Iliac fossa
C – Anterior superior iliac spine
D – Anterior inferior iliac spine
E – Superior ramus
F – Obturator foramen
G – Inferior ramus
H – Pubic arch
I – Ischial tuberosity
J – Symphysis pubis
K – Iliopectineal (iliopubic) line
L – Acetabulum
M – Arcuate line
N – Sacrum
O – Iliac crest
P – Fifth lumbar vertebra

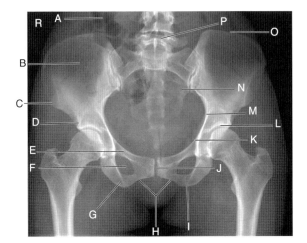

Fig. 8.4 Male pelvis: anteroposterior projection. (From Bruce, Merrill's Atlas of Radiographic Positioning; Procedures: Volume One, 14e, Elsevier)

A – Iliac fossa
B – Anterior superior iliac spine
C – Anterior inferior iliac spine
D – Superior ramus
E – Obturator foramen
F – Inferior ramus
G – Pubic arch
H – Ischial tuberosity
I – Symphysis pubis
J – Iliopectineal (iliopubic) line
K – Acetabulum
L – Arcuate line
M – Sacrum
N – Iliac crest
O – Fifth lumbar vertebra

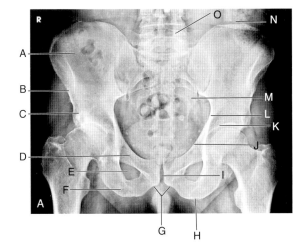

Fig. 8.5 Male pelvis: anteroposterior 3D CT.

A – Iliac crest
B – Iliac fossa
C – Anterior superior iliac spine
D – Anterior inferior iliac spine
E – Superior ramus
F – Obturator foramen
G – Inferior ramus
H – Pubic arch
I – Ischial tuberosity
J – Symphysis pubis
K – Pubic tubercle
L – Acetabulum
M – Arcuate line
N – Sacrum
O – Fifth lumbar vertebra

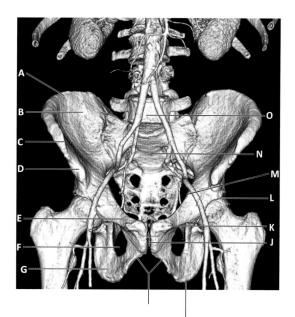

 INSIGHT

There are structural differences between the male and female pelvis; the male pelvis is larger and heavier, whilst the female pelvis is adapted for pregnancy and childbirth. Some of the key differences include:

Feature	Male	Female
General structure	Heavy and thicker	Lighter and thinner
Iliac crest	Curved	Straighter
Pelvic brim (inlet)	Heart-shaped, small	Oval and large
Pelvic outlet	Narrow	Wide
Acetabulum	Large, orientated laterally	Small, orientated more anteriorly
Obturator foramen	Circular	Oval
Pubic arch	<90 degrees	>90 degrees
Greater sciatic notch	Narrow/acute	Wide/less acute
Sacrum	Long, narrow. Straighter anteriorly	Short, wide. Curved anteriorly
Coccyx	Rigid. Straighter anteriorly	Moveable. Curved anteriorly

HIP BONE (FIGS. 8.6, 8.7)

Also known as the *innominate* bones. These are large, irregular bones that are originally three bones – the *ilium, ischium* and *pubis* – that are fused in the mature skeleton. The two hip bones are connected to the sacrum posteriorly at the sacroiliac joints and anteriorly to each other at the symphysis pubis.

Ilium (Figs. 8.6, 8.7)

Type

Flat bone.

Position

Forms the superior aspect of the hip bone, lying mainly above the acetabulum.

Articulations

The *auricular surface* of the ilium with the *auricular facet* of the sacrum to form the sacroiliac joint.
The ilium forms part of the *acetabulum*, which articulates with the head of the femur to form the hip joint.

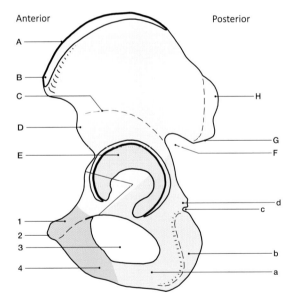

Fig. 8.6 Left hip bone (external aspect).

Ilium
A – Iliac crest
B – Anterior superior iliac spine
C – Inferior gluteal line
D – Anterior inferior iliac spine
E – Acetabulum
F – Greater sciatic notch
G – Posterior inferior iliac spine
H – Posterior superior iliac spine

Pubis
1 – Superior ramus
2 – Pubic tubercle
3 – Obturator foramen (formed by pubis and ischium)
4 – Inferior ramus

Ischium
a – Ischial ramus
b – Ischial tuberosity
c – Lesser sciatic notch
d – Ischial spine

Fig. 8.7 Left hip bone (internal aspect).

Ilium
I – Iliac crest
J – Posterior superior iliac spine
K – Auricular surface
L – Posterior inferior iliac spine
M – Greater sciatic notch
N – Arcuate line
O – Anterior inferior iliac spine
P – Iliopubic (iliopectineal) eminence
Q – Anterior superior iliac spine
R– Iliac fossa

Pubis
5 – Inferior ramus
6 – Obturator foramen
7 – Articular area for symphysis pubis
8 – Pubic tubercle
9 – Superior ramus

Ischium
e – Ischial spine
f – Lesser sciatic notch
g – Body
h – Ischial tuberosity
i – Ischial ramus

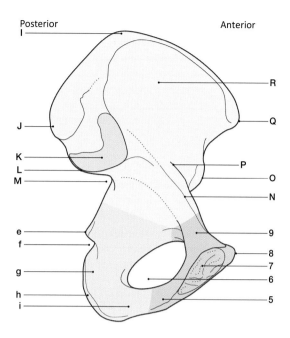

Posterior   Anterior

Main parts

Iliac crest – forms the superior border, which is easily palpated and provides attachment for numerous abdominal muscles. The highest part of the crest lies at the level of the fourth lumbar vertebra.

Anterior superior iliac spine (ASIS) – easily palpated and lies at the lateral end of the iliac crest.

Anterior inferior iliac spine (AIIS) – a bony prominence immediately superior to the acetabulum.

Anterior border – from the ASIS to the acetabulum.

Posterior superior iliac spine (PSIS) – lies at the posterior border of the iliac crest. Easily palpable.

Posterior inferior iliac spine (PIIS) – lies approximately 2.5 cm below the posterior superior iliac spine.

Posterior border – curved border from the posterior superior iliac spine to the posterior border of the ischium.

Greater sciatic notch – lies inferior to the posterior inferior iliac spine. The sciatic nerve leaves the pelvis via the notch.

Internal (medial) surface – divided into two areas, the iliac fossa anteriorly and the sacropelvic surface posteriorly, separated by the arcuate line on the medial border of the ilium.

Iliac fossa – concave surface for the iliacus muscle.

Sacropelvic surface – situated between the arcuate line and posterior border and divided into three areas:

> *Iliac tuberosity* – superior part, roughened for ligament attachment.
> *Auricular surface* – middle part, for articulation with the sacrum.
> *Pelvic surface* – inferior part, forms part of the wall of the true pelvis.

Arcuate line – the border between the 'true' and 'false' pelvis.

Iliopubic (or iliopectineal) eminence – at the junction of the ilium and pubis. Lies at the anterior aspect of the arcuate line.

External (lateral) surface – consists of a large gluteal surface superiorly and a small area inferiorly which forms part of the acetabulum.

Gluteal surface – crossed by three roughened ridges for attachment of the three gluteal muscles.

Ischium (Figs. 8.6, 8.7)

Type — Flat bone.

Position — Forms the posterior and inferior portion of the hip bones.

Articulations — The ischium forms part of the *acetabulum*, which articulates with the head of the femur to form the hip joint.

Main parts — *Body* – forms part of the acetabulum and the greater sciatic notch.

Ischial tuberosity – roughened area on the posterior and inferior aspect of the body; forms attachment for the hamstrings - long head of biceps femoris, semitendinosus and semimembranosus muscles.

Ischial spine – at the inferior end of the greater sciatic notch, insertion for the sacrospinous ligament.

Lesser sciatic notch – inferior to the ischial spine. Contains obturator internus and pudendal nerves and vessels.

Ischial ramus – thin portion of bone on the inferior aspect; is continuous with the pubic ramus to form obturator foramen.

 INSIGHT

The ischial tuberosities are sometimes informally known as the '*sits*' bones as they support one's body weight when sitting.

Pubis (Figs. 8.6, 8.7)

Type — Flat bone.

Position	Forms the inferior, anterior, and medial aspects of the hip bones.
Articulations	The pubis forms part of the *acetabulum*, which articulates with the head of the femur to form the hip joint. The *right* and *left pubic bones* articulate with each other to form the symphysis pubis.
Main parts	*Body* – forms the anterior wall of the true pelvis and articulates with the opposite pubic bone. *Pubic crest* – subcutaneous and easily palpable; forms the superior border of the body. *Pubic tubercle* – on the lateral aspect of the pubic crest, for the inguinal ligament. *Superior ramus* – forms part of the acetabulum and obturator foramen. *Inferior ramus* – extends inferiorly and laterally to join the ramus of the ischium. *Obturator foramen* – large opening formed by the ischium (body and ramus) and the pubis (superior and inferior rami). The foramen is occupied by the obturator membrane and covered by the obturator internus and externus muscles. It permits the obturator nerve and vessels to enter the medial thigh.

Acetabulum (Fig. 8.8)

Cup-shaped socket on the lateral aspect of the hip bone for articulation with the head of the femur. Formed by the pubis (anterior fifth), ischium (posterior two-fifths) and ilium (superior two-fifths).

Acetabular rim – lined with articular hyaline cartilage.

Acetabular notch – gap in the inferior aspect of the acetabular rim. Traversed inferiorly by the transverse acetabular ligament. Contains nerves and vessels for the hip joint.

Acetabular fossa – forms the base of the acetabulum and is non-articular. Attachment site for ligamentum teres to the fovea of the femoral head.

Ossification (Figs. 8.9, 8.10)

Primary centres
Ilium – appears in the eighth week of intrauterine life.
Ischium – age four months.
Pubis – age four to five months.

Fig. 8.8 Acetabulum.

1 – Acetabular rim
2 – Acetabular notch
3 – Acetabular fossa

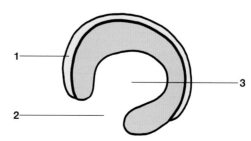

Fig. 8.9 Ossification centres of the pelvis. This image is of a one-year-old (not all ossification centres are present). Note the incomplete fusion between the three parts of the acetabulum (arrows) and of the inferior rami of the pubis and ischium (arrowheads). (From STATdx © Elsevier 2022)

A – Ilium (in utero)
B – Ischium (age four months)
C – Pubis (age six months)
D – Femoral head (age six months)

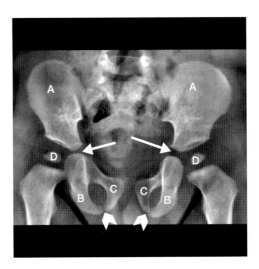

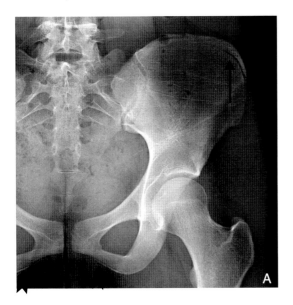

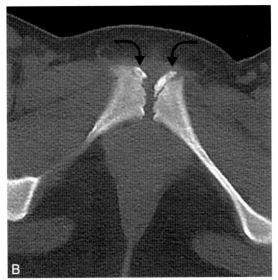

Fig. 8.10 Secondary ossification centres of the pelvis. Anteroposterior pelvis projection (A) and axial CT (B) of a 17-year-old female. Iliac crest (arrow) Ischial tuberosities (arrowheads) Symphysis pubis (curved arrows) All appear during puberty. (From STATdx © Elsevier 2022)

Secondary centres

Ilium – two centres:
   iliac crest appears at puberty;
   AIIS appears at puberty.
Ischium – one centre:
   ischial tuberosity appears at puberty.

> *Pubis* – one centre:
> symphysis pubis appears at puberty.
>
> The hip bone fuses at age 15–25. The iliac crest is one of the last centres in the skeleton to fuse.

FRACTURES

 INSIGHT

The pelvis is another example of a fibro-osseous ring structure; one injury of the pelvic ring most often has a second injury. They may be a combination of bony fracture and dislocation/ diastasis of one of the joints, sacroiliac and/or symphysis pubis.

Fractures that disrupt the pelvic ring are usually caused by high energy trauma and are associated with significant internal soft tissue trauma (consider the organs, large blood vessels, and nerves within the pelvis). Most commonly, there are three main fracture patterns dependent on the mechanism of injury: anterior compression, lateral compression and vertical shear.

Computed tomography (CT) is indicated in suspected pelvis injuries because of its higher accuracy, superior visualisation and the extent of any bony and soft tissue injury.

Anterior compression injury (Figs. 8.11, 8.12)

Diastasis (widening) of the symphysis pubis or fractures of the pubic rami anteriorly associated with vertical fracture of the sacrum or diastasis of the sacroiliac joints posteriorly. Often called *'open-book'* injuries because of the apparent 'opening' of the pelvis.

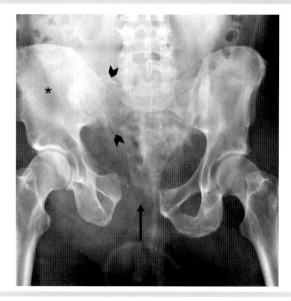

Fig. 8.11 Anterior compression injury of the pelvis; anteroposterior projection. There is diastasis of the symphysis pubis (arrow), a vertical fracture through the sacrum (arrowheads) and lateral rotation of the right hip bone (*). Note the asymmetry of the pelvis. (From STATdx © Elsevier 2022)

Fig. 8.12 Anterior compression injury of the pelvis; 3D CT image. Same patient as Fig. 8.11. CT provides significantly more information on the extent of the injuries and 3D visualisation of the disruption. (From STATdx © Elsevier 2022)

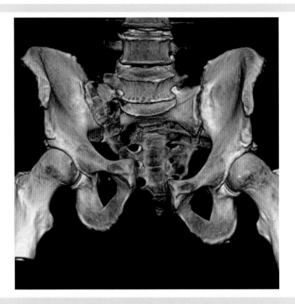

Cause – anterior crushing/compression; typically head on road traffic collisions.
Example of treatment – external fixation until patient stabilised; followed by internal fixation.

Vertical shear injury (Figs. 8.13, 8.14)

Vertical fractures of the pubic rami anteriorly with associated vertical sacral fractures or dislocation of the sacroiliac joint posteriorly. One hemipelvis (half of the pelvic ring) is displaced superiorly, following the direction of force.
Cause – longitudinal force transmits force through limbs into the pelvis, e.g. fall from a height.
Example of treatment – external fixation until patient stabilised; followed by internal fixation.

Fig. 8.13 Vertical shear injury of the pelvis; anteroposterior projection. There are fractures of both the right pubic rami (**arrow**) and left iliac crest (**curved arrow**), as well as diastasis of both sacroiliac joints (**arrowheads**). Note the superior displacement of the left hip bone (*) compared to the right. (From STATdx © Elsevier 2022)

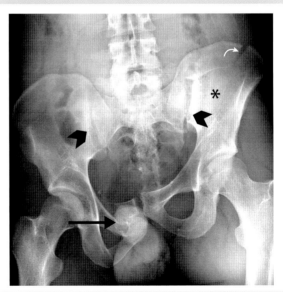

Fig. 8.14 Vertical shear injury of the pelvis; axial CT image. Same patient as Fig. 8.13. Demonstrates marked diastasis (widening) of the left sacroiliac joint (arrow), less so on the right (arrowhead). (From STATdx © Elsevier 2022)

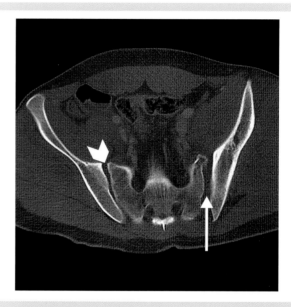

Lateral compression injury (Figs. 8.15, 8.16)

Fractures of the pubic rami, iliac bone and impaction fracture of the sacrum.
Cause – high impact blow from side, e.g., side-impact road traffic collision.

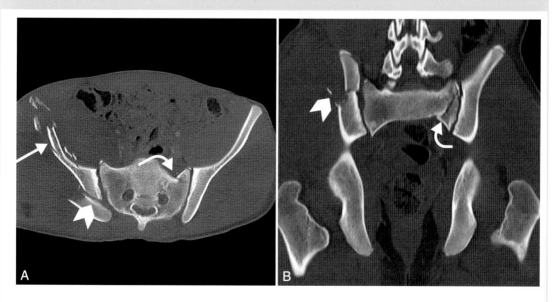

Fig. 8.15 Lateral compression injury of the pelvis. Axial (A) and coronal (B) CT images. Comminuted fracture of the right ilium (arrow), fracture-dislocation of the right sacroiliac joint (arrowhead) and impaction fracture of the left sacrum (curved arrow). (From STATdx © Elsevier 2022)

Fig. 8.16 Lateral compression injury of the pelvis; 3D CT image. Same patient as Fig. 8.15. As well as the previously demonstrated right iliac (arrow) and left sacral (arrowhead) fractures, there are also fracture of both left pubic rami (curved arrows). (From STATdx © Elsevier 2022)

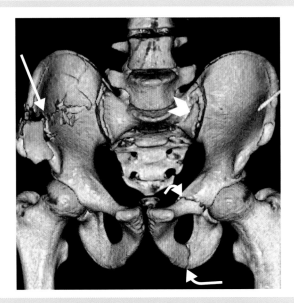

Example of treatment – external fixation until patient stabilised followed by internal fixation.

Avulsion fractures

Isolated avulsion fractures at sites of tendon insertion, particularly at unfused ossification centres. Common examples include:
- ASIS; sartorius muscle
- AIIS; rectus femoris muscle
- Ischial tuberosity; hamstrings
- Iliac crest; oblique abdominal and tensor fasciae latae muscles

Cause – sports (especially kicking) injury in adolescents and young adults.
Example of treatment – usually conservative.

HIP JOINT (FIGS. 8.17, 8.18)

Type   Synovial ball and socket joint.

Bony articular surfaces
The head of the femur with the acetabulum of the hip bone. The articular surfaces are covered with articular hyaline cartilage, except for the fovea of the head of the femur and the acetabular fossa.

Fibrous capsule
Attached medially to the edge of the acetabulum, the acetabular labrum and the transverse acetabular ligament, anteriorly to the intertrochanteric line of the femur, and laterally to the neck of the femur. The capsule is loose inferiorly to allow movement.

Fig. 8.17 Left hip joint
(coronal section).

A – Acetabulum
B – Articular hyaline
    cartilage
C – Synovial membrane
D – Ligament of head of
    the femur (ligamentum
    teres)
E – Transverse acetabular
    ligament (cross-section)
F – Synovial fluid
G – Head of the femur
H – Fibrous capsule
I – Articular hyaline cartilage
J – Acetabular labrum
K – Synovial fluid

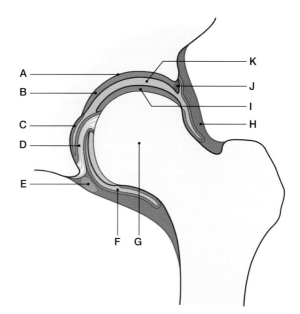

Synovial membrane

Lines the fibrous capsule and covers the ligament of the head of the femur, the intracapsular part of the neck of the femur and the pad of fat in the acetabular fossa. The membrane secretes synovial fluid, which lubricates the joint.

Supporting ligaments

Iliofemoral ligament – triangular-shaped and located anteriorly. The apex is attached to the AIIS and the base to the intertrochanteric line of the femur.
Pubofemoral ligament – anteriorly, from the pubis to the intertrochanteric line. Its fibres blend with those of the fibrous capsule and the iliofemoral ligament.
Ischiofemoral ligament – posteriorly, from the ischium to the intertrochanteric crest.
Ligament of the head of the femur (ligamentum teres) – triangular-shaped. The apex is attached to the fovea of the head of the femur and the base to the acetabular notch and the transverse ligament.
Transverse acetabular ligament – connects the inferior aspect of the acetabular labrum, bridging the acetabular notch.

Intracapsular structures

Acetabular labrum – fibrocartilaginous rim around the acetabulum to deepen the socket.
Pad of fat – lies in the acetabular fossa.

Fig. 8.18 Left hip joint (anterior aspect – A).

A – Iliofemoral ligament
B – Pubofemoral ligament

Left hip joint (posterior aspect – B).
1 – Iliofemoral ligament
2 – Ischiofemoral ligament

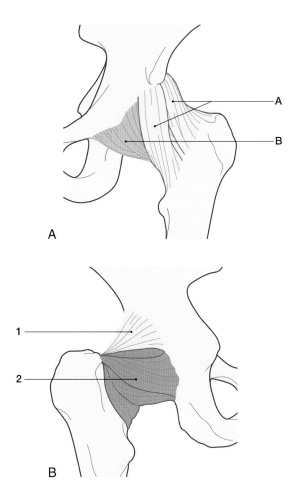

Movements

Flexion by the iliacus and the psoas muscles, assisted by the rectus femoris.
Extension by the gluteus maximus, assisted by the hamstrings.
Abduction by the gluteus medius and the gluteus minimus.
Adduction by the adductor muscles.
Medial rotation by the anterior parts of the gluteus medius, gluteus minimus and tensor fasciae latae.
Lateral rotation by the obturator, gemelli and quadriceps femoris.
Circumduction by a combination of the previously mentioned movements.

Blood supply

Branches of the obturator, gluteal and femoral arteries.

Nerve supply

Branches of the femoral, obturator and gluteal nerves.

Imaging appearances of the hip joint (Figs. 8.19–8.22)

Fig. 8.19 Left hip joint, anteroposterior projection. (From STATdx © Elsevier 2022)

A – Arcuate line
B – Roof of the acetabulum
C – Fovea of the head of the femur
D – Iliopectineal (iliopubic) line
E – Superior ramus
F – Obturator foramen
G – Inferior ramus
H – Lesser trochanter
I – Shaft of the femur
J – Greater trochanter (partially excluded)
K – Neck of the femur
L – Ilium
Solid line – Anterior acetabular rim
Dotted line – Posterior acetabular rim

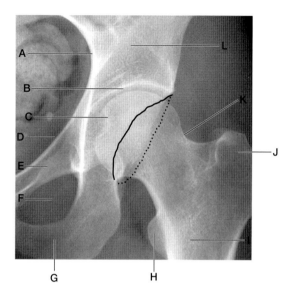

Fig. 8.20 Left hip joint, lateral projection. (From STATdx © Elsevier 2022)

1 – Anterior inferior iliac spine (AIIS)
2 – Anterior acetabular rim
3 – Roof of the acetabulum
4 – Posterior acetabular rim
5 – Ischial tuberosity
6 – Lesser trochanter
7 – Shaft of the femur
8 – Greater trochanter
9 – Head of the femur

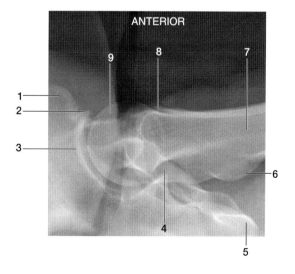

Fig. 8.21 Left hip joint; T1W axial MRI. (From STATdx © Elsevier 2022)

A – Sartorius muscle
B – Iliopsoas muscle
C – Femoral vein and artery
D – Anterior acetabular labrum
E – Ilium
F – Acetabular fossa
G – Ischium
H – Sciatic nerve
I – Gluteus maximus muscle
J – Posterior acetabular labrum
K – Femoral head
L – Gluteus medius muscle
M – Rectus femoris muscle
N – Tensor fascia lata muscle

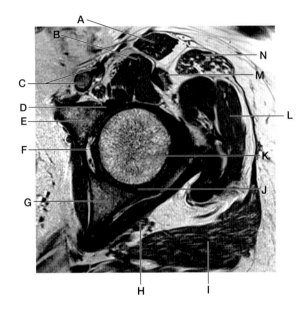

Fig. 8.22 Left hip joint; T1W coronal MRI. (From STATdx © Elsevier 2022)

1 – Ilium
2 – Acetabular fossa
3 – Acetabular labrum
4 – Adductor brevis muscle
5 – Shaft of the femur
6 – Greater trochanter
7 – Acetabular labrum
8 – Gluteus minimus muscle
9 – Gluteus medius muscle
10 – Roof of the acetabulum

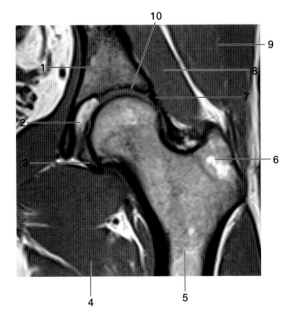

TRAUMA

Posterior dislocation (Figs. 8.23, 8.24)

Ninety percent of hip dislocations (only 10% anterior). Often associated with fractures of the acetabulum or femoral head.

Cause – longitudinal force of the femur on a flexed hip; head on road traffic collisions (dashboard drives the head of the femur posteriorly).

Example of treatment – reduction under anaesthetic. Surgical fixation of fractures.

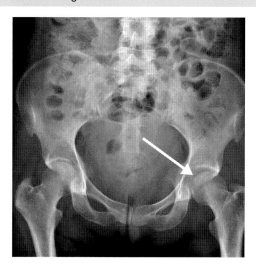

Fig. 8.23 Posterior dislocation left hip; anteroposterior projection. Note widening of the left hip joint space (arrow) and lack of symmetry with the right hip joint. (From STATdx © Elsevier 2022)

Fig. 8.24 Posterior dislocation left hip; axial (A) and 3D (B) CT images. Same patient as Fig. 8.23. The left femoral head (arrow) is dislocated posteriorly from its normal location (*) in the acetabulum. Note in this case that there is no associated fracture. (From STATdx © Elsevier 2022)

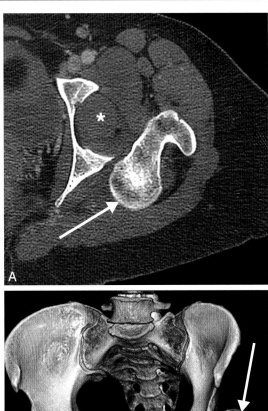

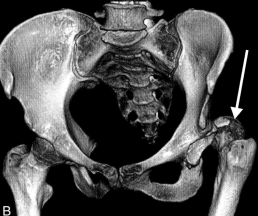

Acetabular fractures (Figs. 8.25-8.27)

May be subtle on radiographs but are usually complex. CT is required for full evaluation and management.

Cause – high energy, forcing the femoral head into the acetabulum (similar to posterior dislocations); road traffic collisions.

Example of treatment – surgical open reduction internal fixation

Fig. 8.25 Right acetabular fracture; anteroposterior projection. Fracture of the posterior acetabulum (arrow) and inferior pubic ramus (arrowhead). (From STATdx © Elsevier 2022)

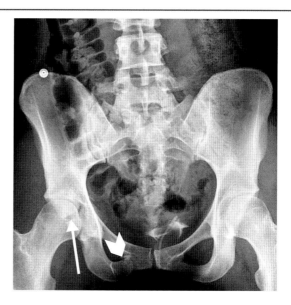

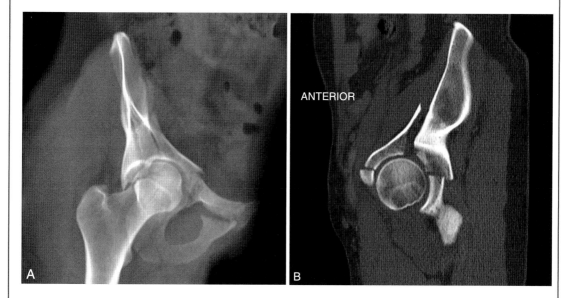

Fig. 8.26 Right acetabular fracture; Oblique (A) and sagittal (B) CT images. Same patient as Fig. 8.25. CT imaging demonstrates the full evaluation of the fractures, not demonstrated on radiographs. (From STATdx © Elsevier 2022)

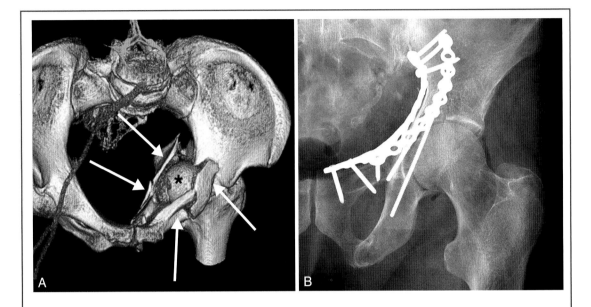

Fig. 8.27 Left acetabular fracture; 3D CT image (A). Note the comminuted fracture of the acetabulum (arrows) and central dislocation of the femoral head (*) into the pelvis. The post-surgery projection (B) demonstrates the extent of the required repair. (From STATdx © Elsevier 2022)

PATHOLOGY

Developmental dysplasia of the hip (DDH) (Figs. 8.28, 8.29)

Abnormal position of the femoral head in relation to the acetabulum. Usually a result of a dysplastic (abnormally developed) shallow acetabulum and ligamentous laxity. Can lead to long-term disability, osteoarthritis and osteonecrosis if not diagnosed and treated early.

Radiological signs – ultrasound indicated in younger infants and radiographs in older infants after ossification of the femoral head. Various lines and angles are measured to assess the congruity of the femoral head and acetabulum and delayed ossification and dislocation of the femoral head.

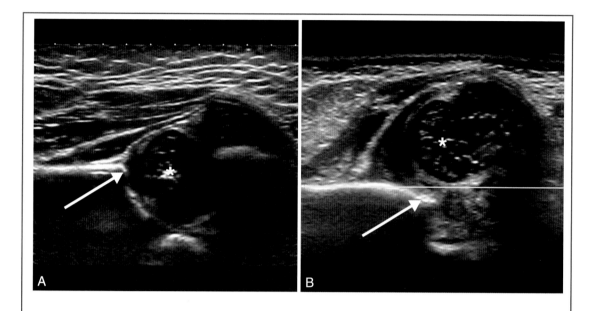

Fig. 8.28 Developmental dysplasia of the hip (DDH); coronal ultrasound images of a normal hip (A) and abnormal hip with dislocation of the femoral head (B). Note the relevant positions of the femoral heads (*) in relation to the acetabulum (arrows). (From STATdx © Elsevier 2022)

Fig. 8.29 Developmental dysplasia of the right hip (DDH); anteroposterior projection. Compared to the normal left hip, the right femoral head (arrow) demonstrates delayed ossification and dislocation from the acetabulum (*). (From STATdx © Elsevier 2022)

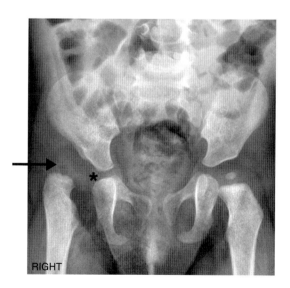

Legg–Calve–Perthes disease (see Chapter 4, Fig 4.7)

Idiopathic osteonecrosis of the femoral head in younger children (typically age four to 12) leading to growth disturbances and early osteoarthritis.
Radiological signs – flattened, sclerotic, and irregular femoral head epiphysis.

Slipped upper (or capital) femoral epiphysis (SUFE) (Fig 8.30)

Cartilaginous fracture of the epiphyseal plate of the proximal femur; the femoral head is displaced posteriorly and medially. Most common in older children (typically age 11-14) until the fusion of the epiphyseal plate. Association with obesity.
Radiological signs – best demonstrated on a 'frog leg' lateral projection. Shortening of the femoral head with medial and posterior displacement in relation to the metaphysis of the femur.

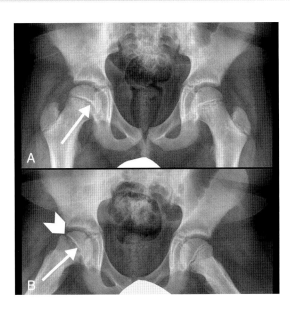

Fig. 8.30 Slipped upper femoral epiphysis (SUFE) right hip; anteroposterior (A) and frog leg (B) projections. The appearances are subtle, with a widening of the epiphyseal plate (arrows) and a slight loss of alignment of the femoral head and metaphysis (arrowhead) compared to the normal left hip. (From STATdx © Elsevier 2022)

SACROILIAC JOINTS (SIJS) (FIG. 8.31)

Very strong, attaching axial skeleton to lower limb and transmission of forces.

Type

Synovial plane joint forms the majority of the joint. Small fibrous syndesmosis portion postero-superiorly.

Sometimes becomes completely fibrous with increasing age.

Orientation

The sacroiliac joints are orientated obliquely to the median sagittal plane; the anterior part is more lateral than the posterior part.

Bony articular surfaces

The auricular surface of the ilium with the auricular facet of the sacrum. The articular surfaces are irregular and interlocking to increase stability.

The articular surface on the sacrum is covered with articular hyaline cartilage and that on the ilium with fibrocartilage.

Fibrous capsule

Attached medially to the sacrum and laterally to the ilium.

Synovial membrane

Lines the fibrous capsule. Secretes synovial fluid, which lubricates the joint.

Fig. 8.31 Sacroiliac joints; axial section.

A – Ilium
B – Synovial aspect of the sacroiliac joint
C – Fibrous syndesmosis aspect of the joint
D – Lumbosacral facet (apophyseal) joint
E – Inferior articular process of the fifth lumbar vertebra
F – Superior articular facet of the first sacral segment
G – Sacral promontory
H – First sacral segment

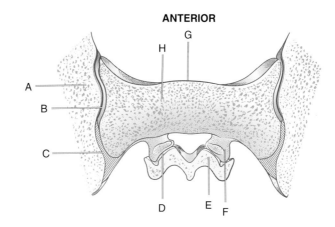

Supporting ligaments

Provide significant strength and stability to the joint.

Ventral (anterior) sacroiliac ligament – covers the anterior and inferior aspects of the joint.

Dorsal (posterior) sacroiliac ligament – covers the posterior aspect of the joint.

Interosseous sacroiliac ligament – short fibres between the two bones; one of strongest ligaments in the body.

Accessory ligaments

Sacrotuberous ligament – from the sacrum to ischial tuberosities.

Sacrospinous ligament – from the sacrum to ischial spines.

Movements

Restricted to *slight anteroposterior rotation* during flexion and extension of the trunk. Increases with hormones released in pregnancy to help facilitate foetus and childbirth.

Radiographic appearances of the sacroiliac joints (Figs. 8.32, 8.33)

Fig. 8.32 Sacroiliac joints; posteroanterior projection.

A – Right sacral ala
B – Ilium
C – Sacroiliac joint
D – Greater sciatic notch
E – Superior ramus
F – Sacral foramina
G – Lumbosacral junction
H – Fifth lumbar vertebra

Note, because of the obliquity of the sacroiliac joints, they are normally better visualised on a posteroanterior projection. (From STATdx © Elsevier 2022)

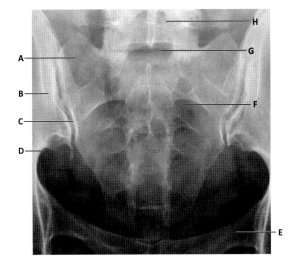

Fig. 8.33 Sacroiliac joints; axial (A) and coronal (B) CT images. (From STATdx © Elsevier 2022)

A – Right sacral ala
B – Right sacroiliac joint
C – Ilium
D – Sacral foramina
E – Fifth lumbar vertebral body
Note the oblique orientation of the sacroiliac joints on the axial image (A)

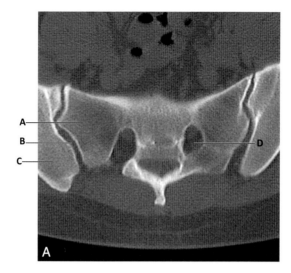

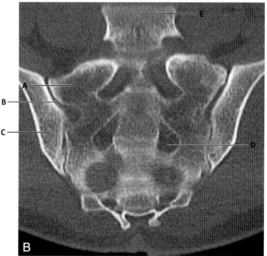

PATHOLOGY

Pathology of the sacroiliac joints is a common cause of lower back pain. Affected by osteo-, inflammatory (e.g. ankylosing spondylitis, see Chapter 4, page 38), and infectious arthritis as well as instability as a result of trauma, childbirth, sports, or spinal deformities (e.g. scoliosis, see Chapter 10, page 296).

SYMPHYSIS PUBIS

Type

Cartilaginous symphysis.

Bony articular surfaces
Right pubic body with left pubic body. The articular surfaces are covered with articular hyaline cartilage.

Supporting ligaments
Superior pubic ligament – covers the superior aspect.
Arcuate (inferior) pubic ligament – covers the inferior aspect.

Intracapsular structures
Interpubic fibrocartilage disc – connects the two bones.

Movements
Minimal movement present. Increases with hormones (relaxin) released in pregnancy to help facilitate childbirth.

Radiographic appearances of the symphysis pubis (Fig. 8.34)

Fig. 8.34 Symphysis pubis; anteroposterior projection. (From STATdx © Elsevier 2022)

A – Superior ramus
B – Obturator foramen
C – Inferior ramus
D – Symphysis pubis
E – Pubic tubercle

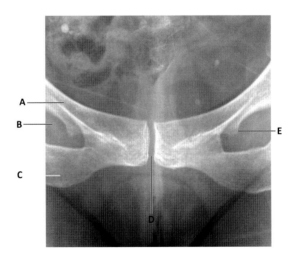

PATHOLOGY

Instability and malalignment may result from previous childbirth, trauma or sports injury.

THORAX

9

CHAPTER CONTENTS

Sternum	221	Costal cartilages	232
Fractures	226	Sternocostal Joints	233
Pathology	227	Interchondral Joints	233
Ribs	228	Trauma	234
Typical ribs	229	Pathology	237
Atypical ribs	230		

The thoracic cage (Fig. 9.1) consists of the ribs and sternum. It is cylindrical in shape with a superior opening to the neck called the *superior thoracic aperture* and a larger *inferior thoracic aperture* to the abdomen. It protects the vital organs within the thorax and upper abdomen, connects the spine and axial skeleton to the upper extremities, and has a role in breathing by acting as a framework for respiratory muscles.

The lower costal margin, which is easily palpable as the inferior part of the thoracic cage, lies at the level of the L3 vertebral body.

STERNUM (FIGS. 9.2, 9.3)

Type

Flat bone.

Position

Lies on the anterior aspect of the thorax in the midline. Known informally as the breast bone.

Articulations

The bilateral *clavicular notches* with the sternal end of the clavicles to form the sternoclavicular joints.
Notches on the lateral aspect of the sternum articulate with the first seven costal cartilages to form the sternocostal joints.

Main parts

Comprises three parts: *manubrium sterni, body*, and *xiphoid process*. The joints between them are cartilaginous symphyses and allow minimal movement during respiration, but they may fuse with age.

Manubrium sterni
Jugular (suprasternal) notch – superior border; subcutaneous, easily palpable, at the level of the second to third thoracic vertebrae.

221

Fig. 9.1 Thoracic cage.

A – First thoracic vertebra
B – First rib
C – First costal cartilage
D – Manubrium sterni
E – Body of the sternum
F – Xiphoid process of the
sternum
G – 11th rib
H – 12th rib
I – Lower costal margin
J – Shared costal cartilage
of the eighth to tenth
ribs
K – Seventh costal cartilage
L – Sixth costal cartilage
M – First intercostal space
N – Superior thoracic
aperture

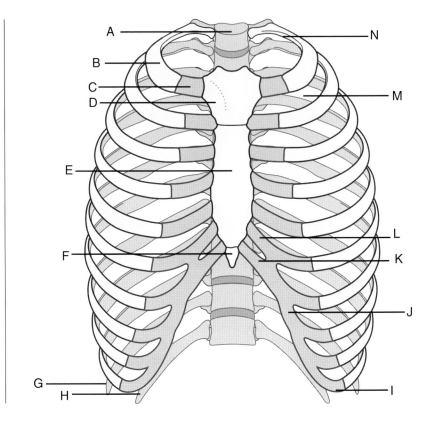

Clavicular notches – either side of the jugular notch; articulate with the clavicles to form the sternoclavicular joints.
Facet for the first costal cartilage – superior end of the lateral border.
Demi-facet for the second costal cartilage – inferior end of the lateral border.
Inferior border – articulates with the body to form the *sternal angle*, at the level of the fourth to fifth thoracic vertebrae, easily palpated.

Body

Four segments – form the long, thin body.
Three ridges – connect the segments.
Four facets – on each lateral aspect for the third to sixth costal cartilages.
Two demi-facets – on each lateral aspect for the second and seventh costal cartilages.

Xiphoid process (Xiphisternum)

Easily palpable at the inferior end of the sternum. Variable in shape.
Superior angle – demi-facet on each side completes the notch for the seventh costal cartilage.
Xiphisternal joint – at the junction of the body and the xiphoid process at the level of the 9th –10th thoracic vertebrae.

Fig. 9.2 Sternum (anterior aspect).

A – Jugular notch (suprasternal notch)
B – Clavicular notch
C – Manubrium sterni
D – Facet for the first costal cartilage
E – Sternal angle
F – Body
G – Xiphisternal angle
H – Xiphoid process
I – Facet for the seventh costal cartilage
J – Facet for the sixth costal cartilage
K – Facet for the fifth costal cartilage
L – Facet for the fourth costal cartilage
M – Facet for the third costal cartilage
N – Facet for the second costal cartilage

Fig. 9.3 Sternum (lateral aspect).

1 – Clavicular notch
2 – Facet for the first costal cartilage
3 – Sternal angle
4 – Xiphisternal angle
5 – Xiphoid process
6 – Facet for the seventh costal cartilage
7 – Facet for the sixth costal cartilage
8 – Facet for the fifth costal cartilage
9 – Facet for the fourth costal cartilage
10 – Facet for the third costal cartilage
11 – Facet for the second costal cartilage

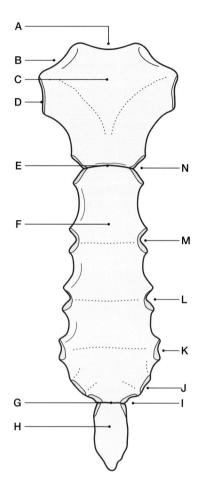

Fig. 9.2

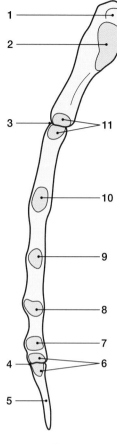

Fig. 9.3

Ossification (Fig. 9.6)

Primary centres

Six centres:

Manubrium – appears in the fifth month of intrauterine life.

Body – four centres (one per segment):

> *first and second segments* – fifth month of intrauterine life.
>
> *third and fourth segments* – fifth to sixth month of intrauterine life.

Xiphoid process – age three (sometimes does not completely ossify until adulthood).

Body begins to fuse after puberty – from the inferior aspect to the superior aspect and continues until complete fusion age 25.

Imaging appearances of the sternum (Figs. 9.4–9.6)

Fig. 9.4 Sternum; posteroanterior projection. (From STATdx © Elsevier 2022)

A – Right first rib
B – Right sternoclavicular joint
C – Manubrium sterni
D – First sternocostal joint
E – Left sternoclavicular joint

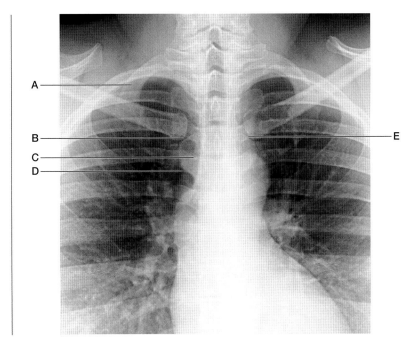

Fig. 9.5 Sternum; sagittal
CT image. (From STATdx ©
Elsevier 2022)

A – Manubrium sterni
B – Body
C – Xiphoid process
D – Heart
E – Thoracic vertebra

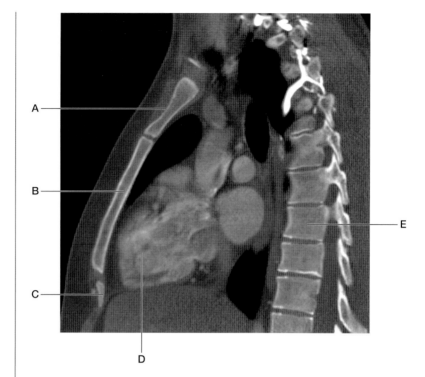

Fig. 9.6 Sternum
ossification centres: lateral
chest projection. Image of
a seven-month-old. Note
the button clothing artefacts
(arrows) (From STATdx ©
Elsevier 2022)

A – Manubrium sterni
(*in utero*)
B – First sternal segment
(*in utero*)
C - Second sternal segment
(*in utero*)
D – Third sternal segment
(*in utero*)
Note, the fourth sternal
segment and xiphoid
process have not yet
ossified significantly enough
to be demonstrated.

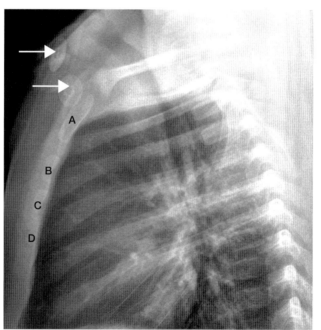

FRACTURES (FIG. 9.7)

High energy injuries that may occur more easily in older persons or those with osteoporosis. Usually transverse and minimally displaced. Best visualised on computed tomography (CT), which can also assess associated significant thoracic injury (e.g., lung, heart, aorta).
Cause – direct blow or deceleration injury (e.g., seatbelt in road traffic collisions).
Example of treatment – often conservative.

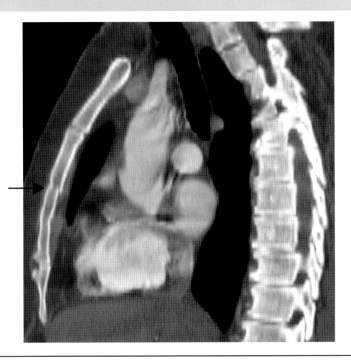

Fig. 9.7 Minimally displaced transverse sternal fracture (arrow); sagittal CT image. (From STATdx © Elsevier 2022)

PATHOLOGY

Pectus excavatum (Fig. 9.8)

Also known as funnel chest. Congenital or developmental abnormality which causes depression and rotation of the sternum with prominence of the anterior ribs.

Fig. 9.8 Pectus excavatum; sagittal (A) and axial (B) CT images. There is posterior displacement of the inferior end of the sternum (arrows). (From STATdx © Elsevier 2022)

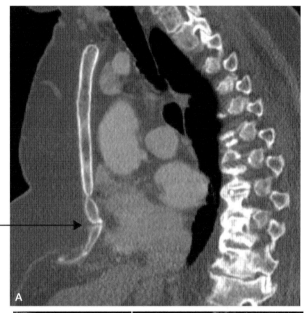

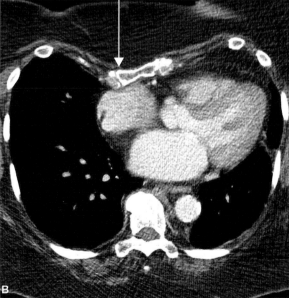

Posterior

Pectus carinatum (Fig. 9.9)

Also known as pigeon chest. Congenital or developmental abnormality which causes abnormal growth of the costal cartilage and prominent protrusion of the sternum.

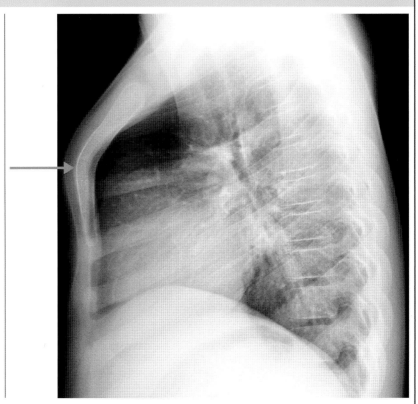

Fig. 9.9 Pectus carinatum; lateral chest projection. There is increased convexity of the sternum (arrow). (From STATdx © Elsevier 2022)

RIBS (FIGS. 9.1, 9.10)

There are 12 pairs of ribs.

One to seven are true ribs as they are directly attached to the sternum by their respective costal cartilages.

Eight to twelve are false ribs; eight to ten are indirectly attached to the sternum by shared costal cartilage; 11 and 12 are floating ribs as they are not attached to the sternum.

Three to nine ribs are considered to be 'typical.'

The ribs increase in size from one to seven and then decrease in size.

The ribs are inclined inferiorly and anteriorly. Therefore, the posterior ends are at a higher level than the anterior ends.

Fig. 9.10 A 'typical' left rib (inferior aspect).

A – Crest
B – Inferior facet of the head
C – Neck
D – Articular part of the tubercle
E – Non-articular part of the tubercle
F – Angle
G – Costal groove
H – Shaft
I – Anterior end

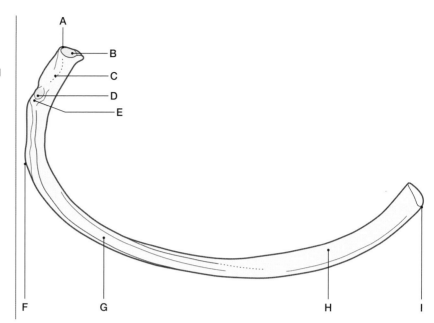

Typical ribs

Type

Flat bone.

Position

Form the thoracic cage.

Articulations

The *anterior end* is connected to the sternum by the costal cartilage to form the sternocostal joints.
The *head* with the demi-facets of the vertebral bodies to form the costovertebral joints.
The *articular part of the tubercle* with the transverse process of the vertebra to form the costotransverse joints.

Main parts

Anterior end – concavity for the costal cartilage.
Head – forms the posterior end with the neck and tubercle.
Crest – divides the head transversely. On either side are an inferior and superior facet for articulation with the corresponding vertebral body and the one above (e.g. the third rib with the second and third thoracic vertebrae).
Neck – narrow portion distal to the head; lies anterior to the transverse process of the corresponding vertebra.
Tubercle – has a medial articular facet for articulation with the vertebra at the transverse process and a lateral non-articular facet.
Angle – near the posterior end of the rib where it changes direction.
Shaft – long and flat.
Costal groove – on the inferior border of the internal surface of the shaft; gives attachment to the intercostal muscle and contains intercostal vessels and nerves.

Ossification

Primary centre
Shaft – eighth week of intrauterine life.

Secondary centres
Three centres:
> *head* – puberty;
> *articular part of the tubercle* – puberty;
> *non-articular part of the tubercle* – puberty.

Fuse with shaft age 20.

Atypical ribs

First rib (Fig. 9.11)
Short, flat, and broad.
Head – single articular facet (articulates only with the body of the first thoracic vertebra).
Tubercle – wide and prominent.
Costal groove – absent.
Scalene tubercle – a ridge across the middle of the superior surface. Separates a posterior groove occupied by the subclavian artery and an anterior groove for the subclavian vein.

Second rib (Fig. 9.12)
Approximately twice the length of the first rib.
Costal groove – shallow.
Rough area – on the lateral surface, for the attachment of the serratus anterior muscle.

Tenth rib
Has only one facet for articulation with the tenth thoracic vertebra.

Eleventh and twelth rib
Short. Have only one facet each for articulation with the 11th and 12th thoracic vertebra, respectively.
> *Tubercle* – absent.
> *Neck* – absent.

Fig. 9.11 Left first rib
(superior aspect).

A – Neck
B – Head
C – Medial border
D – Anterior end
E – Lateral border
F – Tubercle

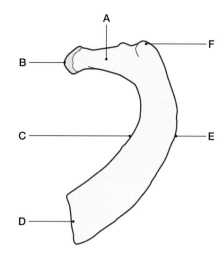

Fig. 9.12 Left second rib
(superior aspect).

1 – Tubercle
2 – Neck
3 – Head
4 – Shaft
5 – Anterior end

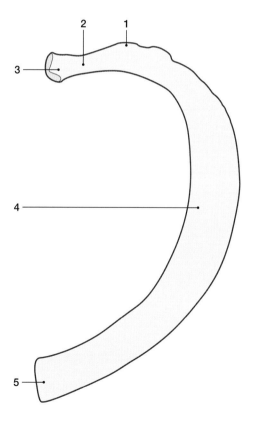

Radiographic appearances of the ribs (Figs. 9.13, 9.14)

Fig. 9.13 Posterior ribs; posteroanterior projection. The posterior part of the ribs is seen to extend from the spine in the midline to the lateral chest wall. (From STATdx © Elsevier 2022)

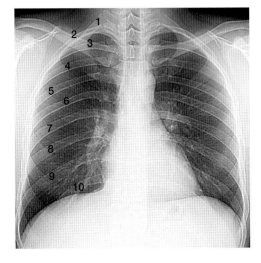

Fig. 9.14 Anterior ribs; posteroanterior projection. The anterior end of the ribs is only visible where they are ossified and do not cross to the midline. (From STATdx © Elsevier 2022)

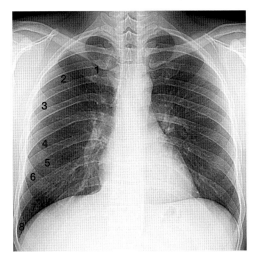

COSTAL CARTILAGES (FIG. 9.1)

Formed by hyaline cartilage. The *base* is attached to the anterior end of the ribs.
Costal cartilages of the:

First–seventh ribs – articulate with the sternum

Eighth–tenth ribs – articulate with the costal cartilage of the rib above

Eleventh and twelfth ribs – end in the muscles of the abdominal wall.

The costal cartilages:
- increase in length from the first to the seventh
- decrease in length from the eighth to the twelth
- decrease in width from the first to the twelth.

STERNOCOSTAL JOINTS (FIG. 9.1)

Type   Second to seventh are synovial plane. The first is cartilaginous synchondrosis.

Articular surfaces
The *hyaline cartilage* at the anterior end of the rib with the corresponding facet (or demi-facet) on the sternum.

Fibrous capsule
Thin between the hyaline cartilage and sternum, reinforced by surrounding sternocostal ligaments. The second sternocostal joint is separated by an intra-articular ligament into two compartments.

Movements
Minimal gliding of the second to seventh during respiration.

Blood supply
Branches of the intercostal vessels.

Nerve supply
Branches of the intercostal nerves.

INTERCHONDRAL JOINTS (FIG. 9.1)

Type   Synovial plane.

Articular surfaces
Between the hyaline cartilages of the sixth to tenth ribs.

Movements
Minimal gliding during respiration.

TRAUMA

Rib Fractures (Figs. 9.15–9.17)

Commonly multiple and of ribs four to nine. May be simple and undisplaced or segmental (more than one fracture per rib). Usually heal with prominent callous.
Cause – direct blow/blunt trauma.
Example of treatment – conservative, pain management.

Fig. 9.15 Multiple rib fractures (arrows); anteroposterior chest projection. There is an associated left pneumothorax (arrowheads) seen as the edge of the lung and lack of peripheral lung markings. Subcutaneous emphysema is also evident in the soft tissue (*). (From STATdx © Elsevier 2022)

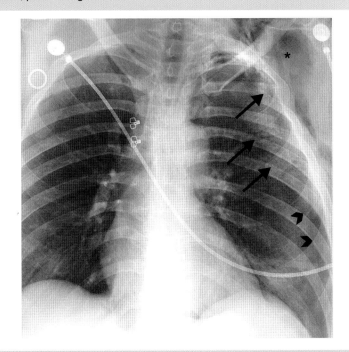

Fractures alone are usually not clinically significant but need to consider associated thoracic/abdominal injury and complications such as:
Haemothorax – blood in the pleural cavity.
Pneumothorax – air in the pleural cavity causing the lung to collapse.
Haemopneumothorax – combination of blood and air in pleural space.
Subcutaneous emphysema – air in the subcutaneous tissue and in the planes between the muscles.
Contusion or laceration – bruising or damage to viscera such as the lungs, liver, or spleen.

Fig. 9.16 Rib fracture (arrow) with associated pneumothorax (arrowheads) and subcutaneous emphysema (*); axial CT image. (From STATdx © Elsevier 2022)

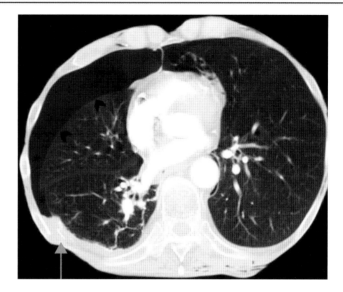

Fig. 9.17 Flail chest; right anteroposterior projection. Multiple segmental rib fractures (arrows) are suspicious for a flail segment. Note the displaced distal clavicle fracture (arrowhead). (From STATdx © Elsevier 2022)

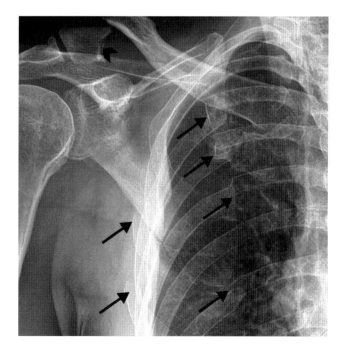

Flail chest (Fig. 9.17)

Associated with major trauma where multiple segmental rib fractures cause a separate '*flail*' segment of the thoracic cage, which moves independently and in opposition to normal movement of the thoracic cage during breathing. High association with significant associated thoracic injury and relatively high mortality rates.

Suspected physical abuse (Fig. 9.18)

Rib fractures are uncommon in children and infants because the ribs are very flexible and elastic. When present in children, rib fractures are highly suspicious of physical abuse, especially if multiple, of varying age, and of the posterior ribs. Most common skeletal injury in suspected physical abuse. Acute injuries often occult on radiographs, subsequent callous formation more prominent.

Fig. 9.18 Suspected physical abuse; anteroposterior chest projection. Posterior rib fractures (arrows) with varying degrees of callous formation in this one-month-old is highly suspicious for suspected physical abuse. (From STATdx © Elsevier 2022)

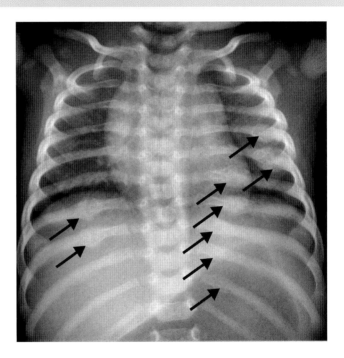

PATHOLOGY

Cervical Rib (Fig. 9.19)

Additional anomalous rib of the 7th cervical vertebra. Can cause compression of neurovascular structures such as the subclavian artery and brachial nerve plexus, with neck/shoulder pain and paraesthesia (numbness) of the forearm and hand, called thoracic outlet syndrome.

Cause – congenital, approximately 0.5% of the population.

Radiographic appearances – variable sized elongation or additional osseous structures related to the transverse processes of the 7th cervical vertebra. Bilateral or unilateral.

Fig. 9.19 Bilateral cervical ribs (arrows); anteroposterior cervical spine projection. (From STATdx © Elsevier 2022)

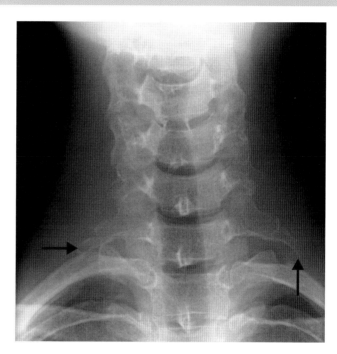

VERTEBRAL COLUMN 10

CHAPTER CONTENTS

A 'Typical' Vertebra	241	Coccyx	270
Cervical Vertebrae	245	Vertebral Curvatures	275
Thoracic Vertebrae	257	Joints of the Vertebral Column	277
Lumbar Vertebrae	262	Trauma	286
Sacrum	268	Pathology	294

The *vertebral column*, or spine, (Figs. 10.1, 10.2) usually consists of:

    Seven cervical vertebrae (movable)
    Twelve thoracic vertebrae (movable)
    Five lumbar vertebrae (movable)
    Five sacral segments (fused)
    Four coccygeal segments (fused to a variable extent).

It acts to protect the spinal cord, support the head, and act as an attachment for the thoracic cage (and in turn, upper limbs), lower limbs through the pelvic girdle, and muscles of the back. It permits movement as a flexible unit.

Fig. 10.1 Vertebral column, lateral view.

A – Cervical spine (seven vertebrae)
B – Thoracic spine (twelve vertebrae)
C – Lumbar spine (five vertebrae)
D – Sacrum and coccyx (five and four segments)

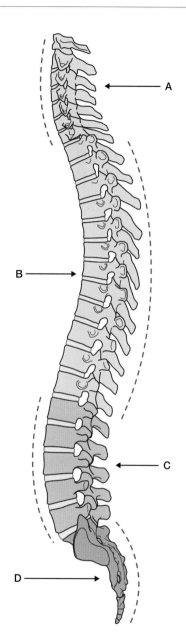

Fig. 10.2 Vertebral column; sagittal T2W MRI. (From STATdx © Elsevier 2022)

1 – Cervical spine (seven vertebrae)
2 – Thoracic spine (twelve vertebrae)
3 – Lumbar spine (five vertebrae)
4 – Sacrum (five segments)
5 – Coccyx (four segments)
6 – Spinal cord

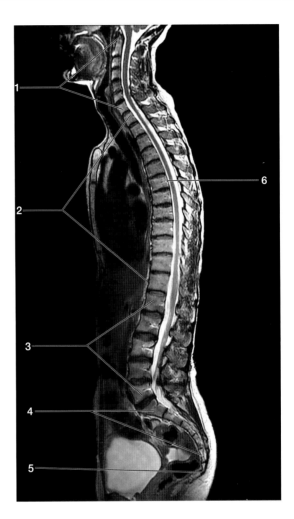

 INSIGHT

Individual vertebrae are often referred to as the first letter of the region of the vertebral column and then the number in that region (from superior to inferior). For example:

First cervical vertebra (atlas) - C1
Fourth thoracic vertebra - T4
Fifth lumbar vertebra - L5
First sacral segment - S1
Lumbosacral joint (between L5 and S1) - L5S1

A 'TYPICAL' VERTEBRA (FIGS. 10.3, 10.4)

The vertebra (plural vertebrae) in each region are slightly different. Some are very specialised, but most have the same typical features.

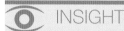

INSIGHT

By learning the parts of a typical vertebra, the majority of the parts of the cervical, thoracic and lumbar vertebrae can be identified. The lumbar vertebrae are often considered 'typical.'

Type   Irregular bone.

Position   Forms part of the central axis of the body.

Articulations   *Superior articular facets* with the inferior articular facets of the vertebra above to form the joints of the vertebral arches (known as *facet* or *apophyseal joints*). *Inferior articular facets* with the superior articular facets of the vertebra below to form the facet (apophyseal) joints of the vertebral arches. *Superior and inferior vertebral endplates* to form the intervertebral joints via the intervertebral discs.

Main parts   Vertebrae are divided into two parts; the anterior *vertebral body*, which is the main weight-bearing portion, and the posterior *vertebral arch*, which

Fig. 10.3 A typical (lumbar) vertebra (superior aspect).

A – Spinous process
B – Superior articular process
C – Transverse process
D – Pedicle
E – Vertebral body (superior endplate)
F – Vertebral foramen
G – Superior articular facet
H – Lamina
The dotted line marks the division between the vertebral body anteriorly and vertebral arch posteriorly.

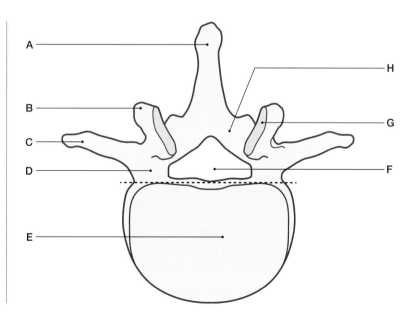

Fig. 10.4 A typical (lumbar) vertebra (lateral aspect).

1 – Vertebral body
2 – Inferior vertebral notch
3 – Inferior articular facet
4 – Spinous process
5 – Pars interarticularis
6 – Transverse process
7 – Superior articular
      process
8 – Superior vertebral notch

The dotted line marks the division between the vertebral body anteriorly and vertebral arch posteriorly.

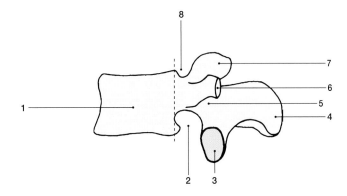

surrounds the spinal cord and has projections that permit movement and muscle attachment.

Vertebral body – cancellous bone covered with a thin layer of compact bone; the anterior surface is convex. Become larger as progress inferiorly down the vertebral column. Anterior and lateral surfaces contain nutrient foramina.

Vertebral endplates, superior and inferior – roughened surfaces of the body to allow attachment of intervertebral discs.

Vertebral arch – formed by two pedicles and two laminae; surrounds the spinal canal.

Pedicles – bilateral; project posteriorly from the posterolateral aspects of the body.

Laminae – bilateral; project posteromedially from the ends of the pedicles; fuse in the midline.

Vertebral foramen – formed by the posterior aspect of the body and the vertebral arch. The vertebral foramen and supporting ligaments form the vertebral canal, which transmits and protects the spinal cord, spinal nerve roots and meninges.

Spinous process – singular; projects posteriorly from the junction of the laminae. In the midline, easily palpable.

Transverse processes – bilateral; project laterally from the junction of the pedicles and laminae.

Superior articular processes – bilateral; projections on the superior aspect of the vertebral arch at the junction of the pedicles and the laminae, which carry the superior articular facets (joint surface).

Inferior articular processes – bilateral; projections on the inferior aspect of the vertebral arch, which carry the inferior articular facets.

Pars interarticularis – joins the superior and inferior articular processes of a vertebra. The junction between the pedicle, lamina, and superior and inferior articular facet on each side of a vertebra.

Vertebral notches; superior and inferior – bilateral; formed between the posterior aspect of the body and the articular processes, superiorly and inferiorly to the pedicles.

Intervertebral foramina – bilateral; formed by the respective vertebral superior and inferior notches between the pedicles of adjacent vertebrae. They transmit the spinal nerves and lie at an angle of 45 degrees to the median sagittal plane and 0–15 degrees to the horizontal.

Ossification

Primary centres

Three centres.

Body – appears between the ninth week of intrauterine life and four months old.

Vertebral arch (two centres, one each side) – between the ninth week of intrauterine life and three months old. Vertebral arch fuses age one to six. Arch fuses with the body at puberty.

Secondary centres

Five centres appear after puberty:

Tip of the spinous process – one centre.

Transverse process – one centre for each process.

Annular plates of the body – one centre superior surface, one centre inferior surface.

Fuse together at age 25.

Imaging appearances of a 'typical' vertebra (Figs. 10.5–10.7)

Fig. 10.5 A 'typical' vertebra; anteroposterior projection of the lumbar spine. (From STATdx © Elsevier 2022)

A – Vertebral body
B – Intervertebral disc space
C – Pedicle
D – Superior articular process
E – Inferior articular process
F – Transverse process
G – Spinous process
H – Facet (apophyseal) joint

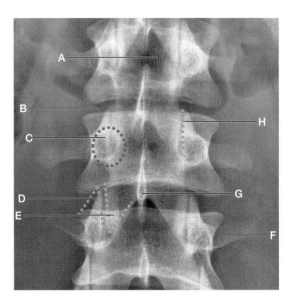

Fig. 10.6 A 'typical' vertebra; lateral projection of the lumbar spine. (From STATdx © Elsevier 2022)

1 – Inferior vertebral endplate
2 – Superior vertebral endplate
3 – Anterior cortical margin
4 – Vertebral body
5 – Intervertebral disc space
6 – Posterior cortical margin
7 – Spinous process
8 – Pedicle
9 – Facet (apophyseal joint)
10 – Pars interarticularis
11 – Superior articular process
12 – Inferior articular process
13 – Intervertebral foramen
14 – Inferior vertebral notch
15 – Rib (not part of typical vertebra)
16 – Superior vertebral notch

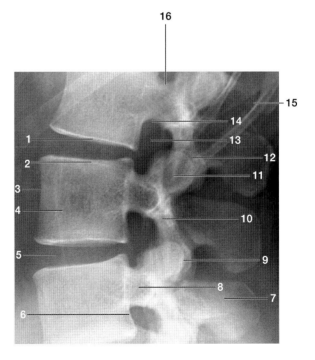

Fig. 10.7 A 'typical' vertebra; sagittal CT image of the lumbar spine. (From STATdx © Elsevier 2022)

A – Superior vertebral endplate
B – Inferior vertebral endplate
C – Superior vertebral notch
D – Inferior vertebral notch
E – Superior articular process
F – Vertebral body
G – Intervertebral disc space
H – Inferior articular process
I – Pars interarticularis
J – Facet (apophyseal) joint
K – Intervertebral foramen
L – Pedicle

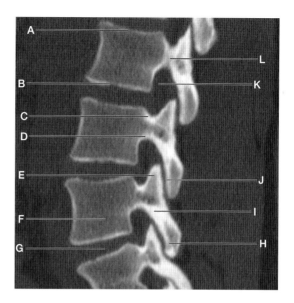

CERVICAL VERTEBRAE

Form the bony structure of the neck. Seven vertebrae; 3rd to 6th are considered 'typical.'

Third to sixth - C3-C6 (typical) (Figs. 10.8, 10.9)

Features

Size – smaller than the thoracic and lumbar vertebrae.
Body – small, oval in shape. Curved into bilateral hook-shaped *uncinate processes* on the superolateral surface.

Fig. 10.8 A typical cervical vertebra (superior aspect).

A – Spinous process (bifid)
B – Lamina
C – Superior articular facet
D – Foramen transversarium
E – Transverse process
F – Vertebral foramen
G – Vertebral body (superior endplate)
H – Uncinate process (edge of the vertebral body)
I – Superior articular process

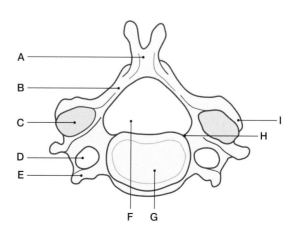

Fig. 10.9 A typical cervical vertebra (lateral aspect).

1 – Vertebral body
2 – Transverse process
3 – Inferior vertebral notch
4 – Inferior articular facet
5 – Inferior articular process
6 – Spinous process
7 – Superior articular facet
8 – Superior articular process
9 – Superior vertebral notch
10 – Uncinate process

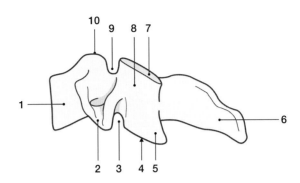

Pedicles – short, round, project posterolaterally at 45 degrees.
Lamina – long and thin.
Vertebral foramen – large and triangular to permit cervical enlargement portion of the spinal cord.
Intervertebral foramen – directed anterolaterally.
Transverse processes – U-shaped in cross-section to carry and protect the cervical nerves. Carry the foramen transversarium for the vertebral arteries towards the head. These divide the processes into anterior and posterior roots, which end in small tubercles.
Superior articular facets – face superoposteriorly.
Inferior articular facets – face inferoanteriorly (to align with opposing superior articular facet of the vertebra below).
Spinous process – short and bifid (divided).

Imaging appearances of the cervical vertebrae (Figs. 10.10–10.15)

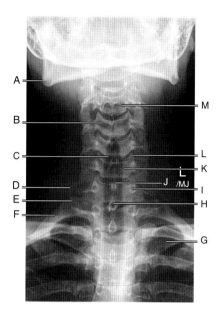

Fig. 10.10 Third to seventh cervical vertebrae: anteroposterior projection. (From Lampignano, Bontrager's Textbook of Radiographic Positioning and Related Anatomy, 10e, Elsevier)

A – Angle of the mandible
B – Body of the fourth cervical vertebra
C – Intervertebral disc space (between the 5th and 6th cervical vertebrae)
D – Transverse process of the 7th cervical vertebra
E – Transverse process of the 1st thoracic vertebra
F – First rib
G – Clavicle
H – Spinous process of the 7th cervical vertebra
I – Pedicle of the 7th cervical vertebra
J – Spinous process of the 6th cervical vertebra
K – Body of the 6th cervical vertebra
L – Uncinate process of the 5th cervical vertebra
M – Body of the 3rd cervical vertebra

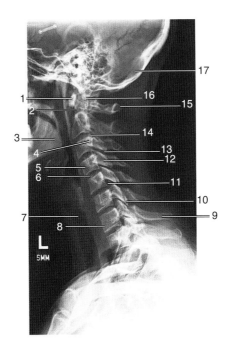

Fig. 10.11 Cervical spine: lateral projection. (From Lampignano, Bontrager's Textbook of Radiographic Positioning and Related Anatomy, 10e, Elsevier)

1 – Anterior tubercle of the atlas
2 – Odontoid process
3 – Mandible
4 – Transverse process of the 3rd cervical vertebra
5 – Body of the 4th cervical vertebra
6 – Intervertebral disc space (between the 4th and 5th vertebral bodies)
7 – Trachea
8 – Body of the 7th cervical vertebra
9 – Spinous process of the 7th cervical vertebra (vertebra prominens)
10 – Inferior articular process of the 6th cervical vertebra
11 – Superior articular process of the 6th cervical vertebra
12 – Lamina of the 4th cervical vertebra
13 – Facet (apophyseal) joint
14 – Intervertebral foramen
15 – Posterior tubercle of the atlas
16 – Atlantooccipital joint
17 – Occipital bone

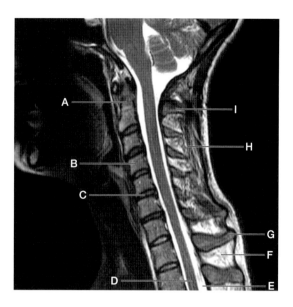

Fig. 10.12 Cervical spine; sagittal T2W MRI. (From STATdx © Elsevier 2022)

A – Odontoid process
B – Body of the 4th cervical vertebra
C – Intervertebral disc between the 5th and
6th cervical vertebrae
D – Spinal cord

E – Cerebrospinal fluid
F – Interspinous ligament
G – Spinous process of the 1st thoracic vertebra
H – Ligamentum nuchae
I – Spinous process of the 2nd cervical vertebra

Fig. 10.13 Fifth cervical vertebra: axial CT image. (From STATdx © Elsevier 2022)

1 – Trachea
2 – Body
3 – Transverse process
4 – Articular processes
5 – Vertebral foramen
6 – Spinous process (bifid)
7 – Lamina
8 – Pedicle
9 – Foramen transversarium (for vertebral artery)
10 – Groove in transverse process for the fifth cervical nerve root

ANTERIOR

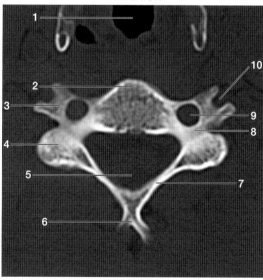

POSTERIOR

Fig. 10.14 Cervical spine; anteroposterior (A) oblique (B) and lateral (C) 3D CT images. (From STATdx © Elsevier 2022)

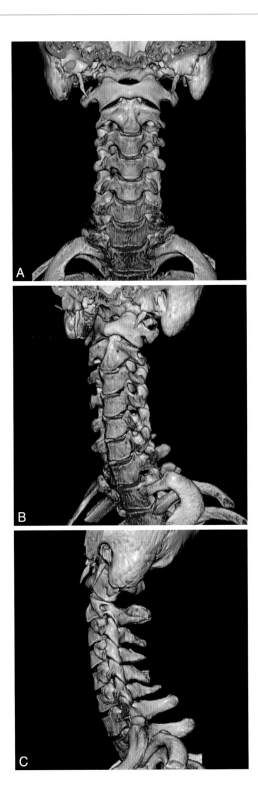

Fig. 10.15 Paediatric cervical spine; lateral projection. Normal appearances. Note the apparent widening of the intervertebral disc spaces (A) and irregularity of the vertebral bodies (B) caused by incomplete ossification of the annular (endplate) parts of the body. (From STATdx © Elsevier 2022)

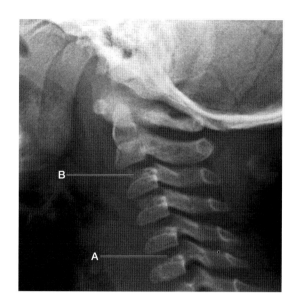

First cervical vertebra - C1 (atlas) (Fig. 10.16)

Articulations

Superior articular facets with the occipital condyles of the skull to form the atlantooccipital joints.

Inferior articular facets with the superior articular facets of the 2nd cervical vertebra to form the lateral atlantoaxial joints.

The facet on the anterior arch with the odontoid process of the 2nd cervical vertebra to form the median atlantoaxial joint.

Fig. 10.16 First cervical vertebra (atlas) - C1 (superior aspect).

A – Anterior tubercle
B – Superior articular facet
C – Foramen transversarium
D – Vertebral foramen
E – Posterior arch
F – Posterior tubercle
G – Groove for the vertebral artery
H – Transverse process
I – Facet for the odontoid process
J – Anterior arch

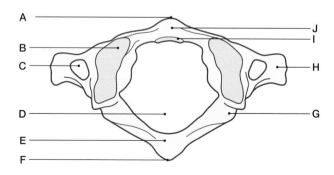

Features

'Ring-shaped' with no body.

Anterior arch – in the midline, there is a projection called the anterior tubercle. On the posterior aspect is a facet for the odontoid process of the second cervical vertebra.

Posterior arch – in the midline, there is a projection called the posterior tubercle, which represents a rudimentary spinous process.

Vertebral foramen – oval.

Lateral masses – either side of the vertebral foramen and carry the superior and inferior articular facets. On the medial aspect is a tubercle for the transverse ligament of the atlas.

Superior articular facets – large and oval.

Inferior articular facets – round and flat.

Transverse processes – long, assist with rotation of the head.

Foramen transversarium – within transverse processes; for passage of vertebral arteries.

Ossification (Fig. 10.24)

Primary centres

Three centres:

Lateral masses/posterior arch (one per side) – seventh week of intrauterine life; fuse age three to four;

Anterior arch – age one; fuse with lateral masses age six to eight.

Second cervical vertebra - C2 (axis) (Figs. 10.17, 10.18)

Articulations

Superior articular facets with the inferior articular facets of the 1st cervical vertebra to form the lateral atlantoaxial joints.

Inferior articular facets with the superior articular facets of the 3rd cervical vertebra to form the facet (apophyseal) joints of the vertebral arches.

Fig. 10.17 Second cervical vertebra (axis) - C2 (anterior aspect).

A – Odontoid process (dens)
B – Facet for the anterior arch of the atlas
C – Superior articular facet
D – Foramen transversarium
E – Transverse process
F – Body
G – Inferior articular facet

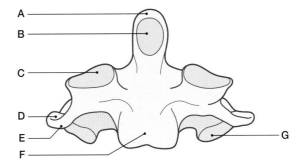

Fig. 10.18 Second cervical vertebra (axis) - C2 (lateral aspect).

1 – Facet for the anterior arch of the atlas
2 – Superior articular facet
3 – Body
4 – Foramen transversarium in the transverse process
5 – Inferior articular facet
6 – Inferior articular process
7 – Spinous process
8 – Lamina
9 – Groove for the transverse ligament of the atlas
10 – Odontoid process (dens)

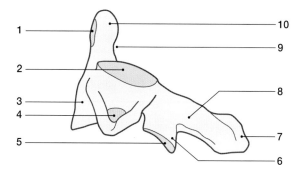

The *odontoid process* with the anterior arch of the 1st cervical vertebra to form the median atlantoaxial joint.
The *body* with the body of the 3rd cervical vertebra to form the intervertebral joint.

Features
Odontoid process (dens) – large tooth/finger-like projection on the superior aspect of the body; has a facet for articulation with the anterior arch of the 1st cervical vertebra. Represents the body of the axis (C2).

Ossification (Fig. 10.24)

Primary centres
Five centres:
   Odontoid process – two centres; sixth month of intrauterine life; fuse together before birth.
   Vertebral arch (one per side) – seventh to eighth month of intrauterine life.
   Body – age four to five months.

Secondary centres
Two centres:
   Tip of the odontoid process – age two; fuses age 12;
   Annular plate – thin round plate inferior to the body; appears at puberty.

Imaging appearances of the first and second cervical vertebrae (Figs. 10.19–10.24)

Fig. 10.19 Upper cervical vertebrae: lateral projection. (From STATdx © Elsevier 2022)

A – Occipital condyles
B – Anterior arch of the 1st cervical vertebra
C – Odontoid process (dens)
D – Mandible
E – Body of the 2nd cervical vertebra
F – Facet (apophyseal) joint
G – Spinous process of the 2nd cervical vertebra
H – Posterior arch of the 1st cervical vertebra
I – External occipital protuberance (of occipital bone)

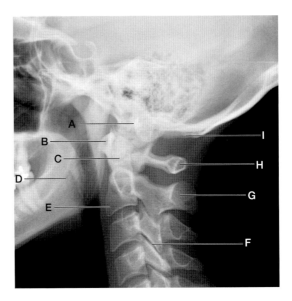

Fig. 10.20 Upper cervical vertebrae: anteroposterior (open mouth) projection. (From STATdx © Elsevier 2022)

1 – Upper teeth
2 – Lateral mass of the 1st cervical vertebra
3 – Lateral atlantoaxial joint
4 – Pedicle of the 2nd cervical vertebra
5 – Lower teeth
6 – Body of the 3rd cervical vertebra
7 – Spinous process (bifid) of the 2nd cervical vertebra
8 – Odontoid process
9 – Occipital bone (superimposed by teeth)

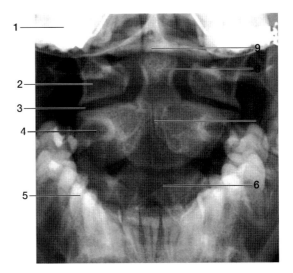

Fig. 10.21 Upper cervical vertebrae: coronal CT image (similar projection to Fig. 10.20). (From STATdx © Elsevier 2022)

A – Occipital condyle
B – Lateral mass of the 1st cervical vertebra
C – Transverse process of the 1st cervical vertebra
D – Body of the 2nd cervical vertebra
E – Intervertebral disc space between the 2nd and 3rd cervical vertebrae
F – Body of the 3rd cervical vertebra
G – Lateral atlantoaxial joint
H – Odontoid process (dens)

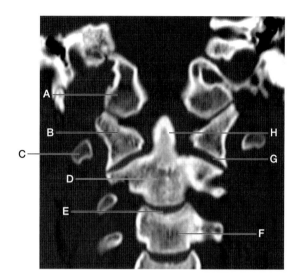

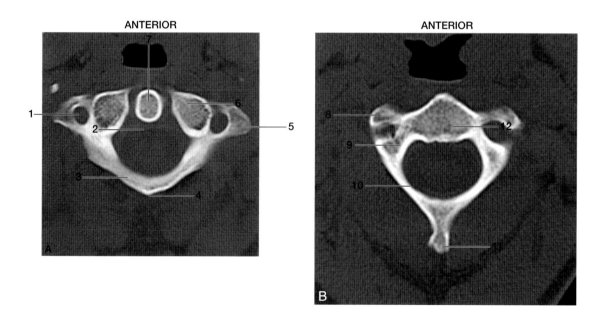

Fig. 10.22 First (A) and second (B) cervical vertebrae: axial CT images. (From STATdx © Elsevier)

1 – Foramen transversarium
2 – Transverse ligament (barely visible)
3 – Posterior arch
4 – Posterior tubercle
5 – Transverse process
6 – Lateral mass
7 – Odontoid process (of the 2nd cervical vertebra)
8 – Transverse process
9 – Pedicle
10 – Lamina
11 – Spinous process
12 – Body

Fig. 10.23 Upper cervical spine; anteroposterior (A), lateral (B) and axial (C) 3D CT images. (From STATdx © Elsevier 2022)

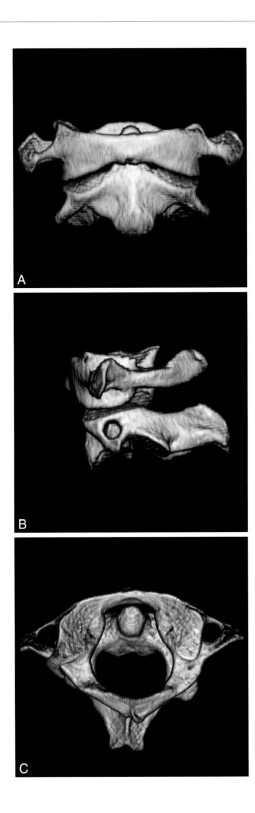

ANTERIOR

ANTERIOR

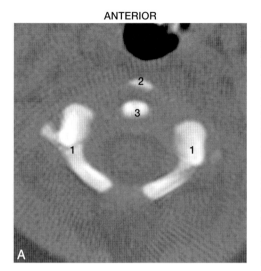

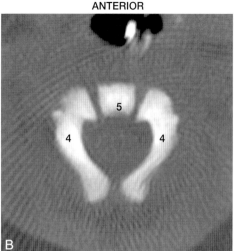

Fig. 10.24 First (A) and second (B) cervical vertebrae ossification centres; axial CT images in a six-month-old. (From STATdx © Elsevier 2022)

1 – Lateral masses (*in utero*)
2 – Anterior arch (age one year)
3 – Odontoid process (*in utero*)

4 – Vertebral arch (*in utero*)
5 – Body (age four to five months)

Seventh cervical vertebra - C7 (vertebra prominens)

Spinous process – long, not bifid; useful bony landmark.
Foramina transversarium – rudimentary or absent; vertebral vessels do not pass through them.
Transverse processes – large.

Ossification

As per a typical vertebra.

Two additional centres for the *costal part of the transverse process* - six months of intrauterine life. Fuse age five to six; occasionally may not fuse and can go on to form cervical ribs (See Chapter 9, page 237).

THORACIC VERTEBRAE

Twelve vertebrae form the upper part of the back. The second to eighth thoracic vertebrae are considered typical.

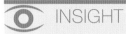 INSIGHT

The body of the thoracic vertebrae lie near the heart and are heart-shaped.

Second to eighth - T2-T8 (typical) (Figs. 10.25, 10.26)

Features

Size – larger than the cervical and smaller than the lumbar vertebrae.

Body – heart-shaped. On each side are two costal (rib) demi-facets. The superior demi-facets are larger and lie at the root of the pedicle, and the inferior demi-facets lie on the inferior border of the body. All four demi-facets articulate with the heads of the ribs, the superior with the corresponding rib and the inferior with the one below.

Pedicles – very short, directed posteriorly. There is virtually no superior vertebral notch.

Laminae – short and wide, overlapping those of the vertebra below.

Vertebral foramen – small and circular.

Transverse processes – thick and strong. Anteriorly there is an oval facet for articulation with the tubercle of the rib.

Superior articular facets – vertical, face posteriorly.

Inferior articular facets – vertical, face anteriorly.

Spinous process – long, slender and directed infero-posteriorly. Easily palpable.

Fig. 10.25 A typical thoracic vertebra (superior aspect).

A – Spinous process
B – Transverse process
C – Superior articular facet
D – Vertebral foramen
E – Superior endplate of the body
F – Pedicle
G – Costal facet for the tubercle of the rib
H – Lamina

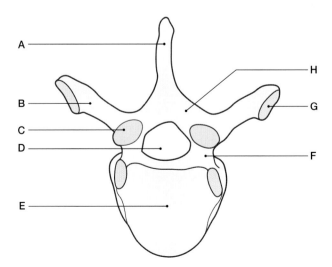

Fig. 10.26 A typical thoracic vertebra (lateral aspect).

1 – Body
2 – Demi-facet for the head of the rib
3 – Inferior vertebral notch
4 – Inferior articular process
5 – Spinous process
6 – Transverse process
7 – Costal facet for the tubercle of the rib
8 – Superior articular facet
9 – Superior articular process
10 – Demi-facet for the head of the rib

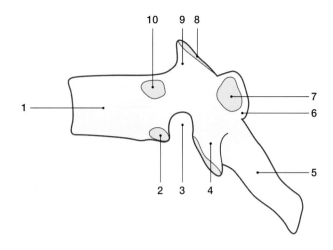

First thoracic vertebra - T1

Special features
Body – full (rather than demi-) superior costal facets are circular and articulate with the first ribs; inferior costal demi-facets are semi-circular and articulate with the second ribs.
Spinous process – thick, long and horizontal.

Ninth thoracic vertebra - T9

Special features
Body – inferior costal demi-facets are sometimes absent.

Tenth thoracic vertebra - T10

Special features
Body – sometimes full (rather than demi-) superior costal facets, oval in shape for articulation with the tenth ribs.
Transverse processes – facet for articulation with the tenth rib may be absent.
Inferior costal facets – absent.

11th and 12th thoracic vertebrae - T11 and T12

Special features
Body – full superior costal facets, oval in shape for articulation with the 11th/12th ribs, respectively.

Transverse processes – small, no costal facets.
Inferior costal facets – absent.

Imaging appearances of the thoracic vertebrae (Figs. 10.27–10.30)

Fig. 10.27 Thoracic vertebrae: anteroposterior projection. (From Lampignano, Bontrager's Textbook of Radiographic Positioning and Related Anatomy, 10e, Elsevier)

A – Body of the first thoracic vertebra
B – Spinous process of the second thoracic vertebra
C – Trachea
D – Pedicle of the fifth thoracic vertebra
E – Costovertebral joint
F – Transverse process of the ninth thoracic vertebra
G – Body of the twelth thoracic vertebra
H – Intervertebral disc space between the sixth and seventh vertebral bodies
I – First rib

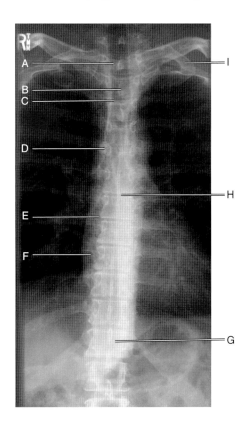

Fig. 10.28 Thoracic vertebrae: lateral projection. (From Lampignano, Bontrager's Textbook of Radiographic Positioning and Related Anatomy, 10e, Elsevier)

1 – Anterior part of the rib
2 – Intervertebral disc space between the eighth and ninth thoracic vertebral bodies
3 – Anterior cortical margin of the tenth thoracic vertebral body
4 – Diaphragm
5 – Body of the twelth thoracic vertebra
6 – Spinous process
7 – Posterior part of the rib
8 – Posterior cortical margin of the eighth vertebral body
9 – Intervertebral foramen
10 – Pedicle

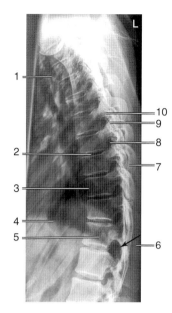

Fig. 10.29 Thoracic vertebrae: median sagittal T1W MRI. (From STATdx © Elsevier 2022)

A – Body of the thoracic vertebra
B – Intervertebral disc
C – Anterior longitudinal ligament (on the anterior cortical edge of the body)
D – Posterior longitudinal ligament (on the posterior cortical edge of the body)
E – Interspinous ligament
F – Supraspinous ligament
G – Spinous process
H – Ligamentum flavum
I – Spinal cord

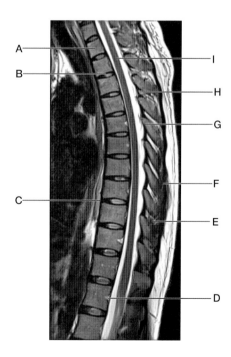

Fig. 10.30 Thoracic vertebrae: sagittal (lateral to the midline) T1W MRI. (From STATdx © Elsevier 2022)

1 – Trachea
2 – Lamina
3 – Intervertebral foramen (and spinal nerve)
4 – Superior articular process
5 – Inferior articular process
6 – Intervertebral facet (apophyseal) joint

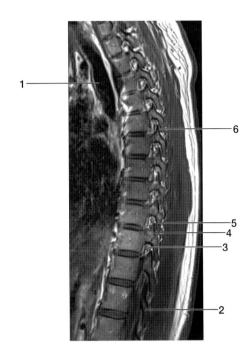

LUMBAR VERTEBRAE

Five vertebrae (normally), forming the lower part of the back. The 1st to 4th lumbar vertebrae are considered typical.

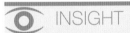 INSIGHT

The lumbar vertebral bodies lie near the kidneys and are kidney-shaped.

First to fourth - L1-L4 (typical) (Figs. 10.3, 10.4)

Features
Size – larger than the cervical and thoracic vertebrae.
Body – large and kidney-shaped. Endplates contain nutrient foramina.
Pedicles – short and thick, set on the superior half of the body.
Laminae – short and thick, inclined inferiorly.
Vertebral foramen – triangular, smaller than the cervical and larger than the thoracic.
Transverse processes – long and thin.
Superior articular processes – have a rough elevation on the posterior border called the mamillary process.

Superior articular facets – vertical, facing medially and posteriorly in opposition to:
Inferior articular facets – vertical, facing laterally and anteriorly.
Pars interarticularis – area between the superior and inferior articular processes at the junction of the pedicle and lamina (important as may fracture either because of trauma or stress).
Spinous process – quadrilateral in shape, thickened on the posterior and inferior margins.

Ossification

Primary centres

Three centres:
Body – between the ninth week of intrauterine life and four months old;
Vertebral arch (one on each side) – between the ninth week of intrauterine life and three months old. Vertebral arch fuses age one to six (the vertebral arch, particularly of L5, does not always fuse).
Arch fuses with the body at puberty.

Secondary centres

Seven centres appear after puberty:
Tip of the spinous process – one centre;
Transverse process – one centre for each process;
Annular surface of the body – one centre superior surface, one centre inferior surface;
Mamillary process – one centre per superior articular process, appears at puberty.
Fuse together at age 25.

Fifth lumbar vertebra - L5

Special features

Body – largest of all vertebrae, deeper anteriorly than posteriorly.
Transverse processes – large, connected to the whole of the pedicle and part of the body.

Imaging appearances of the lumbar vertebrae (Figs. 10.31–10.35)

Fig. 10.31 Lumbar vertebrae; anteroposterior projection. (From Lampignano, Bontrager's Textbook of Radiographic Positioning and Related Anatomy, 10e, Elsevier)

A – Twelth rib
B – Pedicle of the second lumbar vertebra
C – Transverse process of the third lumbar vertebra
D – Spinous process of the fourth lumbar vertebra
E – Sacrum
F – Body of the fourth lumbar vertebra
G – Intervertebral disc space between the third and fourth vertebral bodies
H – Superior articular process of the third lumbar vertebra
I – Facet (apophyseal) joint

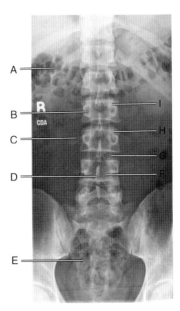

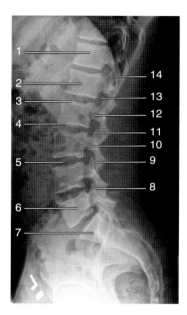

Fig. 10.32 Lumbar vertebrae; lateral projection. (From Lampignano, Bontrager's Textbook of Radiographic Positioning and Related Anatomy, 10e, Elsevier)

1 – Body of the 12th thoracic vertebra
2 – Body of the 1st lumbar vertebra
3 – Superior endplate of the 2nd lumbar vertebra
4 – Inferior endplate of the 2nd lumbar vertebra
5 – Intervertebral disc space between the 3rd and
    4th vertebral bodies
6 – Body of the 5th lumbar vertebra
7 – Sacrum

8 – Facet (apophyseal) joint
9 – Inferior articular process of the 3rd lumbar vertebra
10 – Pars interarticularis of the 3rd lumbar vertebra
11 – Superior articular process of the 3rd lumbar vertebra
12 – Pedicle of the 2nd lumbar vertebra
13 – Intervertebral foramen
14 – 12th rib

Fig. 10.33 Lumbar vertebrae; sagittal T1W MRI. (From STATdx © Elsevier 2022)

A – Body of the 1st lumbar vertebra
B – Anterior longitudinal ligament
C – Intervertebral disc between the 4th and 5th lumbar vertebra
D – Body of the 5th lumbar vertebra
E – 1st segment of the sacrum
F – Epidural fat
G – Supraspinous ligament
H – Spinous process
I – Interspinous ligament
J – Spinal cord

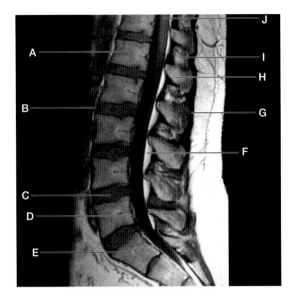

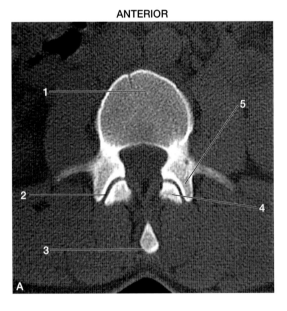

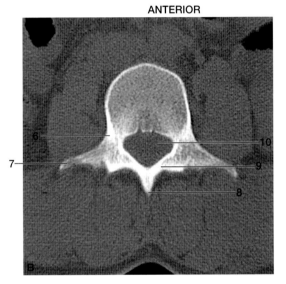

Fig. 10.34 Third lumbar vertebra; axial CT image through the superior (A) and mid (B) part of the vertebra. (From STATdx © Elsevier 2022)

1 – Vertebral body
2 – Facet (apophyseal) joint with the 2nd lumbar vertebra
3 – Tip of the spinous process (of the 2nd lumbar vertebra above)
4 – Inferior articular process (of the 2nd lumbar vertebra)
5 – Superior articular process
6 – Pedicle
7 – Transverse process
8 – Spinous process
9 – Lamina
10 – Vertebral foramen

Fig. 10.35 Lumbar spine; anteroposterior (A), lateral (B) and posterior oblique (C) 3D CT images. (From STATdx © Elsevier 2022)

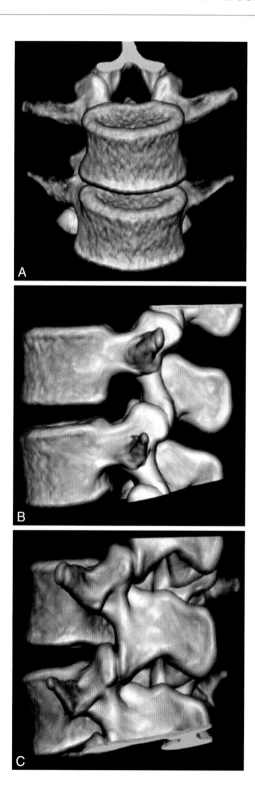

SACRUM (FIGS. 10.36, 10.37)

The sacrum is composed of five sacral segments (S1-S5), which fuse together to form a single bone.

Type

Irregular bone.

Position

Forms the posterior part of the pelvic girdle, between the hip bones.

Articulations

The *base* articulates superiorly with the body of the 5th lumbar vertebra to form the lumbosacral (L5S1) joint or junction.
The *apex* articulates with the base of the coccyx to form the sacrococcygeal joint.
The *auricular facets* articulate with the auricular surface of the bilateral hip bones to form the sacroiliac joints.

Main parts

Base
This is formed by the first sacral segment and has the following features:
Body – large and wide; anterior edge is called the sacral promontory.
Pedicles – short; face posteriorly and laterally.
Laminae – inclined inferiorly, medially and posteriorly.
Transverse processes – project from the body, pedicles and superior articular processes; are fused with the costal element to form the lateral surface, the ala.
Superior articular facets – vertical; face medially and posteriorly.
Spinous tubercle – small spinous process.

Fig. 10.36 Sacrum (anterior aspect).

A – Sacral promontory
B – Pelvic sacral foramen
C – Pedicle
D – Body of the fourth sacral segment
E – Apex: facet for the coccyx
F – Inferior lateral angle
G – Transverse ridge
H – Ala
I – Superior articular facet

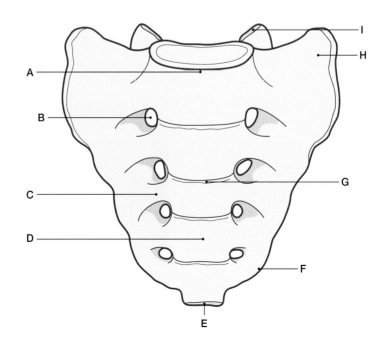

Fig. 10.37 Sacrum and coccyx (lateral aspect).

1 – Sacral promontory
2 – Auricular facet
3 – Lateral border
4 – Sacrococcygeal joint
5 – Coccyx
6 – Coccygeal cornu
7 – Sacral hiatus
8 – Sacral cornu
9 – Dorsal sacral foramen
10 – Intermediate sacral crest
11 – Spinous tubercles
12 – Median sacral crest
13 – Superior articular process

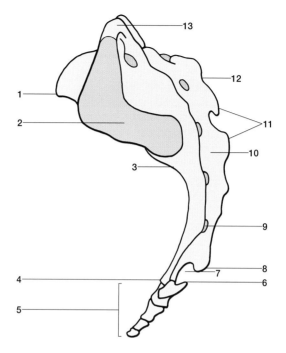

Pelvic surface

This faces inferiorly and anteriorly, is concave, relatively smooth, and has the following features:

Pelvic sacral foramina – four pairs that carry the first four sacral spinal nerves from the sacral canal.

Transverse ridges – four ridges between the pelvic sacral foramina, denoting the fusion of the vertebral bodies (segments).

Dorsal surface

This faces superiorly and posteriorly, is convex and has the following features:

Dorsal sacral foramina – four pairs of foramina that carry the first four dorsal sacral nerves from the sacral canal.

Median sacral crest – raised promontory of bone in the midline representing the fused spinous processes.

Spinous tubercles – four (sometimes three) tubercles on the crest.

Intermediate sacral crests – bilateral; lateral to the median crest and medial to dorsal sacral foramina, formed by four tubercles. Represents the fused articular processes.

Sacral hiatus – the laminae of the 5th sacral segment fail to meet in the midline, forming a gap in the posterior wall of the sacral canal.

Sacral cornua – formed by the inferior articular processes of the 5th sacral segment, either side of the sacral hiatus.

Lateral sacral crests – formed by the fused transverse processes, lateral to the dorsal sacral foramina.

Transverse tubercles – a row of tubercles on the lateral sacral crests.
Sacral canal – Triangular, formed by the vertebral foramina. The superior opening lies obliquely, and the canal terminates at the sacral hiatus.

Lateral surface
Triangular, with the following features:
Auricular facet – 'ear-shaped' surface for articulation with the ilium.
Lateral border – thin, lies inferior to the auricular surface.
Inferior lateral angle – towards the inferior end of the lateral border at the level of the fifth segment.

Apex
The inferior aspect of the fifth sacral segment. It has the following feature:
Oval facet – for articulation with the coccyx.

Ossification (Fig. 10.45)

For each of the sacral segments

Primary centres
Five primary centres
    Body – sixth to eighth month of intrauterine life. Fuse age two to five.
    Costal elements (one centre on each side) – around birth.
    Vertebral arch (one centre on each side) – appear at ten to 12 weeks old.
    Fuse at puberty.
    Arch fuses with the body at puberty.

Secondary centres
Appear after puberty:
    Tip of spinous tubercle – one centre;
    Transverse process – one centre for each process;
    Annular surface of the body – one centre superior surface, one centre inferior surface;
    Fuse together at age 20.

COCCYX (FIGS. 10.37, 10.38)

The coccyx is composed of between three and five segments, partly or totally fused together to form a triangular bone.

Type

Irregular bone.

Position

Lies on the inferior aspect of the sacrum in the midline and forms the base of the spine.

Fig. 10.38 Coccyx (anterior aspect).

A – Coccygeal cornu
B – Rudimentary transverse process
C – Facet for the sacrum
D – First coccygeal segment
E – Second coccygeal segment
F – Third coccygeal segment
G – Fourth coccygeal segment

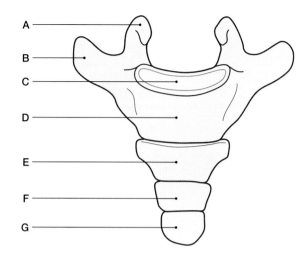

Articulations

The *base* articulates with the apex of the sacrum to form the sacrococcygeal joint.

Main parts

First segment
Largest segment consists of the following features:
Base – formed by the upper surface of the first coccygeal segment; has an oval facet for articulation with the sacrum.
Coccygeal cornua – project superiorly.
Transverse processes – rudimentary; from the body of the first coccygeal segment.

Second to fourth segments
Diminish in size and represent rudimentary vertebral bodies.

Ossification

Primary centres
Body – one centre per body, first present at birth. The rest appear up to age 20. Fuse together up to age 30.

Imaging appearances of the sacrum and coccyx (Figs. 10.39–10.45)

Fig. 10.39 Sacrum: anteroposterior projection. (From STATdx © Elsevier 2022)

A – Transverse process of 5th lumbar vertebra
B – Lumbosacral facet (apophyseal) joint
C – Ilium
D – Sacroiliac joint
E – Pelvic sacral foramen
F – Sacrococcygeal joint
G – Coccyx
H – Inferior lateral angle
I – Body of the 1st sacral segment
J – Spinous tubercle
K – Ala
L – Spinous process of the 5th lumbar vertebra
M – Facet (apophyseal) joint between the 4th and 5th lumbar vertebrae
N – Superior articular process of the 5th lumbar vertebra

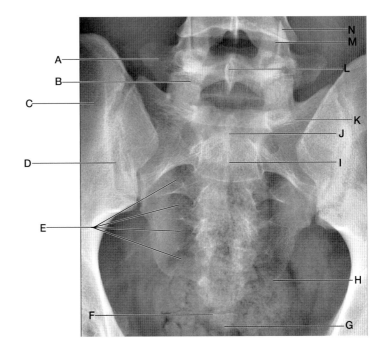

Fig. 10.40 Sacrum; lateral projection. (From Lampignano, Bontrager's Textbook of Radiographic Positioning and Related Anatomy, 10e, Elsevier)

1 – Body of the fifth lumbar vertebra
2 – Intervertebral disc space between the fifth lumbar vertebra and first sacral segment (L5S1)
3 – Promontory
4 – Transverse ridge
5 – Acetabulum
6 – Head of the femur
7 – Coccyx
8 – Sacrococcygeal joint
9 – Sacral canal
10 – Median sacral crest

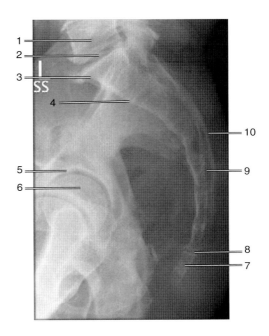

Fig. 10.41 Sacrum and coccyx: sagittal T2W MRI. (From STATdx © Elsevier 2022)

A – Body of the 5th lumbar vertebra
B – Intervertebral disc between the 5th lumbar vertebra and 1st sacral segment (L5S1)
C – Promontory
D – Urinary bladder
E – Rectum
F – Coccyx
G – Sacrococcygeal joint
H – Body of the 3rd sacral segment
I – Body of the 1st sacral segment

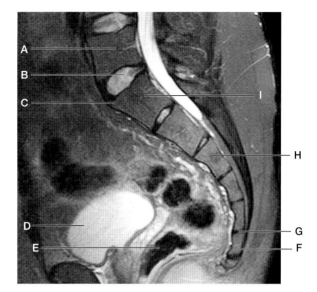

Fig. 10.42 Sacrum: axial CT image. (From STATdx © Elsevier 2022)

1 – Ala
2 – Ilium
3 – Dorsal sacral foramina
4 – Median sacral crest and tubercle
5 – Sacral canal
6 – Sacroiliac joint
7 – Body

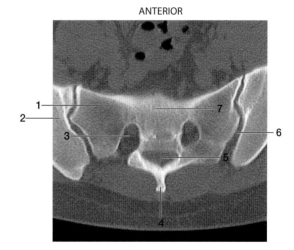

ANTERIOR

Fig. 10.43 Sacrum: anterior oblique 3D CT image. (From STATdx © Elsevier 2022)

A – Body of the fifth lumbar vertebra
B – Intervertebral disc space between the fifth lumbar vertebra and first sacral segment (L5S1)
C – Ala
D – Pelvic sacral foramen
E – Inferior lateral angle
F – Coccyx
G – Transverse ridge
H – Sacroiliac joint
I – Promontory
J – Transverse process of the fifth lumbar vertebra

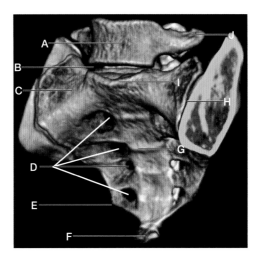

Fig. 10.44 Sacrum: posterior 3D CT image. (From STATdx © Elsevier 2022)

1 – Lamina of the 4th lumbar vertebra
2 – Inferior articular process of the 5th vertebra
3 – Posterior superior iliac spine (PSIS) of the ilium
4 – Dorsal sacral foramen
5 – Sacral cornu
6 – Coccyx
7 – Sacral hiatus
8 – Median sacral crest
9 – Intermediate sacral crest
10 – Lateral sacral crest
11 – Spinous process of the 4th lumbar vertebra

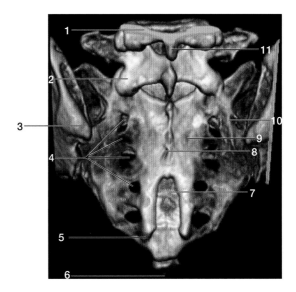

Fig. 10.45 Sacrum ossification centres; axial CT images in a two-year-old. (From STATdx © Elsevier 2022)

A – Body (*in utero*)
B – Costal elements (*in utero*)
C – Vertebral arch (age 10 to 12 weeks)

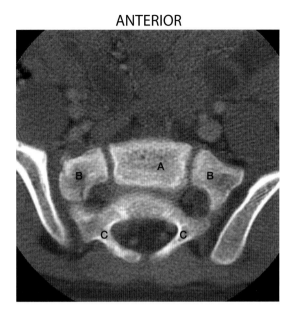

ANTERIOR

VERTEBRAL CURVATURES (FIG. 10.46)

The vertebral column demonstrates normal anteroposterior curves, which can be divided into primary and secondary curves. It develops as two primary curves *in utero* (the foetal position) and then develops two further secondary curves during early childhood to centralise the body's centre of gravity and improve muscular efficiency.

Foetus

Presents with two primary curves:
Thoracic curve – kyphosis (concave anteriorly)
Pelvic (sacrococcygeal) curve – kyphosis (concave anteriorly)

Development of secondary curves

Cervical curve – lordosis (concave posteriorly); accentuated when the child begins to hold its head up and when it sits upright at three to six months.
Lumbar curve – lordosis (concave posteriorly); appears when the child begins to walk at 12–18 months.

Fig. 10.46 Vertebral column (lateral aspect). Normal vertebral curves.

A – Cervical lordosis (secondary curve)
B – Thoracic kyphosis (primary curve)
C – Lumbar lordosis (secondary curve)
D – Pelvic (sacrococcygeal) kyphosis (primary curve)

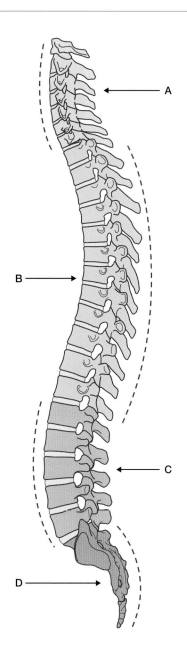

 INSIGHT

The junctions between the curves (i.e. the cervicothoracic, thoracolumbar and lumbosacral), where the spine changes direction, called transition points, are naturally weak and more prone to injury. The curves (lordosis/kyphosis) can become exaggerated or reduced from pathologic conditions.

JOINTS OF THE VERTEBRAL COLUMN

Atlantooccipital joints

Pair of joints connecting the base of the skull with the vertebral column.

Type

Synovial ellipsoid joints.

Bony articular surfaces
Superior articular facets of the atlas with the *condyles of the occipital bone*. Both surfaces are covered with articular hyaline cartilage.

Fibrous capsule
Surrounds the condyles of the occipital bone and the superior articular facets of the atlas; is sometimes absent medially.

Synovial membrane
Lines the fibrous capsule and secretes synovial fluid, which lubricates the joint. May communicate with the synovial bursa between the odontoid process and the transverse ligament of the atlas.

Supporting membranes
Anterior atlantooccipital membrane – from the anterior margins of the foramen magnum to the anterior arch of the atlas.
Posterior atlantooccipital membrane – from the posterior margins of the foramen magnum to the posterior arch of the atlas.

Movements
Flexion/extension – nodding of the head.
Lateral flexion – tilting of the head

Imaging appearances of atlantooccipital joints (Figs. 10.19, 10.21)

Median atlantoaxial joint

Joint between the first (atlas) and second (axis) cervical vertebrae - C1C2

Type

Synovial pivot joint.

Bony articular surfaces
Facet on the anterior part of the odontoid process of the axis and the *facet on the anterior arch of the atlas*. Both surfaces are covered with articular hyaline cartilage.

Fibrous capsule

Surrounds the odontoid process of the axis and the facet on the arch of the atlas. It is weak and loose.

Synovial membrane

Lines the fibrous capsule and the bursa as well as secretes synovial fluid, which lubricates the joint. Posteriorly, there is a bursa between the anterior surface of the transverse ligament and the posterior surface of the odontoid process.

Strengthening ligaments

Transverse ligament of the atlas – posterior to the odontoid process; maintains the odontoid process in contact with the anterior arch of the atlas.

Movements

Rotation – shaking of the head.

Imaging appearances of atlantooccipital joints (Figs. 10.19–10.23)

Intervertebral joints (Fig. 10.47)

Formed between adjacent vertebral bodies, separated by the intervertebral discs. Generally, the more inferior down the spine, the larger the intervertebral disc.

Type

Cartilaginous symphyses.

Bony articular surfaces

The *superior and inferior endplates* of the respective vertebral bodies. Both surfaces are covered with articular hyaline cartilage.

Intracapsular structures

Intervertebral disc – join the vertebrae and act as 'shock-absorbers' against compressive forces. Consists of:

> *Annulus fibrosus* – outer strong, stiff fibrous ring. Arranged in lamellar layers (like an onion) of fibrocartilage.
> *Nucleus pulposus* – inner gelatinous core of the disc; distributes pressure and forces placed upon the disc.
> The nucleus pulposus is located more posteriorly within the disc, so the annulus fibrosis is thinner and weaker posteriorly than it is anteriorly.
> *Sharpey's fibres* – strong connective tissue (mainly collagen) which attach the periphery of the intervertebral discs to the adjacent vertebral bodies (also found elsewhere in the skeleton to attach soft tissue to bone).

Strengthening ligaments

Anterior longitudinal ligament – continuous flowing ligament, extends from the basilar part of the occipital bone to the anterior aspect of the sacrum. It is attached to the anterior margins of the intervertebral discs and vertebral bodies.

Fig. 10.47 Intervertebral joint (disc); sagittal section.

A – Anterior longitudinal ligament
B – Articular hyaline cartilage
C – Annulus fibrosus (note the layers)
D – Vertebral body
E – Nucleus pulposus
F – Posterior longitudinal ligament

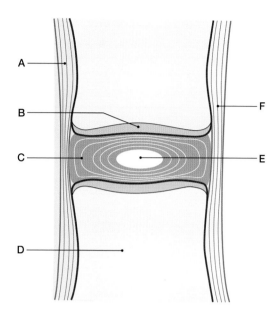

Posterior longitudinal ligament – continuous flowing ligament, extends from the body of the axis to the posterior aspect of the sacrum. It is attached to the posterior aspects of the intervertebral discs and vertebral bodies.

Movements

Each level individually allows a limited degree of:

    Flexion
    Extension
    Lateral flexion
    Rotation

Summated over the length of the spinal column, the movement is considerable.

Imaging appearances of the intervertebral joints (Figs. 10.48, 10.49)

Fig. 10.48 Intervertebral discs; sagittal T2W MRI of the lumbar spine. (From STATdx © Elsevier 2022)

A – Body of the 1st lumbar vertebra
B – Nucleus pulposus (bright signal)
C – Annulus fibrosus (dark signal)
D – Anterior longitudinal ligament
E – Articular cartilage of the superior vertebral endplate
F – Articular cartilage of the inferior vertebral endplate
G – Posterior longitudinal ligament
H – Cauda equina

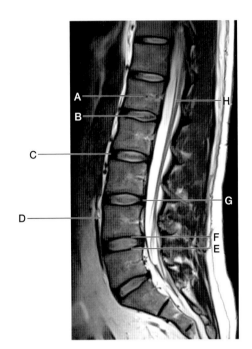

Fig. 10.49 Intervertebral discs; axial T2W MRI of the lumbar spine. (From STATdx © Elsevier 2022)

1 – Inferior vena cava
2 – Annulus fibrosus
3 – Nucleus pulposus
4 – Thecal sac and cauda equina
5 – Lamina
6 – Spinous process
7 – Facet (apophyseal) joint
8 – Psoas muscle
9 – Aorta

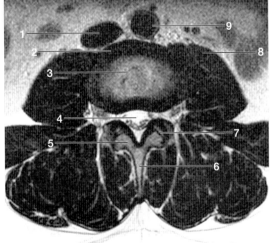

ANTERIOR

Joints of the vertebral arches

Known as the intervertebral facet, or apophyseal, joints.

Type

Synovial plane joints.

Bony articular surfaces
Superior articular facet with the *inferior articular facet* of the vertebra above. Both surfaces are covered with articular hyaline cartilage.

Fibrous capsule
Thin, loose and attached to the margins of the articular facets.

Synovial membrane
Lines the fibrous capsule and secretes synovial fluid, which lubricates the joint.

Strengthening ligaments
Interspinous ligaments – connect adjoining spinous processes.
Supraspinous ligament – connects tips of the spinous processes.
Ligamentum nuchae – only in the cervical region; corresponds to the supraspinous and interspinous ligaments in the rest of the spine. Extends from the external occipital protuberance and crest to the seventh cervical spinous process.
Intertransverse ligaments – connect the transverse processes.
Ligamentum flavum – connects adjoining laminae.

Movements
Gliding.
   Minimal at each level, but summated over the length of the spinal column, the movement is considerable.

Imaging appearances of the joints of the vertebral arches (Figs. 10.50, 10.51)

Fig. 10.50 Facet joints of the vertebral arches; sagittal CT image of the lumbar spine. (From STATdx © Elsevier 2022)

A – Intervertebral disc space
B – Body
C – Superior articular process
D – Inferior articular process
E – Pars interarticularis
F – Facet (apophyseal) joint
G – Intervertebral foramen
H – Pedicle

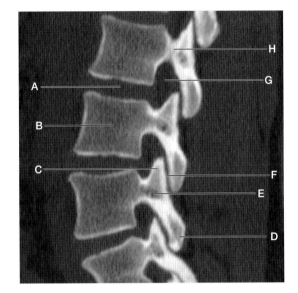

Fig. 10.51 Facet joints of the vertebral arches; axial CT image through the third lumbar vertebra. (From STATdx © Elsevier 2022)

1 – Vertebral body
2 – Pedicle
3 – Superior articular process (of the 3rd lumbar vertebra)
4 – Inferior articular process (of the second lumbar vertebra)
5 – Tip of the spinous process (of the second lumbar vertebra above)
6 – Facet (apophyseal joint) with the 2nd lumbar vertebra
7 – Vertebral foramen

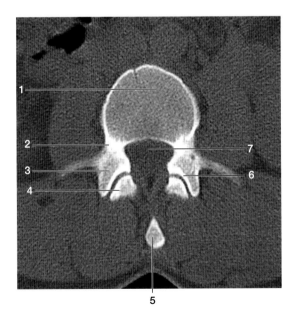

Costovertebral and costotransverse joints

Joints between the ribs and thoracic vertebrae.

Type

Synovial plane joints.

Bony articular surfaces

Costovertebral joints – *Head of the rib* with the *demi-facets* of the corresponding thoracic vertebral body and the one superiorly.
Costotransverse joints – *Facet on the tubercle of the rib* with *the transverse process* of the corresponding thoracic vertebra.
Both surfaces are covered with articular hyaline cartilage.

Fibrous capsule

Surrounds the head of the rib and the margins of the costal facets of the vertebrae.

Synovial membrane

Lines the fibrous capsule and secretes synovial fluid, which lubricates the joint.

Strengthening ligaments

Intra-articular ligament – divides the costovertebral joints into two halves.
Radiate ligament – of the costovertebral joints; between the head of the rib and vertebral body.
Costotransverse ligament – of costotransverse joints; between the neck of the rib and transverse process.

Imaging appearances of costovertebral and costotransverse joints (Figs. 10.52, 10.53)

Fig. 10.52 Costovertebral (A) and costotransverse (B) joints; axial CT images of a thoracic vertebra. (From STATdx © Elsevier 2022)

A – Demi–facet of thoracic vertebra
B – Head of the rib
C – Facet (apophyseal) joint
D – Costovertebral joint
E – Body of thoracic vertebra
F – Tubercle of the rib
G – Transverse process
H – Costotransverse joint

ANTERIOR

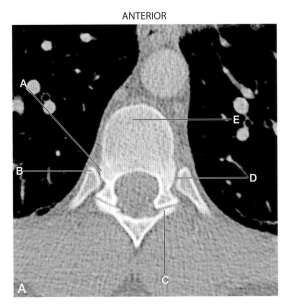

ANTERIOR

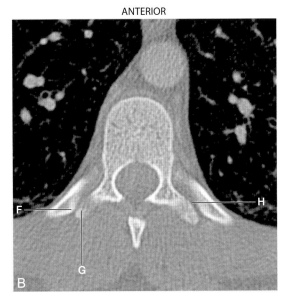

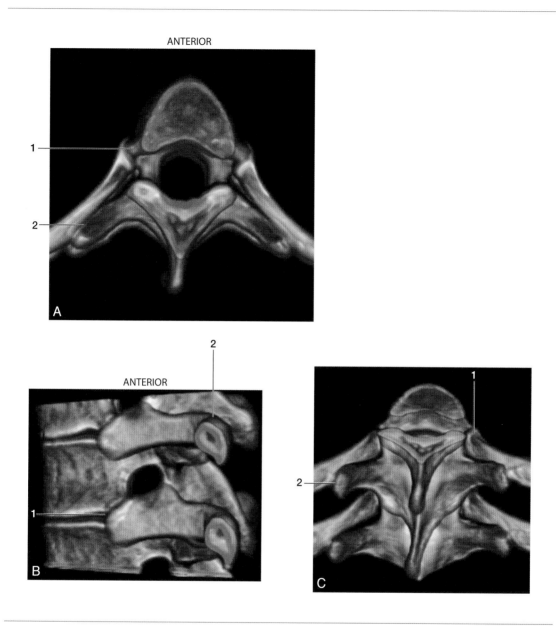

Fig. 10.53 Costovertebral and costotransverse joints; axial (A), lateral (B) and posterior (C) 3D CT images of a thoracic vertebra. (From STATdx © Elsevier 2022)

1 – Costovertebral joint
2 – Costotransverse joint

INSIGHT

When assessing the spine for injury, it is important to assess the normal alignment of a number of spinal lines (Fig. 10.54). These should be smooth and uninterrupted.

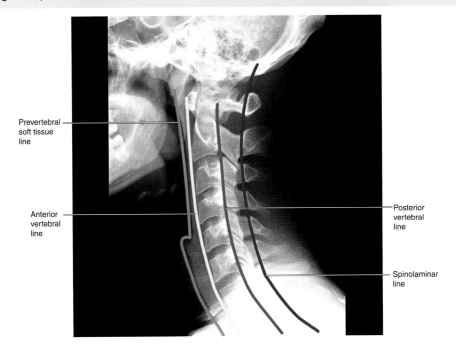

Fig. 10.54 Normal cervical spine alignment; right lateral projection. Assess for normal alignment and smooth, uninterrupted lines. Similar can be demonstrated in the thoracic and lumbar spine. (From STATdx © Elsevier 2022)

C1 (atlas) burst fracture (Fig. 10.55)

Also called the Jefferson fracture. As a ring structure, it fractures in more than one place. Often stable but may cause catastrophic spinal cord injury if unstable. Demonstrated on imaging by widening of the atlas ring.

Cause – axial loading of the head into the spine, e.g., diving headfirst into a swimming pool.

Example of treatment – immobilisation using a rigid collar or 'halo' device.

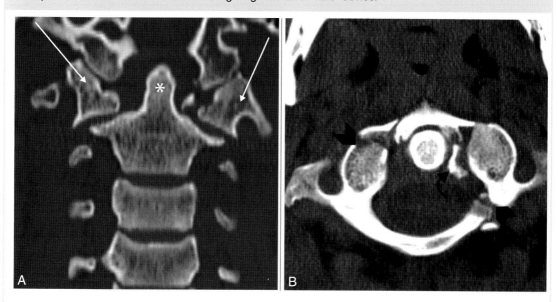

Fig. 10.55 Atlas (C1) burst fracture; coronal (A) and axial (B) CT images. There is a widening of the distances between the lateral masses (arrows) of the atlas and odontoid peg (*) compared to normal (Fig. 10.21). Two fractures of the ring are demonstrated (arrowheads). Note the fracture associated with the avulsion of the transverse ligament (curved arrow). (From STATdx © Elsevier 2022)

Hangman's fracture of C2 (axis) vertebra (Figs. 10.56–10.58)

Bilateral fracture of the pars interarticularis of C2 causes anterior displacement (*spondylolisthesis*) of the skull and atlas. Ranges from stable with no neurological injury to unstable with potentially debilitating spinal cord injury.

Cause – forced hyperflexion (e.g., road traffic collision; almost all cases) or hyperextension with sudden distraction (e.g., execution by hanging).

Example of treatment – immobilisation if stable, fusion if unstable.

Fig. 10.56 Hangman's fracture of C2; right lateral cervical spine projection. Fractures of the pars interarticularis (arrow) with anterior displacement of the body of C2 (*). Note disruption of the anterior and posterior vertebral lines (compared to Fig. 10.54). (From STATdx © Elsevier 2022)

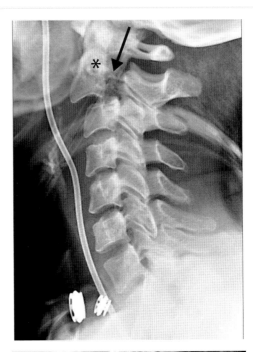

Fig. 10.57 Hangman's fracture of C2; Sagittal T1W MRI. Same patient as Fig. 10.56. There is disruption of the posterior longitudinal (arrow) and interspinous (arrowhead) ligaments. A haematoma (curved arrow) is causing spinal cord compression. (From STATdx © Elsevier 2022)

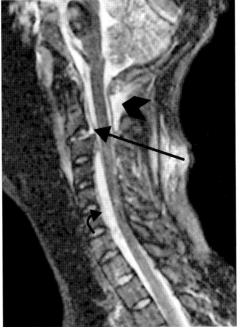

Fig. 10.58 Hangman's fracture of C2; axial (A) and sagittal (B) CT images. This example demonstrates minimally displaced fractures through the pars interarticularis bilaterally (arrows). (From STATdx © Elsevier 2022)

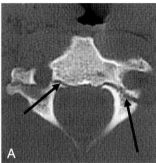

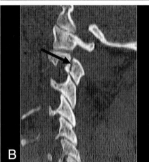

 INSIGHT

The spine can be divided into three columns; anterior, middle and posterior. The involvement of one column usually indicates stable injury. The involvement of two or three columns suggests unstable injury.

Anterior (wedge) compression fracture (Fig. 10.59)

Compression of the anterior part of the vertebral body, middle and posterior aspects spared; so stable. Most common in the thoracic spine, particularly in people with osteoporosis and reduced bone density; causes exaggerated kyphosis if at multiple levels.

Cause – axial loading with flexion (e.g., fall from height); insufficiency in osteoporosis.

Example of treatment – conservative; treatment for underlying osteoporosis.

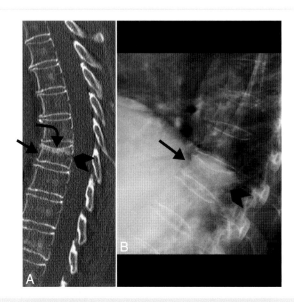

Fig. 10.59 Anterior compression (wedge) fracture; sagittal CT image (A) and right lateral thoracic spine projection (B). In this osteoporotic patient (note the reduced bone density), there is a loss of the anterior vertebral body height (arrow) compared to that posteriorly (arrowhead) and those above and below. There is sclerosis of the superior vertebral body because of the impacted bone (curved arrow). (From STATdx © Elsevier 2022)

Burst fracture (Figs. 10.60–10.62)

Fracture of the vertebral body causing compression anteriorly and fragments displaced posteriorly into vertebral foramen (not seen in simple wedge compression fractures) and compressing the spinal canal. Most common at the thoracolumbar (T12L1) junction; weak transition point.

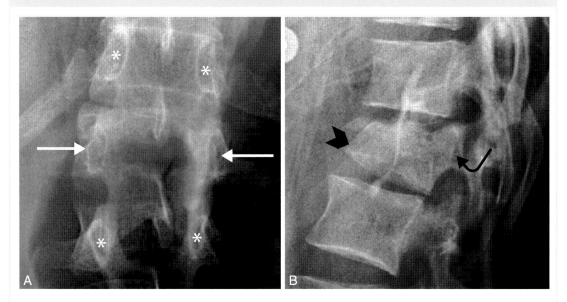

Fig. 10.60 Burst fracture of L1; anteroposterior (A) and right lateral (B) projections. There is a widening of the distance between the L1 pedicles (arrows) compared to those at the level above and below (*) caused by the vertebra 'bursting.' There is loss of the height of the body anteriorly (arrowhead) and loss of the normal posterior contour (curved arrow) than the vertebra above and below. (From STATdx © Elsevier 2022)

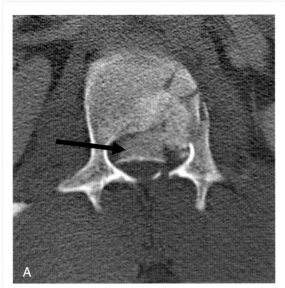 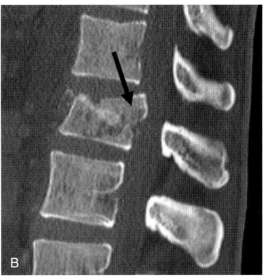

Fig. 10.61 Burst fracture of L1; axial (A) and sagittal (B) CT images. Same patient as Fig. 10.60. There is an osseous fracture fragment (arrow) displaced posteriorly into the vertebral foramen and compressing the spinal cord. (From STATdx © Elsevier 2022)

Fig. 10.62 Burst fracture of L1; sagittal T1W MRI. Same patient as Figs. 10.60 and 10.61. There is an epidural haematoma (arrow) with displacement and compression of the spinal cord (arrowhead). (From STATdx © Elsevier 2022)

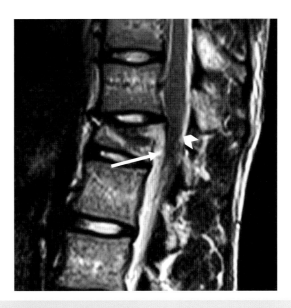

Cause – axial compression, e.g., fall from height.
Example of treatment – surgical fixation, sometimes conservative if no neurological symptoms.

Fracture dislocation (Figs. 10.63, 10.64)

Very significant and unstable injury involving all three spinal columns and a combination of fracture, ligamentous injury and dislocation. High association with spinal cord injury and paralysis.
Cause – high velocity injury (e.g., road traffic collisions); a combination of forces.
Example of treatment – surgical reduction and fixation.

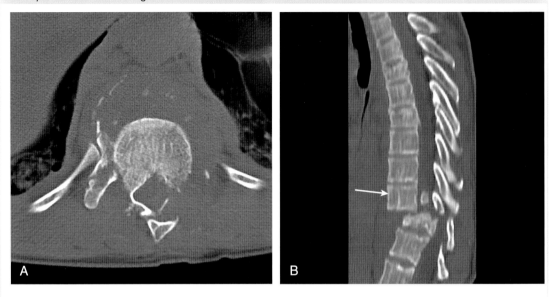

Fig. 10.63 T10–11 fracture dislocation; axial (A) and sagittal (B) CT images. Comminuted fracture of T11 with anterior displacement of T10 (arrow) in relation to T11 below. (From STATdx © Elsevier 2022)

Fig. 10.64 T10–11 fracture dislocation; sagittal MRI. Same patient as Fig. 10.63. There is resultant compression and contusion of the spinal cord (arrow). (From STATdx © Elsevier 2022)

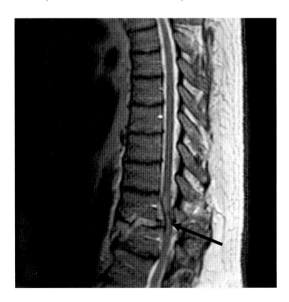

Sacrum fracture (Figs. 10.65, 10.66)

Usually associated with a fracture of the pelvic ring/hip bones (see Chapter 8, page 203) and visceral and neurovascular injury, especially of the sacral nerves. Best evaluated by CT, often missed on radiographs.
Cause – as per pelvic fractures; anterior/lateral compression or vertical shear forces.
Example of treatment – surgical fixation.

Fig. 10.65 Bilateral sacral fracture; axial CT image. Comminuted fracture of the left sacral ala involving the sacral foramen (arrow). A minimally displaced fracture involving the right sacral foramen (arrowhead). These injuries are often very hard to identify on radiographs because of overlying structures. (From STATdx © Elsevier 2022)

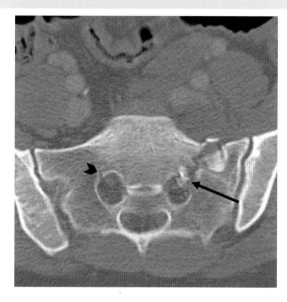

Fig. 10.66 Vertical shear injury; 3D CT image. Displaced longitudinal fracture of the left sacrum (arrow) involving the sacral foramen. Fractures of the superior and inferior pubic rami (arrowheads) and dislocation of the symphysis pubis (curved arrow). (From STATdx © Elsevier 2022)

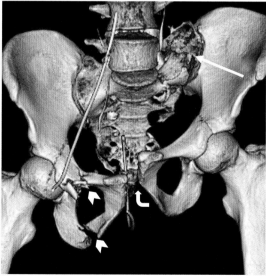

PATHOLOGY

 INSIGHT

Spondylosis is the term used to describe degenerative (wear and tear) changes of the vertebral column by any cause. Most commonly a combination of the intervertebral discs (degenerative disc disease) and facet/apophyseal joints (osteoarthritis). It can be localised by the part of the spine it affects, e.g., lumbar spondylosis.

Facet (apophyseal) joint osteoarthritis

Osteoarthritis of the synovial joints of the spine causing joint space narrowing, sclerosis of the articular surfaces, and *osteophyte* (bone spur) formation. These osteophytes can narrow the intervertebral foramen and impinge on the spinal nerves causing pain and neurological symptoms. Most common in the lower cervical and lumbar spine.

Degenerative disc disease (Figs. 10.67, 10.68)

A common cause of lower back pain. Intervertebral discs degrade and dehydrate, causing cracks in the outer annulus fibrosus. Imaging appearances include intervertebral disc space narrowing, osteophyte formation and radiolucent appearance of discs (called *vacuum phenomenon*).

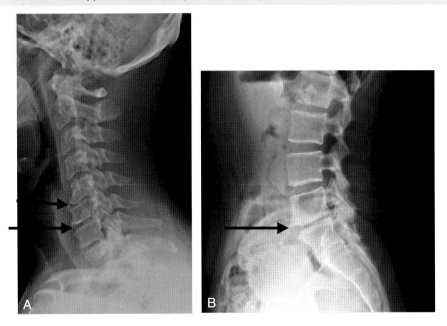

Fig. 10.67 Degenerative disc disease; right lateral cervical (A) and lumbar (B) spine projections. Intervertebral disc space narrowing and osteophyte formation are more evident at affected levels C5/6, C6/7 and L5S1 (arrows) compared to unaffected levels. (From STATdx © Elsevier 2022)

Fig. 10.68 Degenerative disc disease; sagittal CT image lumbar spine. Significant disease at multiple levels shows disc space narrowing, osteophytes, and characteristic vacuum disc phenomenon (arrows). (From STATdx © Elsevier 2022)

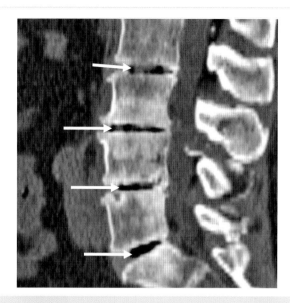

Intervertebral disc herniation (Fig. 10.69)

Also known as a 'slipped' or prolapsed disc. Nucleus pulposus bulges and herniates out of weakness in annulus fibrosus (mostly posterior-laterally) to impinge on spinal nerves and canal; best evaluated on MRI.

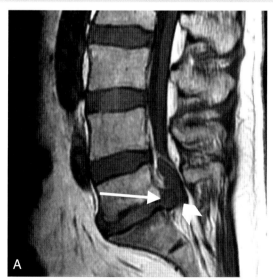

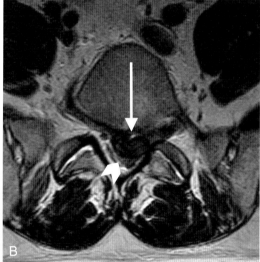

Fig. 10.69 L5S1 intervertebral disc herniation; sagittal T1W (A) and axial T2W (B) MRIs. A large herniation (arrows) is demonstrated, impinging on the spinal canal (arrowheads). (From STATdx © Elsevier 2022)

Cause – chronic (e.g., degenerative disc disease); or acute caused by lifting/twisting injury.
Example of treatment – often conservative. In severe cases, surgical decompression (removal of disc or the lamina of vertebra).

Scoliosis (Fig. 10.70)

Abnormal lateral curvature of the spine with rotation of the vertebrae in more severe cases. Usually of the thoracic and thoracolumbar spine. Mild cases are common, but severe cases develop predominantly in young females and lead to pain, deformities and potential cardiorespiratory problems.
Cause – most common idiopathic (unknown cause) or congenital.
Example of treatment – dependent on severity; from conservative/none to surgical fixation.

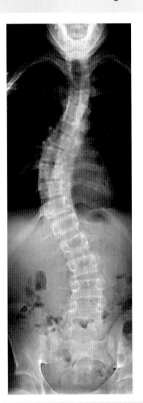

Fig. 10.70 Scoliosis; anteroposterior projection. Lateral curves of the thoracic and lumbar spine in this moderate idiopathic scoliosis are demonstrated. (From STATdx © Elsevier 2022)

Spondylolysis (Fig. 10.71)

A defect (usually bilateral) in the pars interarticularis between the pedicle, lamina and articular processes of a vertebra. Separates the vertebral body from the vertebral arch and may cause displacement of one vertebral body on the one below (*spondylolisthesis*, see following page). Most common in the lower lumbar spine.
Cause – typically stress/repetitive strain, e.g., in gymnasts and weightlifters.
Example of treatment – often conservative.

Fig. 10.71 Spondylolysis; lateral lumbar spine projection (A) and sagittal CT image (B). There is a defect in the pars interarticularis (arrows) bilaterally in this 11-year-old gymnast. The vertebra above (arrowhead) appears normal in comparison. Note that there is currently no associated displacement. (From STATdx © Elsevier 2022)

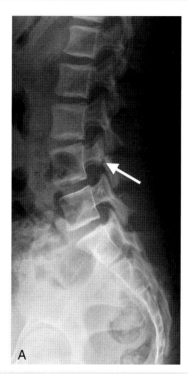

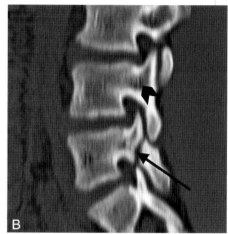

Spondylolisthesis (Fig. 10.72)

Either anterior (*anterolisthesis*) or posterior *(retrolisthesis)* displacement of one vertebral body upon the one below. Visualised by loss of normal alignment of the vertebral bodies.

Cause – degenerative in spondylosis, or because of a defect in the pars interarticularis; either traumatic (fracture) or chronic/repetitive stress (spondylolysis).

Example of treatment –conservative; sometimes surgical fusion.

Fig. 10.72 Spondylo-listhesis; sagittal T2W MRIs. Mild anterior displacement of L4 on L5 (A) and severe anterior displacement of L5 on S1 (B) in these two cases. Both are chronic with no history of trauma. Note the loss of alignment of the anterior and posterior spinal lines. (From STATdx © Elsevier 2022)

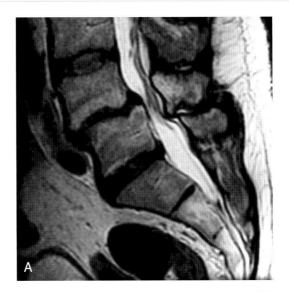

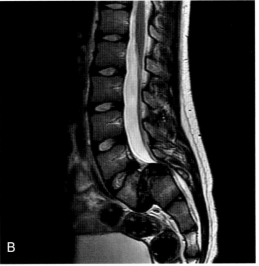

THE SKULL

11

CHAPTER CONTENTS

Skull	299
Individual Bones of the Cranium	308
Frontal bone	308
Parietal bones	310
Occipital bone	311
Temporal bone	313
Sphenoid bone	318
Ethmoid bone	320
Individual Bones of the Face	324
Maxillae	324
Zygomatic bones	326
Palatine bones	327
Nasal bones	329
Lacrimal bones	331

Inferior nasal conchae (turbinates)	331
Vomer	332
Orbital Cavity	336
Nasal Cavity	339
Paranasal Sinuses	342
Maxillary sinuses	342
Frontal sinuses	343
Ethmoidal sinuses	344
Sphenoidal sinuses	344
Mandible	348
Teeth	353
Temporomandibular Joint (TMJ)	357
Hyoid bone	361

SKULL (FIGS. 11.1–11.8)

The skull protects the brain and supports the face and organs for the special senses. It also acts as a muscle attachment for chewing and facial expressions and protects the opening of the respiratory and digestive systems. Consisting of 22 bones in total, joined mainly by *fibrous sutures*, it can be divided into two sections: the cranium and face.

The cranium is composed of the following eight bones:
- Frontal bone
- Parietal bones (two)
- Occipital bone
- Temporal bones (two)
- Sphenoid bone
- Ethmoid bone

The 14 facial bones include:
- Maxillae (two and upper teeth)
- Zygomatic bones (two)
- Nasal bones (two)
- Palatine bones (two)
- Inferior nasal conchae (two)

- Lacrimal bones (two)
- Vomer
- Mandible (and lower teeth)

Although located in the neck, the hyoid bone is also often considered part of the skull because of its close association with the mandible and tongue.

Fig. 11.1 Position of the bones of the skull (anterior aspect).

A – Frontal bone
B – Parietal bone
C – Greater wing of the sphenoid bone
D – Temporal bone
E – Nasal bone
F – Ethmoid bone
G – Maxilla
H – Zygomatic bone
I – Maxilla
J – Mandible
K – Vomer
L – Inferior nasal concha
M – Zygomatic bone
N – Lacrimal bone
O – Greater wing of the sphenoid bone
P – Lesser wing of the sphenoid bone

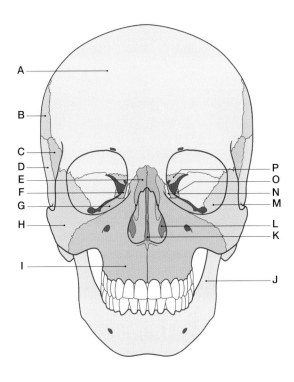

Fig. 11.2 Position of the bones of the skull (lateral aspect).

A – Frontal bone
B – Sphenoid bone (greater wing)
C – Nasal bone
D – Ethmoid bone
E – Lacrimal bone
F – Zygomatic bone
G – Maxilla
H – Mandible
I – Temporal bone
J – Occipital bone
K – Parietal bone

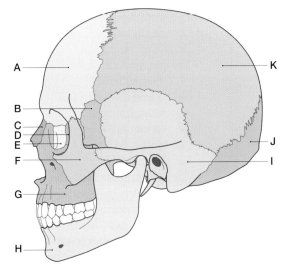

Fig. 11.3 Position of the bones of the skull (cranial cavity) from superior, top of skull removed.

A – Frontal bone
B – Ethmoid bone
C – Sphenoid bone
D – Temporal bone (petrous part)
E – Parietal bone
F – Occipital bone

The floor of the cranial cavity is divided into three distinct sections:
1 – Anterior cranial fossa containing the frontal lobes of the brain.
2 – Middle cranial fossa containing the temporal lobes of the brain and the hypophysis cerebri (pituitary gland).
3 – Posterior cranial fossa containing the cerebellum, pons and medulla oblongata.

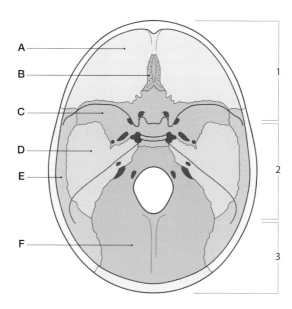

Fig. 11.4 Features of the skull (anterior aspect).

A – Sagittal suture
B – Coronal suture
C – Supraorbital notch (foramen)
D – Superior orbital fissure
E – Middle nasal concha
F – Vomer
G – Inferior nasal concha
H – Mental foramen
I – Zygomatic arch
J – Infraorbital foramen
K – Inferior orbital fissure
L – Optic canal

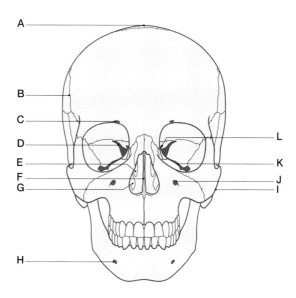

Fig. 11.5 Features of the skull (lateral aspect).

1 – Coronal suture
2 – Glabella
3 – Nasion
4 – Temporal fossa
5 – Zygomatic arch
6 – Anterior nasal spine
7 – Mental foramen
8 – Symphysis menti
9 – Angle of the mandible
10 – Styloid process
11 – Mastoid process
12 – External acoustic (auditory) meatus
13 – External occipital protuberance
14 – Lambdoid suture
15 – Squamosal suture
16 – Pterion

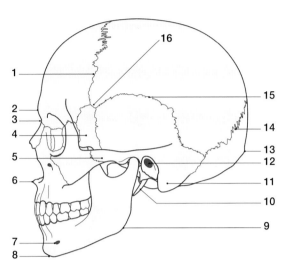

Fig. 11.6 Features of the skull (inferior aspect).

A – Palatine process of the maxilla
B – Zygomatic arch
C – Vomer
D – Foramen ovale
E – Foramen spinosum
F – Styloid process
G – External acoustic (auditory) meatus
H – Stylomastoid foramen
I – Foramen magnum
J – External occipital crest
K – Inferior nuchal line
L – Condylar canal
M – Mastoid process
N – Occipital condyle
O – Jugular foramen
P – Carotid canal
Q – Foramen lacerum
R – Palatine bone

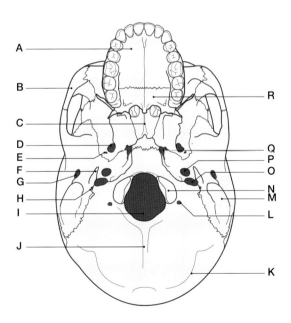

Fig. 11.7 Features in the base of the skull (internal aspect), top of skull removed.

1 – Crista galli of the ethmoid bone
2 – Cribriform plate of the ethmoid bone
3 – Tuberculum sellae of the sphenoid bone
4 – Sella turcica (hypophyseal fossa/ pituitary fossa) of the sphenoid bone
5 – Foramen magnum
6 – Petrous portion of the temporal bone
7 – Dorsum sellae of the sphenoid bone
8 – Anterior clinoid process of the sphenoid bone

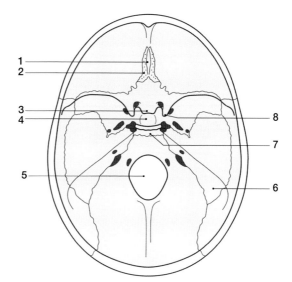

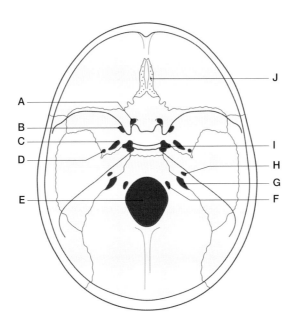

Fig. 11.8 Foramina in the base of the skull (internal aspect).

A – *Optic canal*, for the optic nerve and ophthalmic artery.
B – *Foramen rotundum*, for the maxillary division of the trigeminal nerve.
C – *Foramen ovale*, for the mandibular division of the trigeminal nerve.
D – *Foramen spinosum*, for the middle meningeal artery.
E – *Foramen magnum*, for part of the medulla oblongata, spinal roots of the accessory nerves and vertebral arteries.
F – *Hypoglossal canal*, for the hypoglossal nerve and the meningeal branch of the ascending pharyngeal artery.
G – *Jugular foramen*, for the internal jugular vein, glossopharyngeal, vagus and accessory nerves and the inferior petrosal sinus.

H – *Internal acoustic (auditory) meatus*, for the facial and auditory nerves.
I – *Foramen lacerum*. The inferior part is closed by fibrocartilage; the internal carotid artery crosses it (after entering by the carotid canal).
J – *Cribriform plate*, for the olfactory nerve filaments.

Not visible: *Stylomastoid foramen* – lies on the external aspect between the styloid and mastoid processes of the temporal bone, for the facial nerve.
Superior orbital fissure – concealed by the lesser wing of the sphenoid bone; for the oculomotor, trochlear and abducent nerves, ophthalmic division of the trigeminal nerve and ophthalmic veins.

Imaging appearances of the skull (Figs. 11.9–11.11)

Fig. 11.9 Skull; lateral projection. (From STATdx © Elsevier 2022)

A – Frontal bone
B – Frontal sinus
C – Sphenoid sinus
D – Mandible
E – Sella turcica
F – Petrous part of the temporal bone
G – Mastoid air cells
H – Lambdoid suture
I – External occipital protuberance
J – Anterior clinoid process
K – Dorsum sellae
L – Parietal bone
M – Coronal suture

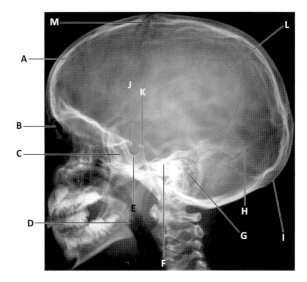

ANTERIOR

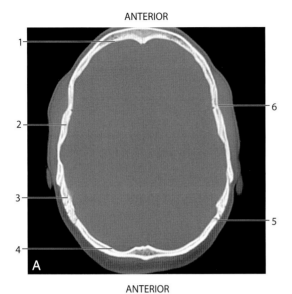

A

ANTERIOR

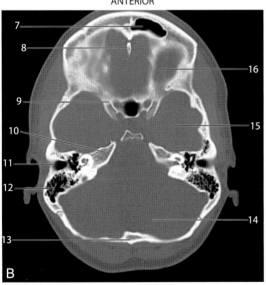

B

ANTERIOR

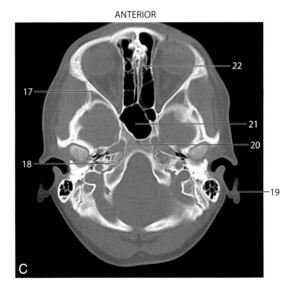

C

Fig. 11.10 Skull; axial CT images of the cranium (A) and superior (B) and inferior (C) base of the skull. (From STATdx © Elsevier 2022)

1 – Frontal bone	**13** – External occipital
2 – Temporal bone	protuberance
3 – Parietal bone	**14** – Posterior cranial fossa
4 – Occipital bone	**15** – Middle cranial fossa
5 – Lambdoid suture	**16** – Anterior cranial fossa
6 – Coronal suture	**17** – Greater wing of the
7 – Frontal sinus	sphenoid bone
8 – Crista galli of the	
ethmoid bone	**18** – Petrous part of the
9 – Anterior clinoid process	temporal bone
10 – Petrous part of the	**19** – Mastoid process
temporal bone	**20** – Clivus
11 – External acoustic	**21** – Sphenoid sinus
(auditory) meatus	**22** – Ethmoid bone and
12 – Mastoid air cells	sinuses

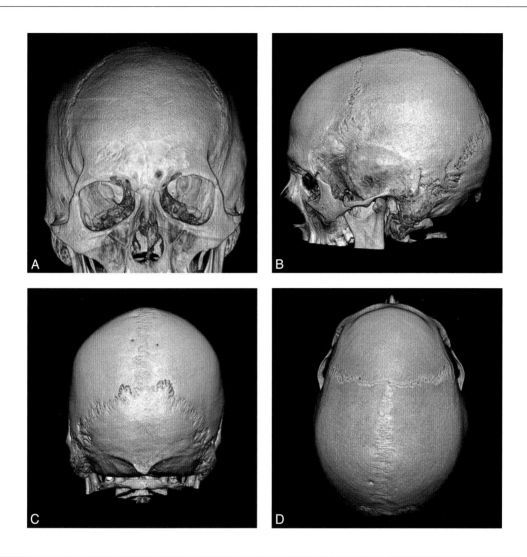

Fig. 11.11 Skull; 3D CT images. Anterior (A), lateral (B), posterior (C) and superior (D). (From STATdx © Elsevier 2022)

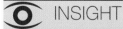 INSIGHT

Most imaging of the skull and head is performed using cross-sectional imaging. Radiographs are still used in certain circumstances, particularly in imaging the facial bones and teeth.

INDIVIDUAL BONES OF THE CRANIUM

The bones which make up the skull vault (frontal, parietal, occipital and temporal) consist of two layers of compact bone separated by the *diploic space;* marrow-containing cancellous bone.

The internal surfaces are lined with the outer (dural) layer of the meninges and contain furrows/ grooves to accommodate vessels.

Frontal bone (Figs. 11.12, 11.13)

Type	Flat bone.
Position	Forms the front (forehead) of the cranium, superior to the orbits.
Articulations	With the maxillae, nasal, lacrimal, ethmoid and sphenoid bones. With the parietal bones at the coronal suture. With the zygomatic bone to form the frontozygomatic suture.
Main parts	***External surface*** – Convex. ***Supraorbital margins*** – Form the superior border of the orbits. ***Supraorbital foramen*** – For the supraorbital vessels and nerves; may be a notch. ***Zygomatic process*** – Lateral end of the supraorbital margin; articulates with the zygomatic bone at the frontozygomatic suture.

Fig. 11.12 Frontal bone (anterior aspect).

A – Superciliary arch
B – Zygomatic process
C – Supraorbital foramen (may be a notch)
D – Nasal notch
E – Nasal spine
F – Glabella
G – Supraorbital margin

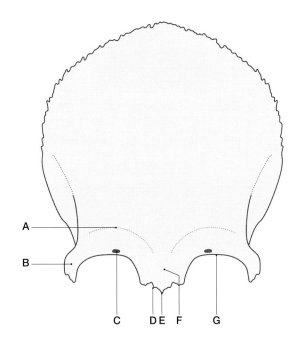

Fig. 11.13 Frontal bone (inferior aspect).

1 – Nasal spine
2 – Frontal sinus
3 – Orbital plate
4 – Roof of the ethmoidal sinuses
5 – Zygomatic process
6 – Fossa for the lacrimal gland
7 – Frontal crest
8 – Supraorbital foramen (may be a notch)

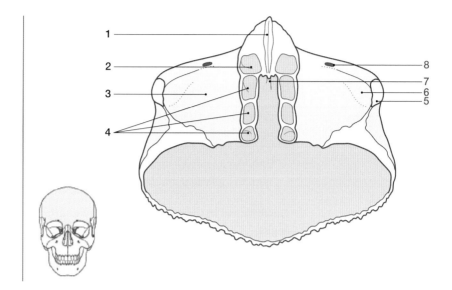

Nasal part – Between supraorbital margins.
Nasal spine – Forms the tip of the nasal part; forms part of the nasal septum.
Nasal notches – Either side of the nasal spine; articulate with the nasal bones.
Superciliary arches – Superior to the supraorbital margins. Eyebrows are located on the lower margin.
Glabella – Junction of the two superciliary arches. Palpable between the eyebrows.

Internal surface – Concave.
Vertical groove – In the midline for the sagittal venous sinus.
Frontal crest – Edges of the vertical groove for attachment of the falx cerebri.
Granular foveolae – Indentations for the arachnoid granulations.
Parietal margin – Articulates with the greater wing of the sphenoid bone.
Orbital plates – Concave; form the roof of the orbit.
Fossa for the lacrimal gland – Anterolateral aspect of the orbital plates for the lacrimal (tear) glands.
Ethmoidal notch – At the junction of the orbital plates, occupied by the cribriform plate of the ethmoid bone.
Frontal sinuses – See paranasal sinuses, p. 342.

Ossification

Intramembranous.
Two primary centres; left and right – appear from the second month *in utero*.
Meet at the *frontal suture* at birth, fuse by six years old but may persist in some when referred to as the *metopic suture*.

Parietal bones (Fig. 11.14)

Type	Flat bones.
Position	Form the sides and roof of the cranium.
Articulations	With the *sagittal border* of the opposite parietal bone to form the *sagittal suture*. With the *frontal bone* to form part of the *coronal suture*. With the *occipital bone* to form part of the *lambdoid suture*. With the *sphenoid and temporal bones* to form the *squamosal suture*.
Main parts	Quadrilateral in shape, each bone has two surfaces, four borders and four angles. ***External surface*** – Convex and has two curved lines, the superior and inferior temporal lines; attachments for the *temporalis fascia* and *muscle*, respectively. ***Internal surface*** – Concave, has grooves for the superior sagittal sinus and meningeal blood vessels and some depressions (*granular foveolae*) for the arachnoid granulations. ***Sagittal border*** – On the superior aspect. Forms the sagittal suture with the opposite parietal bone in the midline. ***Squamosal border*** – On the inferior aspect; articulates with the sphenoid and temporal bones at the squamosal suture. ***Anterior border*** – On the anterior aspect. Forms the coronal suture with the frontal bone.

Fig. 11.14 Left parietal bone (external surface).

A – Anterior angle (bregma)
B – Anterior border
C – Sphenoidal angle
D – Squamosal border
E – Mastoid angle
F – Occipital border
G – Inferior temporal line
H – Occipital angle (lambda)
I – Superior temporal line
J – Sagittal border

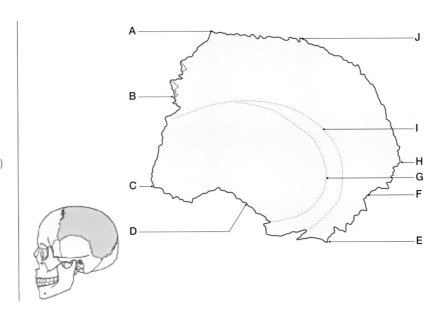

Occipital border – On the posterior aspect. Forms the lambdoid suture with the occipital bone.

Sphenoidal angle – At the junction of the squamosal and frontal borders; has a groove for the frontal branch of the middle meningeal vessels.

Occipital angle – At the junction of the occipital and sagittal borders and therefore at the junction of the sagittal and lambdoid sutures, which is called the *lambda* (back of the skull), so called as it looks like the Greek letter of the same name Λ.

Mastoid angle – At the junction of the occipital and squamosal borders. Meets the mastoid part of the temporal bone.

Anterior angle – At the junction of the sagittal and frontal borders and, therefore, at the junction of the sagittal and coronal sutures, which is called the *bregma* (top of the skull).

Ossification

Intramembranous.
Usually one centre (sometimes two) – eighth week *in utero*.

Occipital bone (Fig. 11.15)

Type

Flat bone.

Position

Forms the posterior part of the base of the skull.

Articulations

The *occipital condyles* with the first cervical vertebra to form the atlantooccipital joints.
The *squamous part* with the temporal bone and the parietal bones to form the *lambdoid suture*.

Main parts

Foramen magnum – Large foramen (literally means *large hole*) for part of the medulla oblongata, the accessory nerves and the vertebral arteries.
The bone can be divided into three areas:

Squamous part
This lies posterior to the foramen magnum. Its features include:
Internal surface – Concave, divided into four fossae by:
- *Horizontal groove* – for the transverse venous sinus; the tentorium cerebelli is attached to the edge of the groove.
- *Sulcus for the superior sagittal venous sinus* – vertically-orientated, situated superior to the horizontal groove; the margins provide attachment for the falx cerebri.
- *Internal occipital crest* – vertically-orientated, inferior to the horizontal groove.

Internal occipital protuberance – Where the horizontal and vertical grooves meet.
External surface – Convex.

Fig. 11.15 Occipital bone (external surface).

A – Squamous part
B – Highest nuchal line
C – External occipital protuberance
D – Superior nuchal line
E – Inferior nuchal line
F – External occipital crest
G – Condylar canal
H – Jugular process
I – Condyle
J – Basilar part
K – Jugular notch
L – Hypoglossal canal
M – Condylar fossa
N – Foramen magnum

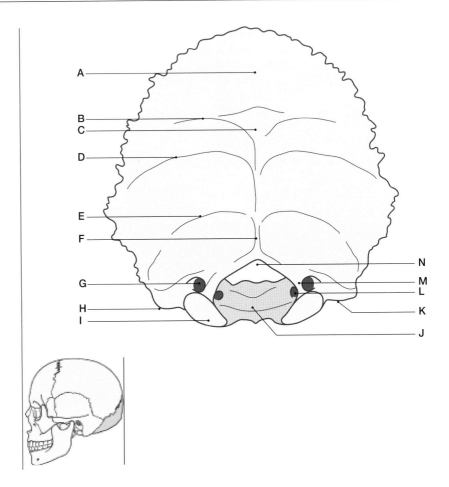

External occipital crest – Midline structure from the foramen magnum to the external occipital protuberance.

External occipital protuberance – Midway between the foramen magnum and the superior aspect of the bone. Easily palpable. The ligamentum nuchae of the spine extend from here to the seventh cervical vertebra.

Nuchal lines

Three pairs of horizontal curved lines provide muscular attachment:

- Superior nuchal lines – run laterally from the external occipital protuberance.
- Highest nuchal lines – faint lines above the superior nuchal lines.
- Inferior nuchal lines – below the superior nuchal lines, running laterally from the external occipital crest.

Basilar part

This lies anterior to the foramen magnum.

Pharyngeal tubercle – Lies on the inferior surface 1 cm anterior to the foramen magnum, in the midline; provides attachment for the pharynx.

Clivus – Means '*slope*.' Lies on the superior surface; runs superiorly and anteriorly forwards from the anterior border of the foramen magnum to the dorsum sellae of the sphenoid; forms attachment for the *membrana tectoria* and *apical ligament*.

Lateral (condylar) parts

These lie on either side of the foramen magnum.

Occipital condyles – Lie on the inferior surface, on either side of the foramen magnum, and articulate with the atlas (C1).

Hypoglossal canal – Situated superior to the condyles on the rim of the foramen magnum; carries the *hypoglossal nerve* and meningeal branch of the ascending pharyngeal artery.

Condylar fossa – Lies posterior to the condyle; receives the superior facet of the atlas (C1) when the head is extended.

Jugular process – Lateral to the condyle.

Jugular notch – On the jugular process, forms the posterior aspect of the jugular foramen.

Jugular tubercle – On the superior surface, above the hypoglossal canal.

Ossification

Intramembranous.

Primary centres

Squamous part – Four centres.
Lateral (condylar) parts – Two centres (one on each side).
Basilar part – One centre.

Appear between six weeks and three months *in utero*. Completely fuse between four and six years.

Temporal bone (Figs. 11.16, 11.17)

Type   Irregular bones. Roughly T-shaped.

Position   Form the lateral aspect of the cranium and part of the base of the skull.

Articulations   *Mandibular fossa* with the head of mandible to form the temporomandibular joint.
The *squamous part* with the parietal bones to form the *squamosal suture*, and the occipital bones to form part of the *lambdoid suture*.
With the *greater wings of the sphenoid* to form the *sphenosquamosal suture*.
With the *zygomatic bone*.

Fig. 11.16 Left temporal bone (external/lateral aspect).

A – Squamous part
B – Zygoma
C – Mandibular fossa
D – External acoustic (auditory) meatus
E – Tympanic plate
F – Styloid process
G – Mastoid process
H – Mastoid part

Fig. 11.17 Left temporal bone (posterior aspect).

1 – Squamous part
2 – Zygomatic process
3 – Mastoid process
4 – Mastoid notch
5 – Styloid process
6 – Petrous part
7 – Internal acoustic (auditory) meatus

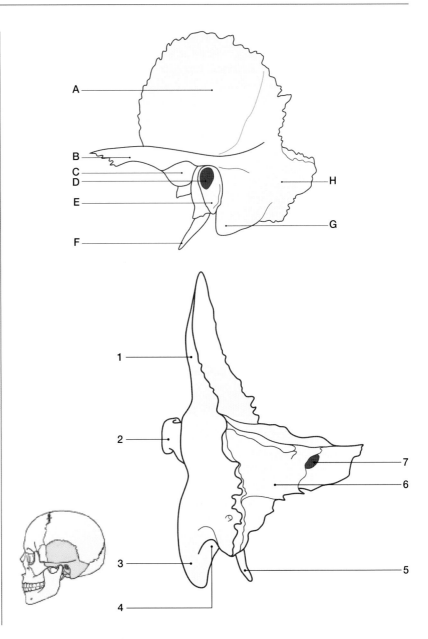

Main parts

The bone is formed by four parts:

Squamous part
Thin and flat. Forms the superoanterior part of the bone and the lateral (temple) part of the cranium.
Temporal surface – Forms part of the temporal fossa.
Zygomatic process (zygoma) – Articulates with the zygomatic bone and forms the mandibular fossa and zygomatic arch (prominent part of cheekbone).

Mandibular fossa – Articulates with the articular disc of the temporomandibular joint. Its posterior aspect is non-articular.

Mastoid part
Forms the posterior aspect of the bone.
Mastoid process – Contains the mastoid air cells, which vary in size from person to person. Easily palpable posterior to the ear lobe. Muscle attachment for the neck.
Mastoid notch – On the medial aspect of the mastoid process.

Tympanic part
This lies anteriorly to the mastoid process and inferior to the squamous part. It forms part of the auditory canal.
External acoustic (auditory) meatus – Mainly lies in the tympanic part; extends to the tympanic membrane (eardrum), which forms the boundary of the middle ear.
Stylomastoid foramen – Between the mastoid and styloid processes and carries the stylomastoid artery and facial nerve.
Styloid process – Tusk-like, lies anterior to the mastoid process and forms attachment for the stylohyoid ligament and other ligaments and muscles of the tongue and neck.

Petrous part
Triangular, lies horizontally between the sphenoid and occipital bones, roughly 90 degrees to the other parts of the temporal bone and forms part of the base of the skull. Contains the middle and inner ear.
Anterior surface – forms part of the floor of the middle cranial fossa.
Posterior surface – forms the anterior aspect of the posterior cranial cavity.
Apex – forms the posterolateral boundary of the foramen lacerum.
Internal acoustic (auditory) meatus – lies on the posterior surface of the petrous part and carries the facial and auditory nerves.
Carotid canal – lies on the inferior surface of the petrous part and carries the internal carotid artery.
Jugular fossa – lies posterior to the opening of the carotid canal. With the jugular notch of the occipital bone, it forms the jugular foramen, which carries the internal jugular vein and glossopharyngeal, as well as the vagus and accessory nerves.

Middle ear
Lies between the external acoustic meatus and inner ear; contains the three auditory ossicles:
Malleus – Hammer-shaped; is in contact with the tympanic membrane (eardrum).
Incus – Anvil-shaped; lies between the malleus and stapes.
Stapes – Stirrup-shaped; lies at the junction of the middle and inner ear. Smallest bone in the body.

Inner ear

Medial to the middle ear, within the petrous part of the temporal bone.

Bony labyrinth – Contains the organs of hearing and balance.

Vestibule – Central part of the cavity, roughly oval in shape.

Semicircular canals – Three canals: superior, posterior and lateral; lie posterosuperior to the vestibule.

Cochlea – Snail-shell-shaped; lies anterior to the vestibule.

Ossification

Part intramembranous, part intracartilaginous.

Squamous part – One centre.

Petrous and mastoid parts – Up to 14 centres.

Tympanic part – One centre.

Styloid process – Two centres.

Centres start to ossify from two months *in utero* until birth. Fusions occur up until after puberty.

Imaging appearances of the temporal bone (Figs. 11.18, 11.19)

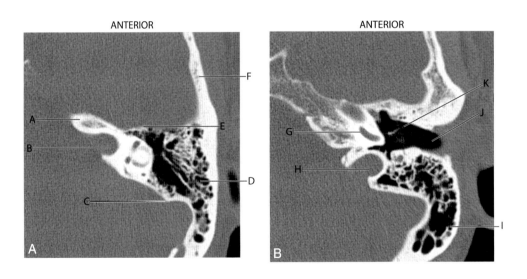

Fig. 11.18 Temporal bone; axial CT images of the superior (A) and inferior (B) aspect of the petrous part. (From STATdx © Elsevier 2022)

A – Petrous apex
B – Internal acoustic (auditory) meatus
C – Posterior surface of the petrous part
D – Mastoid air cells
E – Anterior surface of the petrous part
F – Temporal surface of the squamous part

G – Bony labyrinth in the petrous part
H – Jugular foramen
I – Mastoid process (containing air cells)
J – External acoustic (auditory) meatus/canal
K – Tympanic membrane (faintly seen)

Fig. 11.19 Left temporal bone; coronal CT images of the anterior (A) and posterior (B) aspect of the petrous part. (From STATdx © Elsevier 2022)

1 – Bony labyrinth in the petrous part
2 – Carotid canal
3 – Head of the mandible
4 – Mandibular fossa (temporomandibular joint)
5 – External acoustic (auditory) meatus/canal
6 – Malleus bone (of the middle ear)
7 – Squamous part of the temporal bone
8 – Hypoglossal canal (of the occipital bone)
9 – Occipital condyle
10 – Styloid process
11 – Mastoid process
12 – Mastoid air cells

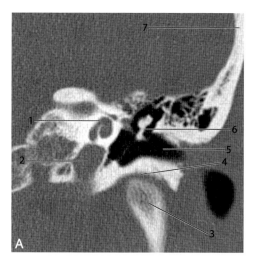

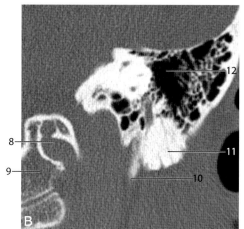

INSIGHT

Within the temporal fossa, a shallow depression on the side of the skull (temple) is an H-shaped point where the temporal, frontal, parietal, and sphenoid bones meet, called the *pterion* (Fig. 11.5). It is clinically important as it is the weakest part of the skull and overlies the middle meningeal vessels. Direct or indirect trauma can fracture this area and damage the vessels leading to an *extradural hematoma* (bleeding between the brain and skull).

Sphenoid bone (Figs. 11.20, 11.21)

Type	Irregular bone, contains a large number of projections and foramen.
Position	Forms the middle part of the base of the skull, lying between the frontal, temporal, parietal and occipital bones.
Articulations	Articulates with all of the cranial bones and the *vomer, ethmoid, occipital, frontal, zygomatic* and *parietal* bones. *The greater wings* with the temporal bone to form the sphenosquamosal suture.
Main parts	Bat-shaped, the bone consists of a body, two pairs of wings (greater and lesser), and two pterygoid processes.

Fig. 11.20 Sphenoid bone (anterior aspect).

A – Lesser wing
B – Superior orbital fissure
C – Sphenoidal crest
D – Foramen rotundum
E – Foramen ovale
F – Vaginal process
G – Lateral pterygoid plate
H – Pterygoid hamulus
I – Sphenoidal rostrum
J – Medial pterygoid plate
K – Spine
L – Orbital surface
M – Temporal surface

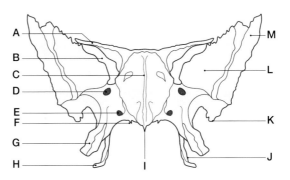

Fig. 11.21 Sphenoid bone (superior aspect).

1 – Greater wing
2 – Lesser wing
3 – Optic canal (foramen)
4 – Superior orbital fissure
5 – Anterior clinoid process
6 – Foramen rotundum
7 – Foramen ovale
8 – Foramen spinosum
9 – Posterior clinoid process
10 – Dorsum sellae
11 – Spine
12 – Sella turcica
13 – Tuberculum sellae
14 – Ethmoidal spine

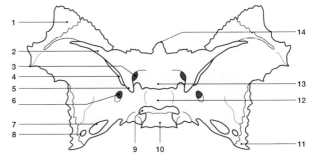

Body

Cube-shaped middle portion.

Superior surface – Articulates with the ethmoid bone.

Optic canal (foramen) – Lateral part of the superior surface for the optic nerve.

Tuberculum sellae – Posterior to the optic canals, forming the anterior boundary of the sella turcica.

Sella turcica – Posterior to the tuberculum sellae. U-shaped, translates as 'Turkish saddle' and contains the *pituitary gland (hypophysis cerebri)*.

Dorsum sellae – Posterior part of the sella turcica.

Clivus – Posterior to the dorsum sellae and articulates with the clivus of the occipital bone.

Middle clinoid processes – Lateral projections on the tuberculum sellae.

Anterior clinoid processes – Lateral to the middle clinoid processes.

Lateral surfaces – Junction of the body and greater wings.

Carotid sulcus – Superior to the lateral surfaces; carries the internal carotid artery and the cavernous venous sinus.

Anterior surface – Articulates with the ethmoid bone.

Sphenoidal crest – On the anterior surface; forms part of the nasal septum.

Sphenoidal sinus – In the body, see paranasal sinuses, p. 342.

Inferior surface – Has several processes:

- *Sphenoidal rostrum* – process in the midline; forms articulation with the vomer.
- *Vaginal processes* – processes on either side of the rostrum.

Greater wings

Two large processes from the sides of the body which form the anterolateral floor of the cranium and part of the lateral wall of the skull.

Sphenosquamosal suture – Junction between the greater wings and squamous part of the temporal bone.

Cerebral surface – Forms part of the middle cranial fossa; presents with three foramina:

- *Foramen rotundum* – on the anteromedial surface, for the maxillary nerve.
- *Foramen ovale* – posterolateral to the foramen rotundum, for the mandibular nerve and accessory meningeal artery.
- *Foramen spinosum* – medial to the foramen ovale, for the middle meningeal artery and meningeal branch of the mandibular nerve.

Orbital surface – Forms the posterolateral wall of the orbit.

Posterolateral border of the inferior orbital fissure – Formed by the inferior border of the orbital surface.

Lateral border of the superior orbital fissure – Formed by the medial border of the orbital surface.

Anterior border of the foramen lacerum – Formed by the posterior border of the junction of the greater wing with the body.

Lesser wings

Smaller triangular plates projecting laterally from the superior surface of the body and anterolaterally to the greater wings. Form part of the floor of the cranium and posterior aspect of the orbit.

Superior surfaces – Support part of the frontal lobe of the cerebrum.

Inferior surfaces – Form part of the roof of the orbit.

Superior border of the superior orbital fissure – Formed by the inferior surface of the lesser wings.

Optic canal – At the junction of the lesser wings and body.

Superior orbital fissure – Carries the oculomotor, trochlear and abducent nerves, and branches of the trigeminal nerves and middle meningeal artery.

Pterygoid processes

'Wing-like' projections inferiorly from the junction of the greater wings and body. Form some of the muscular attachments for the mandible.

Lateral pterygoid plate – Flat plate of bone.

Medial pterygoid plate – Narrow and long, medial to the lateral pterygoid plate.

Pterygoid hamulus – Hook-shaped process on the tip of the medial pterygoid plate.

Pterygoid fissure – At the junction between the two plates.

Ossification

Part intramembranous, part intracartilaginous.

Anterior aspect of the bone – Six centres.

Posterior aspect of the bone – Eight centres.

Centres ossify starting from eight weeks. Fusion of the centres occurs up until about one year old.

Ethmoid bone (Fig. 11.22)

Translates as 'like a sieve' because of numerous air spaces and foramina within it. Forms a prominent role in the structure of the nasal cavity.

Type — Irregular bone.

Position — Posterior to the nasal bones, between the orbits. Forms part of the anterior cranial floor, medial wall of orbits, and superior part of nasal septum and nasal cavity.

Articulations — With the *vomer, maxillae, frontal, palatine, lacrimal,* and *sphenoid* bones.

Main parts — The bone is formed by two plates at 90 degrees to each other and two labyrinths (or masses) on either side.

Fig. 11.22 Ethmoid bone (posterior aspect).

A – Crista galli
B – Ethmoidal labyrinth
C – Orbital plate
D – Medial plate
E – Superior meatus
F – Middle concha
G – Uncinate process
H – Perpendicular plate
I – Superior concha
J – Cribriform plate

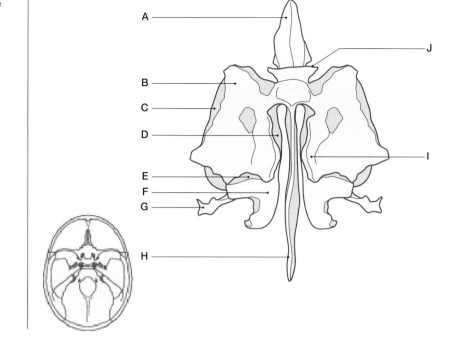

Cribriform plate

Horizontal, lies in the ethmoid notch of the frontal bone and forms the roof of the nasal cavity.
Crista galli – Triangular, superior projection in the midline of the cribriform plate; attachment for the falx cerebri.
Foramina – Perforations in the cribriform plate for the olfactory (smell) nerve filaments.

Perpendicular plate

In the midline and perpendicular to the cribriform plate; projects inferiorly to form the superior part of the nasal septum.

Ethmoidal labyrinths (masses)

Lie at either side of the perpendicular plate.
Ethmoidal air cells – Within the ethmoidal labyrinths, see the paranasal sinuses, p. 342.
Orbital plate – Forms the medial wall of the orbit.
Medial plate – Forms the lateral wall of the nasal cavity.
Superior nasal concha (turbinate) – Thin plate of bone from the cribriform plate, see the nasal cavity, p. 339.
Middle nasal concha (turbinate) – See the nasal cavity, p. 339.
Superior meatus – Space between the superior and middle nasal conchae.

Middle meatus – Space between the middle and inferior nasal concha (which is a separate bone, not part of the ethmoid, page 331).

Ossification

Intracartilaginous.
Perpendicular plate – One centre. Appears in the first year.
Labyrinth – Two centres (one per labyrinth). Appears in the fourth month *in utero*. Centres fuse at two years old.

Imaging appearances of the bones of the cranium (Figs. 11.9–11.11)

FRACTURES

 INSIGHT

When considering trauma and fractures to the skull and cranium, internal brain and vascular injury must be considered. For this reason, cross-sectional imaging, particularly computed tomography (CT), is considered the initial imaging modality of choice.

Cranial fractures (Figs. 11.23, 11.24)

Usually either a longitudinal or a depressed fracture. Almost always associated with haematoma of the scalp, often described as a 'boggy' swelling.

Fig. 11.23 Comminuted depressed skull fracture; axial CT images using brain (A) and bone (B) windows. This patient had been struck with a hammer. In this case, there is no significant underlying brain injury. (From STATdx © Elsevier 2022)

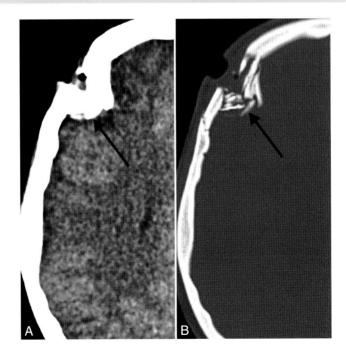

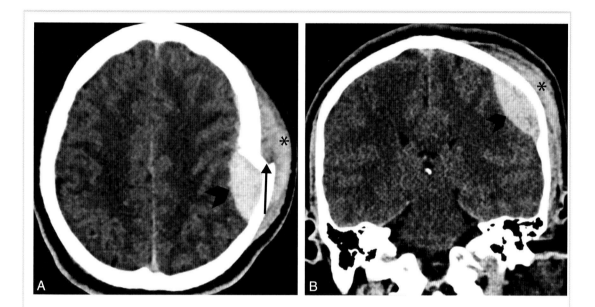

Fig. 11.24 Depressed skull fracture with extradural haematoma; axial (A) and coronal (B) CT images. There is a depressed skull fracture (arrow) and extradural haematoma (arrowhead), which has the classic biconcave lens-shape demonstrating blood collecting between the skull and dural outer layer of the meninges. Note the overlying scalp swelling (*). (From STATdx © Elsevier 2022)

Cause – a direct blow to the head, e.g., a blunt object
Example of treatment – conservative or surgical reduction if displaced; need to treat underlying internal injuries.

Base of skull fractures

Involving the anterior (frontal, ethmoid, anterior sphenoid bones and sinuses), middle (including greater wing and sinus of sphenoid bone), or posterior (petrous part of the temporal bone and occipital bones) cranial fossae. Often associated with facial or other skull fractures and a range of soft tissue injuries, including brain contusion and haematoma, neurovascular injury, leaking of cerebrospinal fluid and *pneumocephalus* (air within the skull).
Cause – range of injuries, including road traffic collisions and falls.
Example of treatment – of associated intracranial injury more so than of fractures

PATHOLOGY

The bones of the cranium are relatively commonly affected by pathologies such as multiple myeloma (see Chapter 4, page 48) and Paget's disease (Fig. 11.25 and also see Chapter 4, page 33)

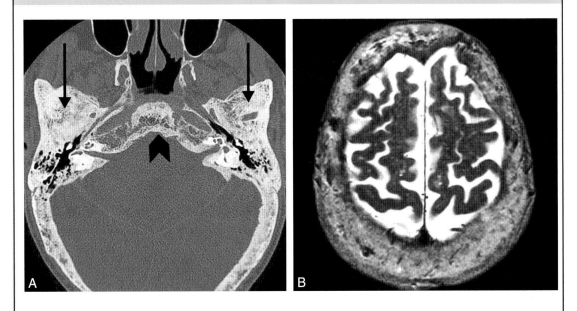

Fig. 11.25 Paget's disease of the skull; axial CT (A) and T2W MRI (B). There is thickening and sclerosis of the temporal (arrows), sphenoid (arrowhead) and cranial bones generally. (From STATdx © Elsevier 2022)

INDIVIDUAL BONES OF THE FACE

Maxillae (Fig. 11.26)

These paired bones form the whole of the upper jaw, part of the orbits, lateral wall and floor of the nasal cavity, and a large amount of the hard palate.

Type   Paired irregular bones.

Position   The upper jaw between the orbits superiorly and the oral cavity inferiorly.

Articulations   With every other bone of the face (except the mandible); the *opposite maxilla*, the *palatine, lacrimal, zygomatic, nasal, ethmoid* and *frontal* bones, the *inferior nasal conchae, vomer* and the *upper teeth.*

Fig. 11.26 Left maxilla
(lateral aspect).

A – Frontal process
B – Infraorbital foramen
C – Anterior nasal spine
D – Canine eminence
E – Maxillary tuberosity
F – Zygomatic process
G – Orbital surface
H – Nasolacrimal groove

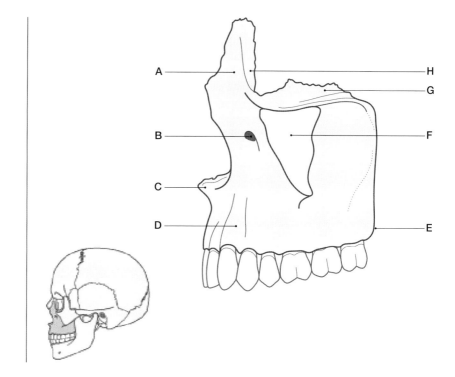

| **Main parts** | Each bone has a body and four processes. |
| | |

Each bone has a body and four processes.

Body – Pyramid-shaped and has four surfaces. It encloses the maxillary sinus, see page 342.

Anterior surface – Directed anteriorly and laterally.

- *Incisive fossa* – depression superior to the incisor teeth.
- *Canine fossa* – depression superior to the canine tooth.
- *Canine eminence* – between the two fossae.
- *Infraorbital foramen* – superior to the canine fossa; for the infraorbital vessels and nerves.
- *Anterior nasal spine* – a pointed process, at the junction of the two bodies.

Infratemporal surface – Convex; lies laterally.

- *Maxillary tuberosity* – lies on the posterior aspect of the roots of the third molar tooth (upper eight).

Orbital surface – forms part of the floor of the orbit.

- *Lacrimal notch* – on the medial border of the orbital surface.
- *Inferior orbital fissure* – the anterior border is formed by the posterior border of the orbital surface.
- *Infraorbital canal* – continuation of the infraorbital foramen.

Nasal surface – Forms the wall of the nasal cavity.

- *Maxillary hiatus* – opening on the posterior part of the nasal surface; leads to the maxillary sinus.

- *Conchal crest* – an oblique ridge on the anterior aspect articulates with the inferior concha bone.

Zygomatic process – Articulates with the zygomatic bone laterally.

Frontal process – Articulates with ethmoid, frontal, nasal and lacrimal bones; forms part of the lateral wall of the nasal cavity.

Alveolar process – Forms articulation with the upper teeth.

Palatine process – Forms part of the floor of the nasal cavity and, therefore, the roof of the mouth. Along with the other palatine process, it forms three-quarters of the bony palate.

Nasal crest – At the junction of the two maxillae, between which is a groove for articulation with the vomer.

Ossification

Intramembranous.

Three primary centres;

One for the main body and two for the alveolar and palatine processes – between six to seven weeks *in utero*

Centres fuse by three months *in utero*.

The two maxillae unite before birth, but the suture between them persists until middle age.

 INSIGHT

The palatine processes of the two maxillae normally unite *in utero*, but when this does not occur, it can leave a defect known as *cleft palate*, an abnormal communication between the oral and nasal cavities. This is also commonly associated with a *cleft* of the upper lip

Zygomatic bones (Fig. 11.27)

Type

Paired irregular bones.

Position

Forms the bony cheek and part of the lateral wall and floor of the orbit.

Articulations

With the *maxilla, temporal, frontal* and *sphenoid* bones.

Main parts

Quadrilateral in shape; each bone has three surfaces, five borders and two processes.

Lateral surface – Convex; projects laterally and anteriorly. Contains *zygomaticofacial foramen* for the nerves/vessels.

Temporal surface – Concave; projects medially and posteriorly. Articulate with the maxilla.

Orbital surface – Concave; forms part of the floor and lateral wall of the orbit.

Orbital border – Concave; forms the inferior and lateral aspects of the orbital margin.

Fig. 11.27 Left zygomatic bone; lateral surface (Source: MOSBY'S DICTIONARY OF MEDICINE, NURSING & HEALTH PROFESSIONS, Eleventh Edition, 2022)

A – Frontozygomatic suture
B – Frontal process
C – Orbital surface
D – Orbital border
E – Maxillary border (forms zygomaticomaxillary suture)
F – Zygomaticofacial foramen
G – Lateral surface
H – Posteroinferior border
I – Temporozygomatic suture
J – Temporal process
K – Temporal border

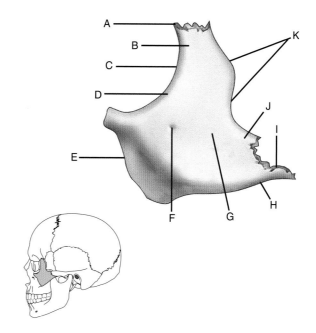

Maxillary border – Articulates with the maxilla at the zygomaticomaxillary suture.
Temporal border – Convex superiorly, concave inferiorly; posterior border of the frontal process and superior border of the temporal process.
Postero-medial border – Articulates with the maxilla inferiorly and the sphenoid bone superiorly. Forms attachment for the masseter muscle.
Postero-inferior border – Forms the inferior aspect of the temporal process.
Frontal process – Articulates with the frontal and sphenoid bone.
Temporal process – Articulates with the temporal bone and together form the *zygomatic arch*, the prominent bony part of the cheek.

Ossification

One primary centre (usually). Appears in the eighth week *in utero*.

Palatine bones (Figs. 11.28, 11.41)

Type

Paired irregular bones.

Position

Lie in the posterior part of the nasal and oral cavities and form the posterior third of the hard palate as well as a small part of the orbital cavity.

Articulations

With the *maxilla, vomer, inferior nasal conchae, sphenoid* and *ethmoid* bones and the other *palatine* bone.

Fig. 11.28 Left palatine bone (anterior aspect).

A – Orbital surface
B – Sphenoidal surface
C – Conchal crest
D – Nasal surface of the horizontal plate
E – Medial border of the horizontal plate
F – Posterior nasal spine (for uvula)
G – Horizontal plate
H – Palatine surface of the horizontal plate
I – Pyramidal process
J – Perpendicular plate
K – Sphenopalatine notch
L – Orbital process

Left palatine bone (medial aspect).
  1 – Sphenopalatine notch
  2 – Sphenoidal process
  3 – Posterior border of the perpendicular plate
  4 – Conchal crest
  5 – Pyramidal process
  6 – Horizontal plate
  7 – Palatine surface of the horizontal plate
  8 – Nasal surface of the palatine plate
  9 – Maxillary process
  10 – Perpendicular plate
  11 – Anterior border of the perpendicular plate
  12 – Ethmoidal crest
  13 – Orbital process

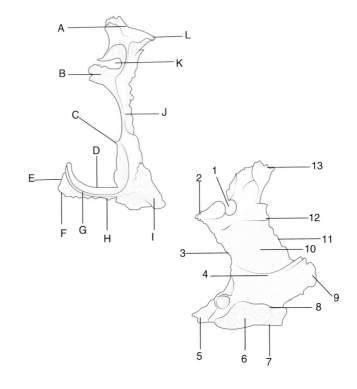

Main parts

The bones are L-shaped, and each has a horizontal and a vertical (perpendicular) plate.

Horizontal plate

Forms part of the hard palate. Has two surfaces and four borders.
Nasal surface – Forms part of the floor of the nasal cavity.
Palatine surface – Forms the posterior part of the bony (hard) palate.
Posterior border – Has a pointed medial end, which forms the *posterior nasal spine*, an attachment for the uvula.
Anterior border – Articulates with the maxilla.
Lateral border – Unites the horizontal and perpendicular plates.

Medial border – Articulates with the other palatine bone, forming the posterior part of the nasal crest.

Perpendicular plate
Has two surfaces and four borders.
Nasal surface – forms part of the inferior meatus of the nasal cavity and has two crests.
- *Conchal crest* – articulates with the inferior nasal concha bone.
- *Ethmoidal crest* – articulates with the middle nasal concha of the ethmoid.
- *Middle meatus* – part of this space lies between the two crests.

Maxillary surface – Articulates with the maxilla and (along with the anterior border of the perpendicular plate) forms part of the medial wall of the maxillary sinus.
Anterior border – Thin and irregular, forms part of the maxillary sinus
Posterior border – Articulates with the medial pterygoid plate of the sphenoid bone.
Superior border – Has two large processes.
- *Orbital process* – articulates with the maxilla and ethmoid; forms part of the floor of the orbit and the inferior orbital fissure.
- *Sphenoidal process* – articulates with the sphenoid bone; forms part of the roof and lateral wall of the nasal cavity.
- *Sphenopalatine notch* – lies between the two processes.

Inferior border – Fused with the lateral edge of the horizontal plate.
- *Pyramidal process* - lies medially of the inferior border at the junction of the horizontal and perpendicular plates; articulates with the maxilla and sphenoid bone.

Ossification

Intramembranous ossification.
One primary centre at the junction of the horizontal and perpendicular plates – eighth week *in utero*.

Nasal bones (Fig. 11.29)

Type

Paired flat bones.

Position

Form the bridge of the nose (most of the structure of the nose is cartilaginous).

Articulations

With the *frontal, maxilla, ethmoid* and other *nasal* bone; is continuous with the cartilage of the nasal septum.

Main parts

The bone has two surfaces and four borders.
External surface – Concave superiorly, convex inferiorly; like a scroll.
Internal surface – Groove for the anterior ethmoid nerve.

Fig. 11.29 Nasal bones; anterior aspect.

A – Superior border (articulates with frontal bone)
B – External surface
C – Inferior border (with the nasal septum)
D – Lateral border (with the maxilla)
E – Medial border (internasal suture)

Right lacrimal bone; lateral and medial aspects.
1 – Lateral (orbital) surface
2 – Lacrimal crest
3 – Descending process
4 – Lacrimal hamulus
5 – Fossa for the lacrimal sac
6 – Anterior border (articulates with the maxilla)
7 – Inferior border (with the maxilla)
8 – Medial (nasal) surface
9 – Posterior border (with the ethmoid)
10 – Superior border (with the frontal bone)

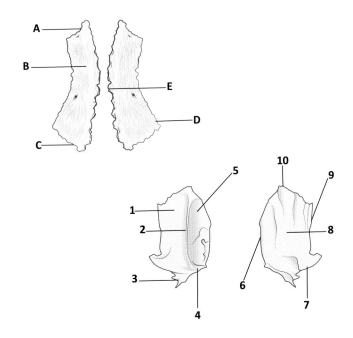

Superior border – Articulates with the frontal bone at the nasion.
Inferior border – Articulates with the cartilage of the nasal septum.
Lateral border – Articulates with the maxilla.
Medial border – Articulates with the ethmoid, frontal and other nasal bone at the *internasal suture*.

Ossification

Intramembranous.
One primary centre – third month *in utero*.

 INSIGHT

The absence of ossified nasal bones is associated with Down's syndrome. It may be assessed on prenatal ultrasound.

Lacrimal bones (Fig. 11.29)

Type   Paired irregular bones. Shape and size of a fingernail, smallest facial bone.

Position   Lie on the medial wall of the orbits.

Articulation   With the *maxilla, ethmoid* and *frontal* bones and the *inferior nasal concha*.

Main parts   The bones have two surfaces and four borders each.
Lateral or orbital surface – Is divided by the vertical *lacrimal crest* posteriorly.
Fossa for the lacrimal sac – Formed where the crest articulates with the maxilla; forms part of the canal for the nasolacrimal duct.
Lacrimal hamulus – A hook at the end of the crest.
Descending process – For articulation with the inferior nasal concha.
Medial or nasal surface – Forms the middle meatus of the nasal cavity and articulates with the ethmoid bone.
Anterior border – Articulates with the maxilla.
Posterior border – Articulates with the ethmoid bone.
Superior border – Articulates with the frontal bone.
Inferior border – Articulates with the maxilla.

Ossification

Intramembranous.
One primary centre – 12th week *in utero*.

Inferior nasal conchae (turbinates) (Fig. 11.30)

Type   Paired irregular bones.

Position   Lie on the lateral walls of the nasal cavity, inferior to the superior and middle conchae of the ethmoid bone. Project into the nasal cavity.

Articulations   With the *maxilla, ethmoid, palatine* and *lacrimal* bones.

Main parts   Each bone has two surfaces, two borders and two ends.
Medial surface – Convex. Contains grooves and foramen for numerous blood vessels.
Lateral surface – Forms part of the inferior meatus of the nasal cavity.
Superior border – Thin and irregular, the middle of which presents three processes:
   • *Lacrimal process* – forms part of the nasolacrimal canal.
   • *Ethmoidal process* – articulates with the ethmoid bone.
   • *Maxillary process* – forms part of the medial wall of the maxillary sinus.

Fig. 11.30 Right inferior nasal concha; lateral aspect.

A – Ethmoidal process
B – Maxillary process
C – Posterior end (articulates with the palatine bone)
D – Inferior border
E – Anterior end (with the maxilla)
F – Lateral surface (inferior meatus)
G – Lacrimal process
H – Superior border

Vomer; left lateral aspect.
1 – Superior surface/border (articulates with the sphenoid and palatine bones)
2 – Anterior border (with the ethmoid bone and septal cartilage)
3 – Inferior border (with the maxillae and palatine bones)
4 – Posterior border
5 – Alae

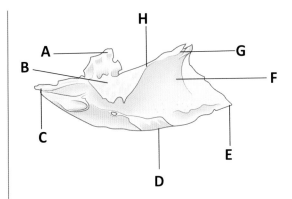

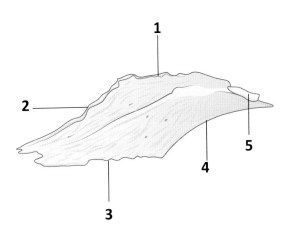

Inferior border – Thicker, non-articular, lies within the nasal cavity.
Ends (extremities) of the bone – *Anterior* and *posterior*; pointed.

Ossification

Intracartilaginous.
One primary centre – fifth month *in utero*.

Vomer (Fig. 11.30)

Type   Flat bone. Quadrilateral, 'plough'-shaped.

Position   Forms the posteroinferior aspect of the bony nasal septum.

Articulations   With the *maxilla*, *sphenoid*, *ethmoid* and *palatine* bones and the cartilage of the nasal septum.

Main parts

The bone has two surfaces and four borders.

Superior surface – Has small grooves for the blood vessels and nerves.

Inferior surface – Has small grooves for the blood vessels and nerves.

Superior border – Thick, and has a deep furrow.

    Alae – Projections from the superior border; articulate with the sphenoid and palatine bones.

Inferior border – Articulates with the nasal crest of the maxillae and palatine bones.

Anterior border – Slopes anteroinferiorly, articulates with the ethmoid and nasal septum (cartilaginous part).

Posterior border – Thick and bifid superiorly, thinner inferiorly. Separates the posterior nasal apertures of the nasal cavity (called *choanae*). No articulations.

Ossification

Intramembranous.

Two primary centres; thin left and right plates – eighth week *in utero*.

Fused in puberty.

Imaging appearances of the facial bones (Figs. 11.31, 11.32)

Fig. 11.31 Facial bones; occipitomental projection. (From Bruce, Merrill's Atlas of Radiographic Positioning; Procedures: Volume Two, 14e, Elsevier)

A – Supraorbital rim
B – Lesser wing of the sphenoid
C – Infraorbital foramen in the infraorbital rim
D – Zygomatic bone
E – Zygomatic arch
F – Maxillary sinus
G – Petrous part of the temporal bone
H – Mastoid air cells
I – Angle of mandible
J – Odontoid process of axis (C2)
K – Vomer
L – Perpendicular plate of the ethmoid
M – Nasal bone
N – Frontozygomatic suture
O – Frontal sinus

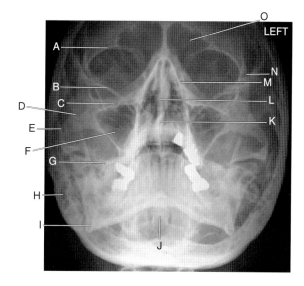

Fig. 11.32 Facial bones; 3D CT image. (From STATdx © Elsevier 2022)

1 – Frontozygomatic suture
2 – Infraorbital rim
3 – Zygomatic bone
4 – Anterior nasal spine of the maxillae
5 – Canine eminence on the alveolar ridge of the maxillae
6 – Mandible
7 – Mastoid process of the temporal bone
8 – Condylar process of the mandible
9 – Vomer
10 – Zygomatic arch
11 – Infraorbital foramen
12 – Perpendicular plate of the ethmoid
13 – Nasal bones

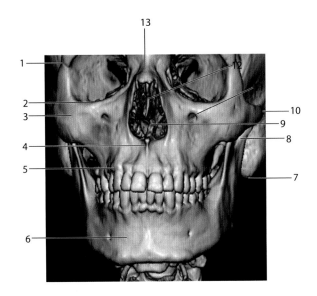

FRACTURES

Nasal bones

Most common facial bone fracture. May be isolated or associated with other more complex injuries. Typically diagnosed clinically, there is no need for imaging except if another associated injury is suspected.
Cause – direct blow, e.g., punching injury.
Example of treatment – conservative, manual reduction if displaced.

Zygomaticomaxillary complex (ZMC) fracture (Fig. 11.33)

Previously known as tripod fractures as involve three structures: the zygomatic arch, frontozygomatic suture, and wall of the maxillary sinus. Normally more than three fractures so now referred to as ZMC fractures.
Cause – a direct blow to the cheek, e.g., punching injury.
Example of treatment – surgical reduction and fixation.

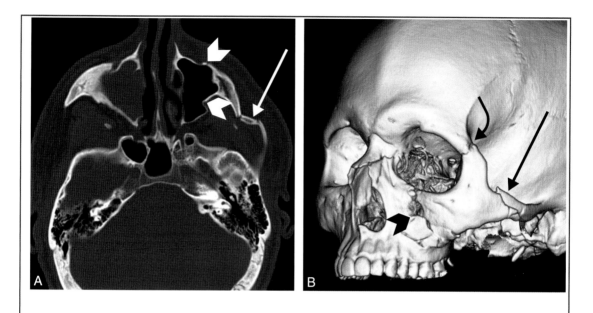

Fig. 11.33 ZMC fracture; axial (A) and 3D (B) CT images. Fractures of the zygomatic arch (arrows), walls of the maxillary sinus (arrowheads) and lateral wall of the orbit (curved arrow). (From STATdx © Elsevier 2022)

Transfacial (Le Fort) fractures (Fig. 11.34)

Classification of fractures involving the bones of the face and pterygoid plates of the sphenoid bone which lead to separation of the maxilla from the rest of the skull. Usually complex and bilateral and associated with intracranial and orbital injuries.
Cause – blunt facial trauma, e.g., road traffic collisions or assaults.
Example of treatment – surgical reduction and fixation.

Fig. 11.34 Transfacial (Le Fort) fracture; 3D CT image. Multiple fractures of the bones of the face result in the separation of the maxilla. (From STATdx © Elsevier 2022)

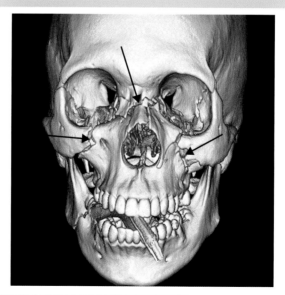

ORBITAL CAVITY (FIG. 11.35)

Bones forming the orbital cavity

The orbital cavity contains the eyeball - its muscles, nerves and blood vessels - and the lacrimal (tear) gland.

Sphenoid bone – The greater and lesser wings.

Zygomatic bone – Orbital surface and border.

Ethmoid bone – Orbital plate.

Palatine bone – Orbital process.

Frontal bone – Supraorbital margin and the orbital plate.

Lacrimal bone – Orbital surface.

Maxilla – Orbital surface.

Features of the orbital cavity

Superior orbital fissure – Transmits the oculomotor, trochlear and abducent nerves, ophthalmic division of the trigeminal nerve and the ophthalmic veins.

Inferior orbital fissure – Transmits the maxillary nerve.

Supraorbital foramen (or notch) – Transmits the supraorbital vessels and nerves.

Optic foramen – Opening of the optic canal.

Optic canal – Transmits the optic nerve and ophthalmic artery.

Infraorbital groove – Contains the infraorbital nerve before it passes through the infraorbital canal to the infraorbital foramen.

Lacrimal groove – In which the lacrimal sac is situated.

Nasolacrimal canal – Carries the nasolacrimal duct from the lacrimal gland to the nasal cavity.

Fig. 11.35 Bones forming the left orbit (anterior aspect).

A – Ethmoid bone (orbital plate)
B – Lacrimal bone (orbital surface)
C – Palatine bone (orbital process)
D – Maxilla (orbital surface)
E – Zygomatic bone (orbital surface and border)
F – Sphenoid bone (greater and lesser wings)
G – Frontal bone (supraorbital margin and orbital plate)

Structures associated with the left orbit (anterior aspect):
1 – Optic canal (foramen)
2 – Inferior orbital fissure
3 – Superior orbital fissure
4 – Supraorbital foramen (notch)

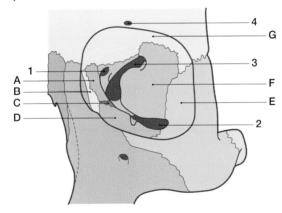

Imaging appearances of the orbital cavity (Figs. 11.36–11.38)

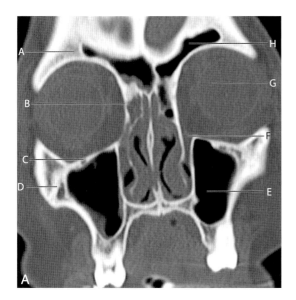
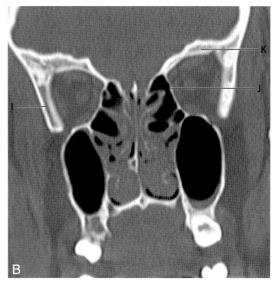

Fig. 11.36 Orbital cavity; coronal CT images of the anterior (A) and mid (B) orbit. (From STATdx © Elsevier 2022)

A – Frontal bone (supraorbital ridge)
B – Lacrimal bone
C – Infraorbital canal
D – Zygomatic bone
E – Maxillary sinus
F – Nasolacrimal duct
G – Eyeball
H – Frontal sinus
I – Zygomatic bone
J – Ethmoid bone (orbital plate)
K – Frontal bone (orbital plate)

Fig. 11.37 Orbital cavity; axial CT image. (From STATdx © Elsevier 2022)

1 – Ethmoid bone (orbital plate)
2 – Zygomatic bone
3 – Sphenoid bone (greater wing)
4 – Sphenoid sinus
5 – Superior orbital fissure
6 – Eyeball
7 – Lacrimal bone

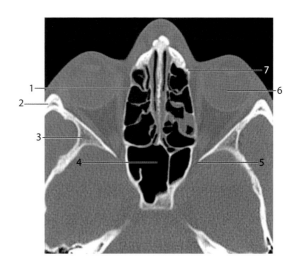

Fig. 11.38 Orbital cavity; 3D CT image. (From STATdx © Elsevier 2022)

A – Frontal bone
B – Supraorbital rim
C – Frontozygomatic suture
D – Greater wing of the sphenoid bone
E – Inferior orbital fissure
F – Zygomatic bone
G – Infraorbital foramen
H – Lacrimal bone
I – Ethmoid bone (orbital plate)
J – Superior orbital fissure
K – Optic nerve canal
L – Lesser wing of the sphenoid bone
M – Supraorbital notch

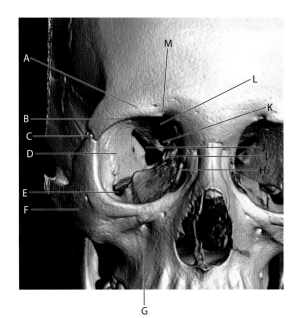

FRACTURES

Blowout fracture (Fig. 11.39)

Fracture of the floor or medial wall of the orbit, which allows herniation of soft tissue structures of the orbit into the maxillary or ethmoid sinus. Classically the inferior rectus muscle drops into the maxillary sinus and becomes trapped in the fracture meaning the patient cannot look down. This creates the typical 'teardrop' sign on imaging.

Cause – direct blow to the orbit, e.g., punching injury or from a ball, causes an increase in pressure in the orbital cavity and the floor to fracture.

Example of treatment – surgical reconstruction.

Fig. 11.39 Blowout fracture right orbit; coronal CT image. There is a fracture of the floor of the orbit with resultant herniation of the inferior rectus muscle into the maxillary sinus (arrow); the classic 'teardrop' sign. (From STATdx © Elsevier 2022)

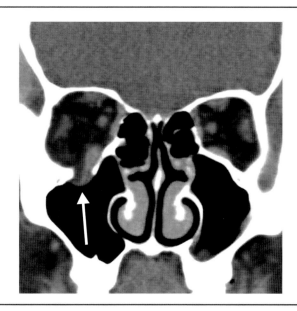

NASAL CAVITY (FIGS. 11.40, 11.41)

Large vault-like structure forming the upper part of the respiratory tract. Irregular in shape.

Roof

Formed by:
Nasal septum of the frontal and nasal bones.
Cribriform plate of the ethmoid bone, perforated (contains receptors for smell).
Body of the sphenoid bone.

Floor

Forms the division between the oral and nasal cavities. Formed by:
Palatine process of the maxilla (anterior).
Horizontal plate of the palatine bone (posterior).

Medial wall (septum)

Referred to as the *nasal septum*, which divides the nasal cavity into left and right. Formed by:
Vomer.
Perpendicular plate of the ethmoid bone.
Septal cartilage.

Lateral wall

Irregular as it forms the three nasal conchae. Formed by:
Nasal surface of the maxilla.
Perpendicular plate of the palatine bone.
Ethmoidal labyrinth.
Inferior nasal concha bone.

Fig. 11.40 Nasal cavity; coronal section.

1 – Superior nasal concha of the ethmoid
2 – Middle nasal concha of the ethmoid
3 – Inferior nasal concha bone
4 – Vomer bone
5 – Inferior meatus
6 – Middle meatus
7 – Superior meatus
8 – Spheno-ethmoidal recess
9 – Perpendicular plate of the ethmoid bone

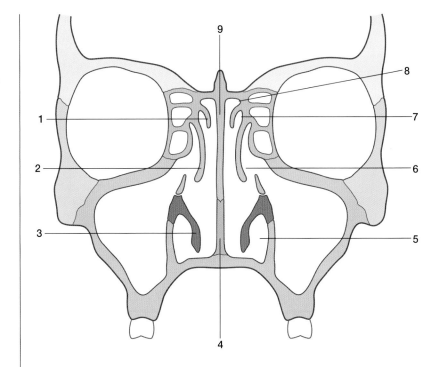

Fig. 11.41 Nasal cavity (lateral wall); sagittal section.

A – Nasal bone
B – Superior concha of the ethmoid bone
C – Middle concha of the ethmoid bone
D – Inferior concha bone
E – Palatine process of the maxilla
F – Horizontal plate of the palatine bone
G – Inferior meatus (palatine bone in red)
H – Middle meatus
I – Spheno-ethmoidal recess
J – Sphenoidal sinus
K – Cribriform plate of the ethmoid bone

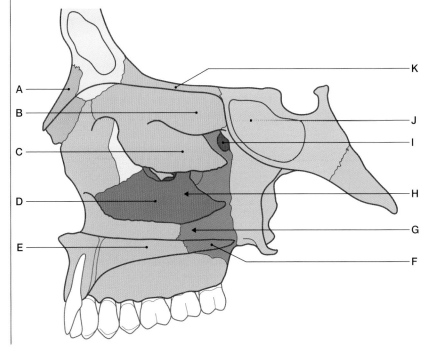

Conchae

Also known as *turbinates*. Scroll-shaped bony projections on the lateral wall of the nasal cavities. Increase surface area of the nasal cavity and disturb airflow to help warm and moisten inhaled air and trap microbes and foreign particles in the mucosa covering the nasal cavity.

Superior nasal concha – Projection from the ethmoid bone.
Middle nasal concha – Projection of the ethmoid bone.
Inferior nasal concha – A separate bone.

Spaces between the conchae known as *meati*.
Spheno-ethmoidal recess – Superior and posterior to the superior concha. Communicates with the *sphenoidal sinus*.
Superior meatus – Lies between the superior and middle nasal conchae. Communicates with the *posterior ethmoidal sinuses*.
Middle meatus – Lies between the middle and inferior nasal conchae. Communicates with the *anterior* and *middle ethmoidal sinuses, frontal sinus* and *maxillary sinus*.
Inferior meatus – Lies inferior to the inferior nasal concha. Communicates with the orbit via the *nasolacrimal canal*.

Imaging appearances of the nasal cavity (Fig. 11.42)

Fig. 11.42 Nasal cavity; coronal CT image. (From STATdx © Elsevier 2022)

A – Superior concha
B – Middle concha
C – Inferior concha
D – Vomer bone
E – Inferior meatus
F – Middle meatus
G – Superior meatus
H – Ethmoid air cells
I – Perpendicular plate of the ethmoid bone
Note the thick mucosal lining surrounding the bones of the nasal cavity, particularly the middle and nasal conchae and vomer.

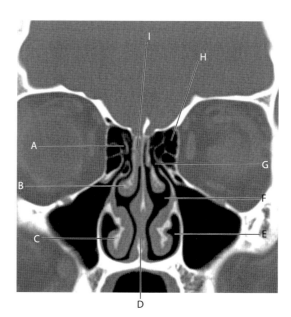

PARANASAL SINUSES (FIGS. 11.43, 11.44)

Hollow air-filled spaces in the bones of the skull. Consist of four pairs on left and right, named after the bone in which they are located:

Maxillary sinuses
Frontal sinuses
Ethmoidal sinuses (three groups)
Sphenoidal sinuses

The sinuses are lined with mucous membrane, which is continuous with the nasal cavity and forms a similar role in protecting the respiratory tract from microbes and particles. The mucous drains into the nasal cavity through holes called *ostia*.

Additional functions

To lighten the skull.
To add resonance to the voice.

Maxillary sinuses (Fig. 11.43)

Shape

Pyramidal cavities.

Position

They lie on either side of the nasal cavity, inferior to the orbits, within the maxillae.

Fig. 11.43 Paranasal sinuses and associated structures (coronal section).

A – Ethmoidal sinuses
B – Maxillary sinus
C – Nasal cavity
D – Orbital cavity

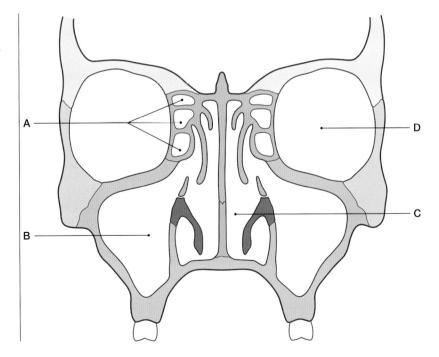

Fig. 11.44 Paranasal sinuses and associated structures (sagittal section). Arrows show sinus drainage.

A – Frontal sinuses
B – Spheno-ethmoidal recess
C – Opening for the ethmoidal sinuses
D – Opening for the maxillary sinuses
E – Hard palate
F – Inferior meatus
G – Middle meatus
H – Opening for the ethmoidal sinuses
I – Superior meatus
J – Sphenoidal sinuses
K – Sella turcica (hypophyseal fossa/ pituitary fossa)

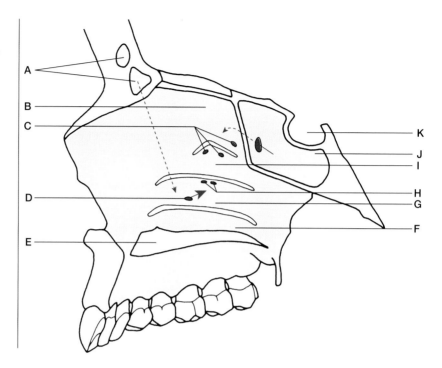

Structure	Largest of the paranasal sinuses.

Structure

Largest of the paranasal sinuses.
Base – Medially, formed by the lateral wall of the nasal cavity.
Apex – Projects superolaterally into the zygomatic process of the maxilla.
Floor – Inferiorly, formed by the alveolar process of the maxilla.
Roof – Superiorly, formed by the floor of the orbit.

Communication

With the middle meatus of the nasal cavity via the antral ostium.

Frontal sinuses (Fig. 11.44)

Shape

Irregular.

Position

In the midline of the frontal bone, superior to the nasal cavity and the orbits. Anterior to the anterior cranial fossa, posterior to the superciliary arches.

Structure

Vary in size and shape from person to person. They are divided from each other by a septum near the midline.

Communication

With the middle meatus of the nose via the frontonasal canal or ethmoidal infundibulum.

Ethmoidal sinuses (Fig. 11.43)

Shape	Numerous small cavities, irregular in shape.
Position	Situated in the ethmoid labyrinths between the medial wall of the orbit and nasal cavity and inferior to the anterior cranial fossa.
Structure	Divided into three groups: anterior, middle and posterior. *Orbital plate* – Forms the boundary between the sinus and medial wall of the orbit. *Medial plate* – Forms the boundary between the sinus and lateral wall of the nasal cavity.
Communication	*Anterior and middle groups* – Via the spheno-ethmoidal recess superior to the superior conchae of the nasal cavity. *Posterior group* – With the superior meatus of the nasal cavity.

Sphenoidal sinuses (Fig. 11.44)

Shape	Cuboidal.
Position	In the body of the sphenoid bone inferior to the sella turcica, hypophysis cerebri (pituitary gland) and hypothalamus of the brain. Superior and posterior to the nasal cavity and ethmoidal sinuses.
Communication	With the spheno-ethmoidal recess in the nasal cavity.

Imaging appearances of the paranasal sinuses (Figs. 11.45–11.47)

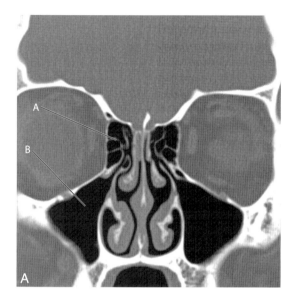
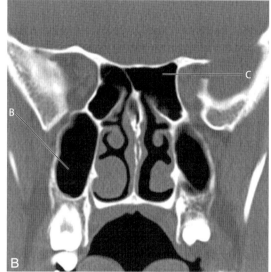

Fig. 11.45 Paranasal sinuses; coronal CT images anteriorly (A) and posteriorly (B). (From STATdx © Elsevier 2022)

A – Ethmoid sinuses
B – Maxillary sinuses
C – Sphenoid sinuses

Fig. 11.46 Paranasal sinuses; sagittal CT image. (From STATdx © Elsevier 2022)

1 – Frontal sinus
2 – Maxillary sinus
3 – Sphenoid sinus
4 – Posterior ethmoid air cells
5 – Middle ethmoid air cells
6 – Anterior ethmoid air cells

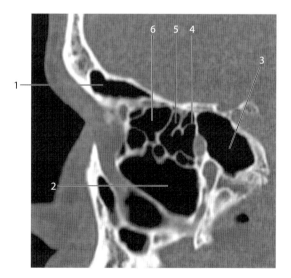

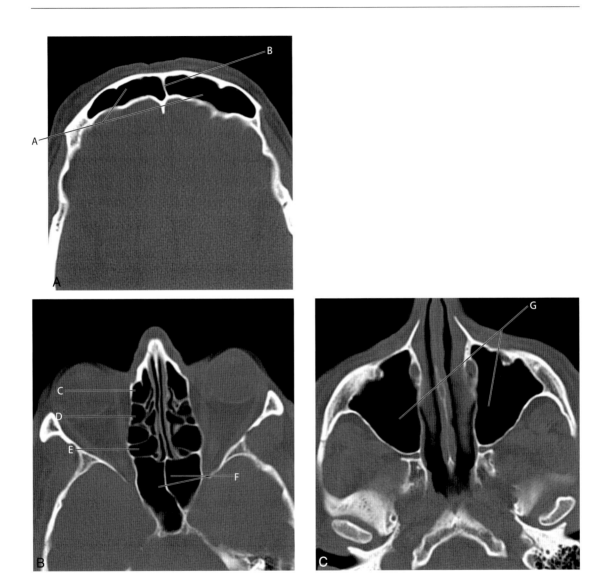

Fig. 11.47 Paranasal sinuses; axial CT images superior (A), mid (B) and inferior (C). (From STATdx © Elsevier 2022)

A – Frontal sinuses
B – Frontal sinus septum
C – Anterior ethmoid air cells
D – Middle ethmoid air cells
E – Posterior ethmoid air cells
F – Sphenoid sinuses
G – Maxillary sinuses

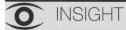 INSIGHT

The paranasal sinuses may fill with blood following trauma or associated fracture. Where the fluid collects during imaging is dependent on the position of the patient because of gravity.

PATHOLOGY

Rhinosinusitis (Fig. 11.48)

Caused by inflammation of the mucosa of the paranasal sinuses. Presents with facial pain and pressure, nasal discharge and blocked nose. Causes include infections and inflammation; may be chronic or acute. Imaging demonstrates thickened mucosa, fluid levels and sclerosis of the sinus walls (when chronic).

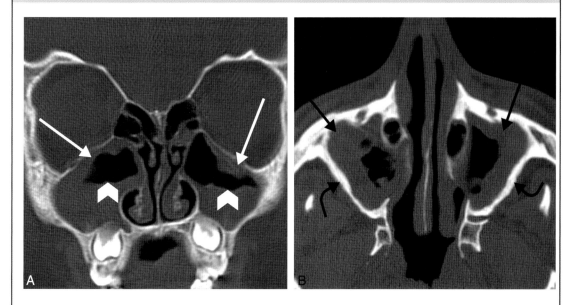

Fig. 11.48 Chronic rhinosinusitis; coronal (A) and axial (B) CT images. There is mucosal thickening (arrows), fluid (arrowheads), and sclerotic bone formation (curved arrows) of both maxillary sinuses. (From STATdx © Elsevier 2022)

MANDIBLE (FIGS. 11.49, 11.50)

Largest and strongest bone in the face. Only moveable bone in the skull (except for the auditory ossicles in the ear).

Type

Irregular bone.

Position

Forms the lower jaw.

Articulations

The *head of the mandible* with the mandibular fossa of the temporal bone to form the temporomandibular joint.
With the *lower teeth* via the alveolar sockets.

Fig. 11.49 Left mandible (external aspect).

A – Coronoid process
B – Symphysis menti
C – Mental protuberance
D – Mental foramen
E – Oblique line
F – Angle
G – Ramus
H – Condylar process
I – Head of the mandible

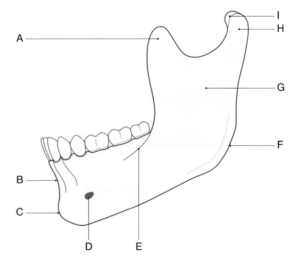

Fig. 11.50 Left mandible (internal aspect).

1 – Head of the mandible
2 – Condylar process
3 – Neck
4 – Mylohyoid line
5 – Submandibular fossa
6 – Angle
7 – Body
8 – Mental protuberance
9 – Symphysis menti
10 – Sublingual fossa
11 – Mandibular foramen
12 – Coronoid process

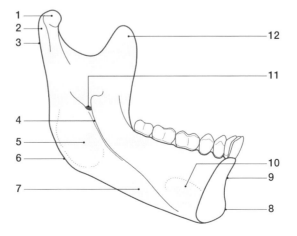

Main parts

The bone is formed by a central body and two rami.

Body
The horseshoe-shaped aspect of the bone.
External surface – Convex and subcutaneous.
Symphysis menti – In the midline, where the two halves of the body join.
Mental protuberance – Base of the symphysis menti; the chin.
Mental foramen – Inferior to the second premolar tooth (lower four); carries the mental nerve and vessels.
Oblique line – Continuation of the anterior border of the ramus.
Alveolar ridge – Contains the alveoli sockets for the lower teeth.
Internal surface – Concave.
Mylohyoid line – Oblique ridge for the attachment of the muscles of the pharynx.
Submandibular fossa – Lies inferior to the mylohyoid line, for the submandibular salivary glands and lymph nodes.
Sublingual fossa – Superior to the mylohyoid line, for the sublingual salivary glands.

Ramus (plural rami)
Flat plate of bone at right angles to the body, one on each side.
Mandibular foramen – On the medial aspect, and is the opening of the mandibular canal.
Mandibular canal – Carries the mental nerve and vessels. Divided into two canals:
  * *Mental canal* – opens at the mental foramen.
  * *Incisive canal* – opens at the incisor teeth.
Angle of the mandible – Junction of the body and ramus.
Coronoid process – Triangular; forms the anterior aspect of the superior border of the ramus.
Condylar process – Posterior aspect of the superior border of the ramus.
Head of mandible – Expanded part of the condylar process; articulates with the mandibular fossa of the temporal bone at the temporomandibular joint.
Neck – Narrow portion inferior to the head.

Ossification

Intramembranous.

Primary centres
Body – Two centres; *left and right.* - sixth week *in utero*.
  The mandible is initially a paired bone but unites early. The symphysis menti between the bodies ossifies in the first year.

Secondary centres
Ramus – Four centres; *left and right condylar and coronoid processes*. Fuse with the body before birth.

Radiographic appearances of the mandible (Figs. 11.51, 11.52)

Fig. 11.51 Mandible; panoramic tomogram/ orthopantomogram (OPG/ OPT). (From Spratt, Weir; Abrahams' Imaging Atlas of Human Anatomy, 6e, Elsevier)

A – Head
B – Neck
C – Rami
D – Mental protuberance
E – Body
H – Angle
G – Temporomandibular joint (TMJ)
H – Mandibular fossa of the temporal bone
I – Maxillary sinus
J – Vomer
K – Hard palate
L – Coronoid process

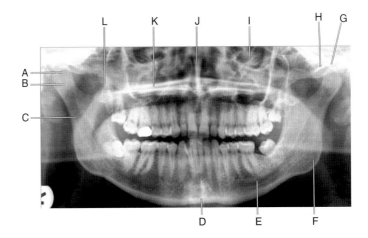

Fig. 11.52 Mandible; 3D CT image of the left lateral aspect. (From STATdx © Elsevier 2022)

1 – Coronoid process
2 – Alveolar ridge
3 – Mental foramen
4 – Mental protuberance
5 – Body
6 – Oblique line
7 – Angle
8 – Ramus
9 – Neck
10 – Condylar process

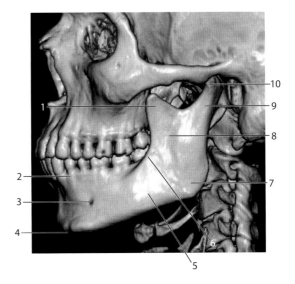

FRACTURES

 INSIGHT

Due to the rigidity of the temporomandibular joints, the mandible can be considered a ring structure. A fracture of the mandible will often result in a second fracture of the mandible or a fracture-dislocation of the temporomandibular joint on the contralateral (opposite) side.

Mandible fracture (Figs. 11.53, 11.54)

Second most common facial bone fracture. If fractures extend into the root of teeth, it is considered an open fracture with a high risk of infection (*osteomyelitis*).
Cause – a direct blow to the jaw, e.g., assault or road traffic collision.
Example of treatment – surgical fixation common.

Fig. 11.53 Mandible fracture; axial (A) and 3D (B) CT images. Fracture of the right ramus (arrows) and left body involving the lower teeth (arrowheads); therefore, an open fracture. (From STATdx © Elsevier 2022)

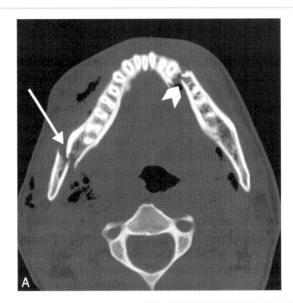

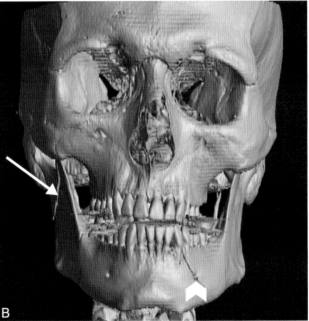

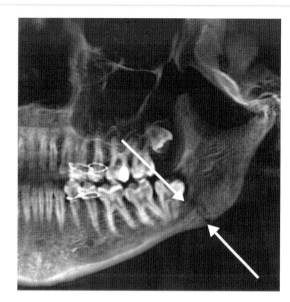

Fig. 11.54 Mandible fracture; panoramic projection. Open fracture of the left angle involving the lower third molar. (From STATdx © Elsevier 2022)

TEETH (FIG. 11.55)

Position	Lie in the alveolar ridges of the maxillae and mandible.
Articulations	*Fibrous gomphosis* joints between the teeth and alveoli (sockets) in the maxillae and mandible.
Main parts	***Crown*** – Area above the gum. ***Neck*** – Constriction between the root and crown at the level of the gum. ***Root*** – Embedded in the alveoli in the mandible and maxillae. ***Pulp cavity*** – Central canal(s) of the tooth.
Structure	***Enamel*** – Dense (densest material in body), white, avascular structure covering the crown; approximately 1.5 mm thick, mainly formed by calcium phosphate (hydroxyapatite). ***Dentine*** – Hard, yellow or white avascular structure, similar to bone. Small canals from the dentine open into the pulp cavity. ***Dental pulp*** – Connective tissue with blood vessels, nerves and lymphatic vessels; found in the pulp cavity. ***Apical foramen*** – At the apex of the root; for the passage of blood vessels and nerves. ***Cement*** – Layer of bone-like tissue, continuous with the enamel and covering the root.

Fig. 11.55 Lower premolar tooth (coronal section). (From STATdx © Elsevier 2022)

A – Enamel
B – Dentine
C – Pulp cavity
D – Cement
E – Periodontal membrane
F – Lamina dura
G – Apical foramen
H – Nerve and vessels

1 – Crown
2 – Neck
3 – Root

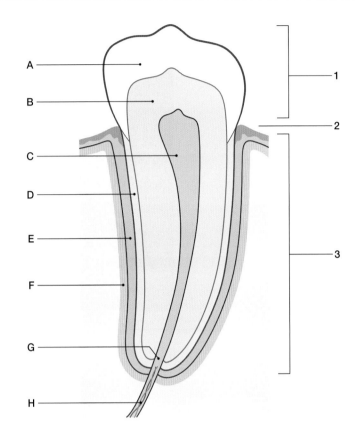

Periodontal membrane (ligament) – Attaches the cement to the alveoli root socket.

Lamina dura – A thin layer of compact bone forming the cortex of the alveoli socket in which the tooth lies.

Types of teeth (Fig. 11.56)

Incisors
Sharp, chisel-shaped crown, single root.
> *Function* – biting and cutting food.

Canines
Blunt, pointed crown, single root.
> *Function* – grasping and tearing food.

Premolars
Two cusps: one labial (lip side) and one lingual (tongue side). Usually a single, grooved root, but the upper four often have two roots.
> *Function* – grinding and chewing food.

Fig. 11.56 Permanent teeth – right upper and lower quadrants.

1 2 – Incisors
3 – Canine
4 5 – Premolars
6 7 8 – Molars

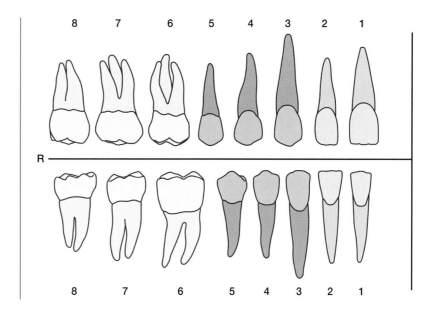

Molars

Largest teeth; occlusal surface cuboidal with three or four cusps. The upper molars have three roots; the lower have two roots.

Function – grinding and chewing food.

Dentition

Deciduous (baby/milk) teeth

Children have a full dentition of 20 teeth: two incisors, one canine and two molars in each quadrant of the mouth.

Permanent teeth

Adults have a full dentition of 32 teeth: two incisors, one canine, two premolars and three molars in each quadrant.

Dental formulae (Fig. 11.56)

To identify the different teeth in the mouth, a formula is used. Numbers are used to identify permanent teeth:

Upper: R 87654321 | 12345678 L
Lower: R 87654321 | 12345678 L

Letters are used to identify deciduous teeth:

R edcba | abcde L
R edcba | abcde L

INSIGHT

To identify an individual tooth, part of the grid and the tooth are given, e.g.

The upper right one would be

1 |

The lower left four would be:

4

Radiographic appearances of the teeth (Fig. 11.57)

Fig. 11.57 Teeth; mandible; panoramic tomogram/ orthopantomogram (OPG). (From Spratt, Weir; Abrahams' Imaging Atlas of Human Anatomy, 6e, Elsevier)

A – Incisors
B – Canine
C – Premolars
D – Molars
E – Third molars (unerupted)
F – Crown
G – Pulp cavity
H – Root

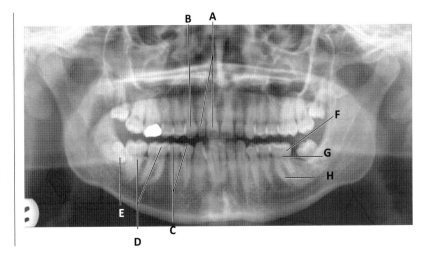

PATHOLOGY

Dental caries (Fig. 11.58)

Known informally as tooth decay or cavities. Demineralisation of the tooth structures leads to erosions and exposure of the nerves, leading to sensitivity and pain symptoms. Best seen on radiographs, although up to 40% of mineralisation needs to be lost before visible. May lead to an abscess if it proceeds to erode and infect the underlying bone socket.
Cause – acid within the diet and produced by bacteria in the mouth.
Example of treatment – replacement of caries with a filling, tooth extraction in advanced cases.

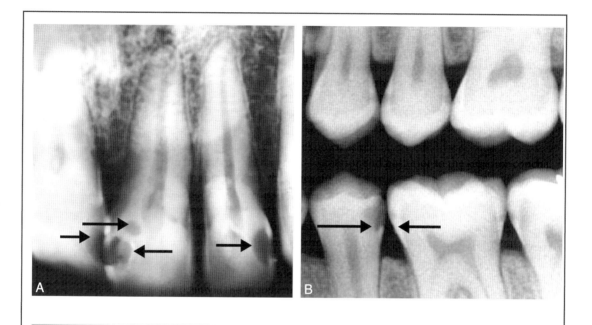

Fig. 11.58 Dental caries; periapical (A) and bitewing (B) radiographs. Lucencies are seen within the structure (arrows). (From STATdx © Elsevier 2022)

TEMPOROMANDIBULAR JOINT (TMJ) (FIG. 11.59)

Type   Synovial bicondylar joint (two joints work as one functional unit).

Bony articular surfaces
Articular tubercle and the *anterior aspect of the mandibular fossa* of the temporal bone superiorly, with the *head of the condyle* of the mandible inferiorly. The articular surfaces are covered with fibrocartilage.

Fibrous capsule
Surrounds the joint; it is attached to the articular tubercle and the circumference of the mandibular fossa and the neck of the mandible. The capsule is loose superiorly and tight inferiorly.

Synovial membrane
Lines the fibrous capsule. The membrane secretes synovial fluid, which lubricates the joint.

Fig. 11.59 Left
temporomandibular joint
(sagittal section).

A – Fibrocartilage
B – Synovial fluid
C – Articular disc
D – Lateral pterygoid
ligament
E – Fibrous capsule
F – Fibrocartilage
G – Head of mandible
H – Synovial fluid
I – Synovial membrane
J – External acoustic
meatus
K – Venous plexus
L – Mandibular fossa of the
temporal bone

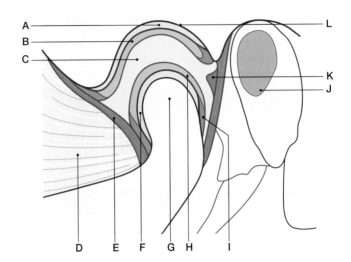

Supporting ligaments

Lateral (temporomandibular) ligament – From the zygoma to the neck of the
mandible.
Sphenomandibular ligament – From the spine of the sphenoid to the lingula of
the mandibular foramen.
Stylomandibular ligament – From the styloid process to the angle and ramus of
the mandible.

Intracapsular structure

Articular disc – Fibrous tissue, divides the joint cavity horizontally into two
sections and is fused with the capsule.

Movements

Depression by the lateral pterygoid muscle.
Elevation by the temporalis, masseter and medial pterygoid muscles.
Protrusion by the lateral and medial pterygoid muscles.
Retraction by the temporalis muscle.
Lateral movement by the medial and lateral pterygoid muscles.
   When the mouth opens, the head of the mandible moves antero-inferiorly
from the mandibular fossa onto the articular tubercle. The articular disc moves
with the head to protect the articular surfaces.

Blood supply

Superficial temporal and maxillary arteries.

Nerve supply

Branches of the mandibular nerve.

Imaging appearances of the temporomandibular joint (Figs. 11.60, 11.61)

Fig. 11.60 Left temporomandibular joint; sagittal (A) and 3D (B) CT images. (From STATdx © Elsevier 2022)

A – Articular tubercle of the temporal bone
B – Coronoid process of the mandible
C – Ramus of the mandible
D – Angle of the mandible
E – Mastoid process
F – Neck of the mandible
G – External acoustic (auditory) meatus
H – Head of mandible
I – Mandibular fossa of the temporal bone

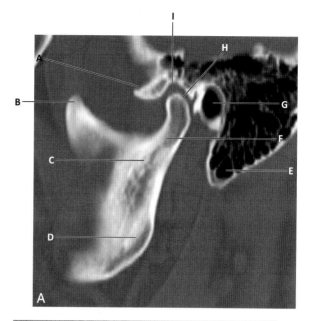

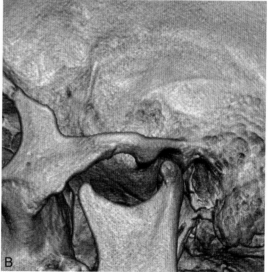

Fig. 11.61 Left temporomandibular joint; sagittal T2W MRI with the mouth closed (A) and open (B). Note how the head of the mandible and articular disc move anteriorly out of the mandibular fossa on opening the mouth. (From STATdx © Elsevier 2022)

1 – Articular tubercle of the temporal bone
2 – Articular disc
3 – Head of the mandible
4 – Mandibular fossa of the temporal bone

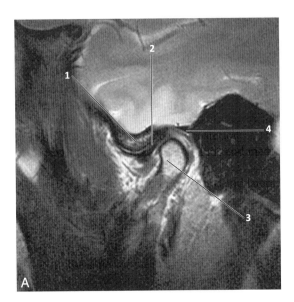

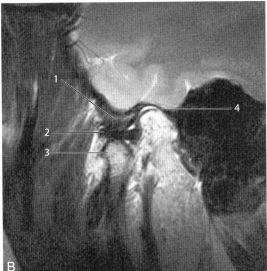

HYOID BONE (FIG. 11.62)

Fig. 11.62 Hyoid bone; anterior aspect. (Source: MOSBY'S® MEDICAL DICTIONARY, Eleventh Edition, 2022)

A – Greater cornu (horn)
B – Lesser cornu (horn)
C – Body

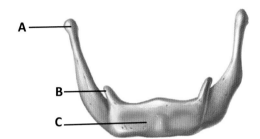

Not strictly a facial bone, it gives attachment for muscles of the mouth, tongue and middle constrictor muscle of the pharynx.

Through attachments has an important role in a number of processes:
- Mastication (chewing)
- Deglutition (swallowing)
- Respiration
- Phonation (production of sounds)
- Posture of neck

Type

Irregular bone.

Position

Lies anteriorly in the neck, at the root of the tongue. Superior to the thyroid cartilage of the larynx at the level of the angle of the mandible and third and fourth cervical vertebra.

Articulations

The bone is suspended from the *styloid process of the temporal bone* by the stylohyoid ligament. It is unique in that it does not directly articulate with any other bone

Main parts

Consists of a body and two pairs of horns (*cornu*).
Body – Convex, horseshoe-shaped.
Greater cornua – Project posterolaterally from the body.
Lesser cornua – Project superiorly at the junction between the body and greater cornua.

Ossification

Six primary centres.
Body – Two centres - in utero close to birth.
Greater cornua – Two centres (one each side) - in utero close to birth.
Lesser cornua – Two centres (one each side) - between one and two years old.
Initially connected by cartilaginous synchondroses, the bone finally fuses in middle age.

Imaging appearances of the hyoid bone (Fig. 11.63)

Fig. 11.63 Hyoid bone; 3D CT image. (From STATdx © Elsevier 2022)

A – Lesser cornu
B – Body
C – Greater cornu
Note that the cartilaginous synchondrosis between the body and greater cornu has not yet fused.

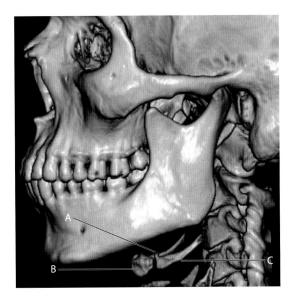

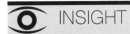 INSIGHT

The hyoid bone is often fractured during strangulation, so it is considered important in forensics.

GLOSSARY

Please note that many of these terms might have wider meanings beyond the skeletal system.

A- Absence of.

Abduction To move away from the midline, usually a limb.

Abscess A cavity containing pus.

Achondroplasia Genetic disease of cartilage development causing lack of bone growth, particularly the limbs.

Acromegaly Excessive secretion of growth hormone causing thickening of the bones and soft tissues, usually caused by a tumour of the pituitary gland.

Acute Short, sudden onset and duration.

Adactyly Congenital absence of fingers or toes.

Adipose Relating to fatty tissue.

Adduction To move towards the midline, usually a limb.

Aetiology Cause, or origin, of disease.

Amelia Congenital absence of a limb/limbs.

Amphiarthroses Type of joint with minimal movement; mainly cartilaginous symphyses.

Anastomosis Joining of different vessels which would normally diverge.

Androgens Male sex hormones produced by the adrenal glands and testes; steroids, include testosterone and androsterone.

Ankylosing spondylitis Inflammatory disorder, predominantly of the axial skeleton, leading to bony ankylosis of the spinal column and other large joints.

Ankylosis Fusion or immobility of a joint caused by disease; may be bony or fibrous.

Anterior Nearer the front of the body.

Apophysis A secondary ossification centre, typically an elevation or projection, at the site of ligament or tendon attachment. Usually fuses with skeletal maturity.

Arthr Relating to a joint.

Arthropathy Disease or pathologic condition involving a joint.

Arthritis Inflammation of a joint.

Atlas First cervical vertebra.

Auricular Ear-shaped.

Autoimmune Body's immune system attacking itself.

Avascular Necrosis (AVN) 'Bone death' results from blood supply loss to the area; now more commonly known as osteonecrosis.

Axial plane Horizontal or transverse plane of the body; divides the body into top and bottom.

Axis Second cervical vertebra.

Benign Not malignant, does not spread/metastasise.

Bi Two or twice.

Biaxial Movement around two axes/planes.

Bipartite In two parts.

Brachi Relating to the arm.

Brachy Short.

Brodie's abscess Chronic collection of pus/infection within bone.

Buccal Relating to the cheek of the mouth.

Bursa Sac of synovial membrane found around joints to reduce friction.

Calcification The deposition of mineral salts, mainly calcium phosphate, in tissue.

Calcitonin Hormone produced in the thyroid gland. Involved in calcium homeostasis by reducing the rate of bone resorption by osteoclasts.

Callus The temporary new bone formation as part of fracture healing.

Canal Bony tunnel.

Canaliculi Channels carrying nutrient fluid between lacunae in the Haversian systems.

Cancellous bone Lighter than compact bone found at the ends of long bones and in the middle of other bones. Formed by a lattice of trabeculae. Also known as spongy bone.

Caries Tooth decay, demineralisation of teeth.

Cartilaginous joint Bones joined by a layer of fibro- or hyaline cartilage with minimal/no movement; synchondroses, symphyses.

Caudal Towards the feet.

Cephalic Relating to the head.

Cervical rib An anomalous extra rib, usually of the seventh cervical vertebra.

Chondro Relating to cartilage.

Chondrocytes Cartilage cells.

Chondrosarcoma A primary malignant tumour of cartilage cells.

Chronic Longstanding.

Circumduction Combination of movements to make a circle, usually with a limb.

Circumferential lamellae Rings of bone around the inner and outer circumference of compact bone.

Collagen Strong fibrous protein, a major component of connective tissue and the organic matrix (osteoid) of bone tissue.

Colles' fracture Fracture of the distal end of radius with posterior displacement of the distal fragment.

Comminuted Broken into small pieces; type of fracture with more than two parts/fragments.

Compact bone Dense, hard cortex of bones. Made of organised Haversian systems.

Compression Crushed/pressed together; type of fracture.

Concave Depressed, hollowed out, curved inward.

Condyle Smooth, rounded area; often form the articular surface of synovial joints.

Congenital Existing at birth; developmental or genetic.

Convex Elevated, curved outward.

Contralateral On the opposite side of the body.

Contrecoup An injury caused by a blow to the opposite side of an area.

Coronal (plane) Dividing the body into anterior and posterior (front and back).

Cortex Outer layer of an organ; compact bone in the skeleton.

Cortisol Steroid hormone produced by the adrenal glands; anti-inflammatory properties.

Costal Associated with the ribs.

Coxa Relating to the hip.

Coxa vara Deformity of the proximal femur when the angle between the neck and the shaft is reduced, resulting in medial angulation and shortening of the leg.

Cranial Towards the head.

Crepitus Grating or cracking sound/sensation.

Crest A sharp ridge.

CT Computed tomography.

Cusp Rounded projection of a tooth.

Cytes Cells.

Dactyly Related to the phalanges of the digits (fingers and toes).

Deep Further from the surface.

Delayed union When a fracture heals more slowly than expected.

Demi Half.

Depression Moving inferiorly.

Diarthroses Type of joint which is freely moveable; synovial joint.

Diastasis Separation, or widening, of a joint.

Dislocation Complete displacement of two bones in a joint; articular surfaces are no longer opposing.

Distal Further away from the attachment/origin; the lower end of a bone.

Dorsal The posterior (back) surface of the body.

Dorsiflexion Moving the foot superiorly at the ankle joint.

Dys Abnormal, difficult, painful.

Dysplasia Abnormal growth.

Dystrophy Abnormal activity of cells because of poor or defective nutrition.

Ecchymosis Bruising.

Edentulous Without teeth.

Effusion Abnormal fluid collection within a joint cavity.

Elastic cartilage Flexible type of cartilage which gives structure; not found in the skeleton or joints.

Elevation Moving superiorly.

Emphysema, subcutaneous Air or gas within the subcutaneous tissues.

Emphysema, surgical Air or gas within the subcutaneous tissues, as above but usually iatrogenic (because of surgical treatment/intervention).

Enchondroma A benign tumour of mature cartilage cells.

Endocrine Relating to hormones and the glands that produce them.

Endosteum Thin vascular membrane lining the inner, medullary surface of a long bone.

Enthesis Site of attachment of ligament or tendons on bone.

Enthesophyte Bony growth or ossification of the insertion of a ligament or tendon.

Epi Above, upon.

Epicondyle An elevation/projection of a bone above its condyle.

Epinephrine Hormone produced by the adrenal glands; previously known as adrenaline.

Epiphysis End of a long bone, upon the physeal growth plate, where bone growth occurs. The secondary ossification centre of long bones.

Epiphyseal plate Physeal plate or physis. Site of growth for the length of a bone; located between the metaphysis and epiphysis. Primary cartilaginous synchondrosis. Fuse at skeletal maturity.

Ewing's sarcoma Malignant primary bone tumour, usually affecting long bones or the pelvis of children and adolescents.

Exostosis Bone growth on the surface of the bone.

Extension Straightening of a joint. Increasing the angle between bones at a joint.

External Outside.

External rotation Turn outwards.

Eversion Moving externally/laterally, commonly the foot/ankle.

Facet Smooth flat area, often articular.

Fibroblastic Producing fibrous connective tissue.

Fibrocartilage Very strong type of cartilage that gives support and rigidity between bones.

Fibrosarcoma Malignant tumour of the fibroblasts in fibrous tissue.

Fibrous dysplasia Benign condition causing abnormal growth of fibrous tissue in place of normal bone.

Fibrous joint Bones joined by strong connective tissue with minimal/no movement; sutures, gomphoses, and syndesmoses.

Fissure Narrow slit.

Flexion Bending a joint; decreasing the angle between bones at a joint.

FOOSH Acronym standing for 'fall on outstretched hand.' A common mechanism of injury.

Foramen Hole; plural foramina.

Foreign body Any external substance or material that enters the body. Can cause infection or inflammation.

Fossa Wide depression or hollow.

Fragility fracture Caused by normal forces on abnormal bone (e.g. osteoporosis); insufficiency fracture.

Galeazzi's fracture Fracture of the distal third of radius with dislocation of the head of the ulna at the inferior radioulnar joint.

Genu Relating to the knee.

Genu valgus 'Knock knees.' Lateral bowing of the lower legs at the knee joints.

Genu Varus Medial bowing of the lower legs at the knee joints. Often seen in severe osteoarthritis.

Gigantism Excessive growth because of abnormal secretion of growth hormone by the pituitary gland.

Gingivitis Inflammation of gums.

Gliding Sliding; one articular surface sliding smoothly over another.

Glossal Relating to the tongue.

Gout A metabolic disorder and type of arthritis resulting in high uric acid levels in the blood and urate crystal in and surrounding joints; causes intense inflammation and pain.

Granulation tissue New connective tissue and blood vessels formed as part of the inflammatory and healing process of wounds and certain infections.

Greenstick fracture An incomplete fracture in children; one cortex of the bone fractures, the other buckles or bends.

Groove Uncovered passage.

Growth hormone Produced by the anterior pituitary gland. Influences the growth and replacement of bone.

Haem Pertaining to blood.

Haemarthrosis Collection of blood within a joint.

Haematogenous Carried by the blood.

Haematoma Abnormal collection of blood outside a vessel; normally traumatic.

Haematopoiesis The process of blood cell formation in red bone marrow.

Haemophilia Inherited disorder of blood clotting. Causes excessive bleeding, which can result in bleeding into joint cavities.

Haemothorax Blood in the pleural cavity, outside the lung.

Hallux The big toe.

Hallux valgus Lateral angulation of the great toe at its metatarsophalangeal joint.

Hamulus Hook-like projection.

Haversian canal Channel in the centre of a Haversian system containing blood, lymphatic vessels and nerves.

Haversian systems The microscopic structural units of compact bone. Also known as osteons.

Hemi One side/half of the body.

Hemivertebra Congenital abnormality causing one-half, or side, of a vertebra not to develop.

Heterogeneous Of different/non-uniform appearance, structure or composition.

Homeostasis Processes involved in ensuring a steady state, or equilibrium, within living tissue.

Homogeneous Of the same/uniform. appearance, structure or composition.

Hyaline cartilage Smooth, avascular connective tissue found on articular surfaces and from which most bones of the skeleton form.

Hydroxyapatite The main mineral salt that forms the hard inorganic matrix of bone made up of calcium and phosphate.

Hyper More, high, above normal.

Hyperparathyroidism Endocrine disorder causing overproduction of parathormone in the parathyroid glands; leads to increased absorption of calcium from bones into the blood.

Hypo Less, low, deficient.

Idiopathic Of unknown cause.

Ilizarov frame External fixation device used for complex fractures, particularly the lower leg.

Impacted One item pushed into another, or within itself; type of fracture.

Inferior Below; lower.

Inflammatory Relating to inflammation and the body's immune response.

Infra Below.

Inorganic Not living, or not containing carbon. In bone this relates specifically to the mineralised (e.g., calcium phosphate) components of the intercellular matrix.

Innervate Supply with nerves.

Innominate bone Hip bone or hemipelvis; comprised of the ilium, ischium and pubis.

Insufficiency fracture Caused by normal forces on abnormal bone (e.g., osteoporosis); fragility fracture.

Inter Between.

Intermediate Between two other structures.

Internal Inside.

Internal rotation Turn inwards.

Interstitial lamella The spaces between the Haversian systems in compact bone.

Intra Within.

Intracartilaginous ossification Main process of bone formation from a hyaline cartilage model of the bone.

Intramembranous ossification Process of bone formation from mesenchyme, particularly of bones of the cranium.

In utero In the womb; stage of growth of an embryo and foetus.

Inversion Moving internally/medially, commonly the foot/ankle.

Ipsilateral On the same side of the body.

Ischaemia Insufficient blood supply.

Kyphosis Anterior curve of the spine, concave anteriorly; usually used to describe excessive thoracic spine curvature.

Labial Relating to the lips.

Labrum Ring of fibrocartilage surrounding some articular surfaces to increase the congruity of a joint.

Lacunae Space between the lamellae of compact bone, contain osteocyte cells.

Lamellar Arranged in layers or plates, like layers of an onion.

Lamellae Microscopic rings of bone around a Haversian canal.

Lamina Thin plate; forms part of the vertebral arch of a vertebra.

Lateral Away from the midline of the body.

Leukaemia Cancer of leukocytes; uncontrolled production of immature white blood cells.

Leukocytes White blood cells.

Lipo Pertaining to fat.

Lipohaemarthrosis Collection of fat and blood within a joint cavity indicates an intra-articular fracture. Most common in the knee.

Line Long, low, narrow ridge.

Lingual Relating to the tongue; also referred to as glossal.

Lordosis Posterior curve of spine; concave posteriorly.

Macro Large.

Malignant Invasive, destructive and prone to spread (metastasise) to other tissues; cancer.

Malunion When a fracture heals to leave a residual deformity of the bone.

Matrix The intercellular system, or network, of structures between cells. In bone, this is a mixture of organic (osteoid) and inorganic mineralised material.

Meatus Narrow passage.

Mechanism of Injury (MoI) The method, manner, or force by which and injury occurred. A good predictor for the likely injuries sustained.

Medial Nearer the midline of the body.

Median sagittal plane (MSP) Dividing the body into left and right sides directly down the middle.

Megaly Abnormally enlarged.

Mesial Nearer the midline of the mouth. Alternative (less commonly used) term for medial.

Mesenchyme The embryonic framework of fibrous tissue from which all connective tissues, including the musculoskeletal system, form.

Metabolic Relating to metabolism, the physical and chemical processes within all living tissues;

in bone particularly relates to bone density and mineralisation.

Metaphysis Part of a long bone between the epiphysis (and physeal plate) and diaphysis.

Metastasis(e) A secondary tumour; spread to a site remote from the original, usually through blood or lymph vessels.

Monteggia's fracture Fracture of the proximal third of ulna with dislocation of the head of the radius.

MRI Magnetic resonance imaging. Uses non-ionising radiation, a magnet and radio waves to provide diagnostic images, particularly of soft tissue structures.

Multiaxial Movement round more than two axes/planes of the body.

Multipartite More than two parts.

Multiple Myeloma(tosis) Malignant tumour of the blood plasma cells in bone marrow.

NAI Non-accidental injury. Previously used term for suspected physical abuse.

Neural Relating to a nerve/the nervous system.

Neuralgia Pain in the region, or distribution, of a nerve.

Neuropathy Disease or pathologic condition of nerves; may cause pain, numbness, or weakness.

Neoplastic 'New growth'; relating to tumours (benign or malignant).

Non-union When the ends of a fractured bone fail to unite.

Notch Large groove.

Occlusal Biting edge of a tooth.

Occult Not visible on imaging.

Organic Living, or contains carbon. In bone this relates specifically to the collagenous protein components (osteoid) of the intercellular matrix.

Osgood–Schlatter's disease Fragmentation of the tibial tuberosity in adolescents.

Ossicle A tiny bone, usually refer to the auditory ossicles in the ear.

Ossification The formation of bone from connective tissue.

Osteo Relating to bone.

Osteoarthritis Degenerative joint disease; caused by degradation and thinning of articular hyaline cartilage. Informally known as 'wear and tear' arthritis.

Osteoblastoma Benign bone-forming tumour of the osteoblasts.

Osteoblasts Bone cells which build bone. Produce the organic osteoid matrix and initiate its mineralisation to the inorganic matrix.

Osteochondroma Benign tumour of bone and cartilage cells. Grows away from a bone, also known as an exostosis.

Osteochondrosis Osteonecrosis of the ossification centres of the immature skeleton.

Osteoclasts Bone cells which destroy, break down and shape bone.

Osteoclastoma Benign tumour of the osteoclasts; also known as a Giant-cell tumour.

Osteocytes Mature bone cells. Maintain bone tissue. Formed from osteoblasts.

Osteogenic cells Stem cell of bone; precursor to osteoblasts.

Osteoid The collagenous, organic, uncalcified matrix of bone. Predominantly collagen.

Osteology Study of bones.

Osteolytic Area of bone loss, destruction, or reduced density.

Osteoma Benign bone-forming tumour on the bone surface involving the osteoblast cells; exostosis.

Osteomalacia Decrease of bone mineralisation and bone softening because of lack of vitamin D; the adult form of Rickets.

Osteomyelitis Infection of bone.

Osteon The microscopic structural units of compact bone. Also known as Haversian systems.

Osteonecrosis Ischaemic loss of blood supply to bone leading to the death of the bone tissue; previously referred to as avascular necrosis.

Osteopaenia Reduction in bone density or mineralisation by any cause.

Osteopetrosis 'Marble bones.' Rare, hereditary metabolic condition causing a deficiency of osteoclast activity resulting in an increase in immature bone, density and fragility.

Osteophyte Spur, or outgrowth, of bone adjacent to a joint surface. Common in osteoarthritis.

Osteoporosis 'Porous bones.' Loss of mineralised inorganic bone matrix causing reduced bone density and insufficiency (fragility) fractures.

Osteosarcoma Malignant tumour of bone, usually arising from osteoblasts so bone-forming tumour.

Osteosclerosis Increase in bone density and mineralisation by any cause. Opposite of osteopaenia.

Paget disease of bone Also known as 'osteitis deformans.' Metabolic disease causing altered bone remodelling, typically with enlarged, deformed, sclerotic and weak bones.

Palatal Related to the palate.

Palmar Relating to the palm/anterior/volar aspect of the hand.

Paraesthesia Abnormal sensation, e.g., tingling, 'pins and needles.'

Parathyroid hormone/ Parathormone Hormone produced in the parathyroid glands. Involved in calcium homeostasis by increasing the rate of bone resorption by osteoclasts.

Pathology Study of disease.

Pathological fracture Caused by any underlying pathologic condition, e.g., tumour or osteoporosis.

Pathophysiology The study of the structural and functional changes caused by a disease/ pathologic condition, i.e., what it actually does to the body.

Pedunculated Attached by a stalk.

Periodontal Around a tooth; relating to the structures surrounding the teeth.

Periosteum Fibrous membrane, which covers bone surfaces, except the articular surfaces.

Perthes disease Osteochondrosis of the head of the femur epiphysis; leads to flattening, sclerosis and growth disturbance. Full name is Legg-Calve-Perthes disease.

Pes planus Flat foot, loss of the longitudinal arch of the foot.

PET Positron emission tomography, imaging method using radiopharmaceuticals to demonstrate functional information of an abnormality.

PET-CT Combining (or fusing) PET and CT images to demonstrate accurate anatomical and functional information of an abnormality.

Plantar Relating to the sole of the foot.

Plantar flexion Moving the foot inferiorly at the ankle joint (pointing the toes).

Pneumothorax Air in the pleural cavity, outside the lung.

Pollex The thumb.

Poly More; multiple.

Polydactyly More than the normal number of digits.

Posterior Nearer the back of the body.

Process Localised projection.

Pronation Rotating the arm internally, so the palm faces posteriorly; or the foot by rotating the plantar aspect (sole) laterally/externally.

Prone Lying on the anterior (front) of the body.

Prosthesis Artificial replacement, such as a joint replacement.

Proximal Closer to the attachment/origin; the upper end of a bone.

Pseudo False; resembling something else.

Radiculopathy Symptoms radiated by an abnormality of the root of a nerve. Symptoms usually remote from the nerve route, including pain, weakness and paraesthesia.

Radiolucent Appears darker/less opaque on X-ray/CT.

Radiopaque Appears brighter, or sclerotic, on X-ray/CT.

Remodelling The continuous turnover of bone by resorption and deposition by osteoclasts and osteoblasts, a process in equilibrium in normal bone.

Rheumatoid arthritis Chronic autoimmune inflammatory disease causing, amongst other systemic problems, inflammation and deformity of joints.

Rickets Decrease in bone mineralisation of the paediatric skeleton; similar to osteomalacia in adults.

Sagittal plane Dividing the body into left and right on either side of the median sagittal plane.

Sclerotic Denser; brighter. Increase in bone.

Sciatica Paraesthesia/pain relating to the sciatic nerve, usually round the buttock, hip or thigh.

Septic arthritis Infection within a joint.

Sesamoid bones Bones that develop in tendons, usually found around a joint.

Sessile Attached by a broad base.

Sharpey's fibres Strong connective collagen tissue which connects soft tissues to bone.

Sinus Hollow cavity; channel.

Skeletal maturity Fusion of the epiphyseal growth plates of a bone/the skeleton.

Smith's fracture Fracture of the distal end of the radius with anterior displacement of the distal fragment. Also known as reverse Colle's fracture.

SPECT Single-photon emission computed tomography, demonstrates functional abnormality. Similar principle to PET; cheaper but poorer image quality.

SPECT-CT Combining (or fusing) SPECT and CT images to demonstrate anatomical and functional information of an abnormality.

Spina bifida Incomplete fusion of the neural/vertebral arches or neural tube *in utero*.

Spine Long process; the vertebral column.

Spondyl Relating to a vertebra.

Spondylolisthesis Displacement of one vertebra on another, anterior or posterior.

Spondylolysis Fracture (acute or chronic) of the pars interarticularis of a vertebra.

Squamous Scale-like; thin, flat.

Sub Below; under.

Subchondral sclerosis Increased bone density and thickening deep to articular cartilage in a joint. Usually a response to degenerative disease.

Subluxation Incomplete or partial dislocation. Articular surfaces displaced but still partly opposing.

Sulcus Groove or furrow.

Superficial Closer to the surface.

Superior Above; towards the head.

Supination Rotating the arm externally, so the palm faces anteriorly, or the foot by internally rotating the plantar aspect (sole) medially.

Supine Lying on the posterior (back) surface of the body.

Supra Above; on top of.

Synarthroses Joints which demonstrate very minimal/no movement.

Syndesmophyte Ossification of the ligaments and intervertebral discs of the spine.

Synostosis Fusion of adjacent bones into one.

Synovial joint Bones are separated by a cavity and surrounded by a capsule lined with a synovial membrane; diarthroses, allow movement.

Trabeculae Lattice of thin columns of bone tissue making up cancellous bone.

Trochanter Large, rounded elevation. Specifically of the proximal femur.

Trochlea Pulley-shaped surface.

Tubercle Small, rounded elevation.

Tuberculosis Contagious infection caused by the Mycobacterium tuberculosis; predominantly affects the lungs but can affect any system, including bones.

Tuberosity Large, rounded elevation.

Uniaxial Movement round one axis/plane of the body.

Valgus Abnormal angulation at a joint where the distal bone is angled laterally.

Varus Abnormal angulation at a joint where the distal bone is angled medially.

Vascular Relating to or containing blood vessels.

Ventral The anterior (front) surface of the body.

Volar The anterior (front) surface of the body, especially the hand.

Volkmann's canals Connect adjoining Haversian canals and contain nerves and blood, and lymphatic vessels.

Woven bone Immature irregular matrix of new bone tissue formed as part of early fracture healing; provisional callus.

INDEX

Page numbers followed by "*f*" indicate figures, "*t*" indicate tables, and "*b*" indicate boxes.

A

Abduction, 16
Abscess, tooth, 356*b*
Accessory ligaments, 15
Acetabular fossa, 20
Acetabular fractures, 212
Acetabular labrum, 207
Acetabular notch, 20
Acetabulum, 198, 201, 201*f*
Achilles tendon, 183*f*
Achondroplasia, 53
ACL. *See* Anterior cruciate ligament (ACL)
Acromegaly, 53, 53*f*
Acromial angle of scapula, 105
Acromial end of clavicle, 102
Acromioclavicular joint (AC joint), 122–124
  right acromioclavicular joint, 122*f*, 123*f*, 124*f*
  trauma, 123*b*
  type, 122–123
    blood supply, 123
    bony articular surfaces, 122
    fibrous capsule, 122
    intracapsular structure, 122–123
    movements, 123
    nerve supply, 123
    supporting ligaments, 122
    synovial membrane, 122
Acromioclavicular ligament, 122
Acromion fractures, 110*b*
Acromion process, 105, 110

Additive diseases, 33
Adduction, 16
Adductor tubercle of femur, 129
Adrenal glands, 54–56
Age, fracture healing and, 26–27
Alae of vomer, 333
Alveolar process, 325
Alveolar ridge of mandible, 349
Amphiarthroses, 19
Anatomical neck of humerus, 63
Androgens, 54
Angle of mandible, 349
Ankle joint, 179–188
  achilles tendon, 183*f*
  fractures, 184*b*
  left ankle joint, 179*f*
  maisonneuve injury, 186*f*
  ossification centres around ankle, 182*f*
  pilon fracture, 187*f*
  pilon fracture right ankle, 188*f*
  right ankle joint, 181*f*, 183*f*
  type, 179–182
    blood supply, 179
    bony articular surfaces, 180–181
    fibrous capsule, 181
    movements, 182
    nerve supply, 179
    supporting ligaments, 182
    synovial membrane, 181–182
  Weber classification of ankle fractures, 185*f*
Ankylosing spondylitis, 38–39, 38*f*, 39*f*
Ankylosis, 37

Annular ligament, of elbow joint, 86
Annulus fibrosus, 278
Anterior, definition of, 12
Anterior angle, of parietal bones, 311
Anterior arch, 1st (atlas) cervical vertebrae, 252
Anterior atlantooccipital membrane, 277
Anterior border
  of fibula, 144
  ilium, 199
  of lacrimal bones, 331
  of parietal bones, 310
  of radius, 71
  of tibia, 143
  of ulna, 72
  of vomer, 333
Anterior compression
  fracture, 289*b*–293*b*, 290*f*
  injury, 203–204
    of pelvis, 203*f*
    3D CT image, 204*f*
Anterior cruciate ligament (ACL), 168
  tears, 176, 177*f*
Anterior dislocation of shoulder joint, 116–118, 116*b*, 116*f*
Anterior inferior iliac spine (AIIS), 199
Anterior longitudinal ligament, 278
Anterior oblique ligament, 97
Anterior sternoclavicular ligaments, 125
Anterior superior iliac spine (ASIS), 199

Anterior surface, 152
　of ethmoid bone, 320–324
　of femur, 129
　of maxillae, 325
　of radius, 71
　of ulna, 72
Anterior talofibular
　　ligament, 182
Anterior tubercle, 252
Antero-lateral surface, 65
Antero-medial surface, 65
Apex of patella, 136
Apical foramen, teeth, 353
Apophyseal joint osteoarthritis.
　　See Facet joint
　　osteoarthritis
Apophyseal joints. *See*
　　Facet
Apophysis, 7
Appendicular skeleton, 8
Arches of foot, 157–158
Arcuate line, 200
Arcuate popliteal
　　ligament, 168
Arcuate pubic ligament, 220
Arthritis, 57–61
　gout, 61
　osteoarthritis, 59–60
　rheumatoid, 60–61
　septic, 56
Arthrology, 14
Arthroses, 14
Articular (hyaline) cartilage,
　　14, 15*f*
Articular fat pads, 16
Articular surfaces of sternocostal
　　joints, 233
Articulating bones, 14–15
Atlantooccipital joints, 277
Atlas, 251*f*, 252
Atypical ribs, 230–232
　first rib, 230, 231*f*
　　eleventh and twelfth rib,
　　　230–232
　　tenth rib, 230
　　second rib, 230, 231*f*

Auricular, definition of, 11
Auricular facet, 270
Auricular surface, 200
Avascular necrosis, 35
Avulsion fractures, 22, 206
Axial skeleton, 8
Axis, 252–254, 252*f*

B

Ball and socket joints,
　　synovial, 18
Benign bone tumours, 33
Bennett's fracture-dislocation, 98
Bicipital groove, 63
Bicondylar joints, synovial, 17
Bifurcate ligament, 189
Blood supply, 5, 27
　of AC joint, 123
　of ankle joint, 179
　of bones, 5
　of carpometacarpal joint, 98
　of distal tibiofibular joint, 179
　of elbow joint, 86
　of intertarsal joints, 189
　of knee joint, 169
　of MTPJs and IPJs, 100
　of proximal tibiofibular
　　joint, 178
　of SC joint, 125
　of shoulder joint, 115
　of sternocostal joints, 233
　of wrist joint, 93
Blood vessels, 5, 15
Blowout fracture, 338
　blowout fracture right
　　orbit, 339*f*
Body, 221
　hyoid bone, 361
　ischium, 200
　pubis, 201
　of scapula, 105
　of sphenoid bone, 319
　　anterior clinoid processes,
　　　319
　　anterior surface, 319
　　inferior surface, 319

Body *(Continued)*
　　lateral surfaces, 319
　　middle clinoid
　　　processes, 319
　　superior surface, 319
Body fractures of scapula, 110,
　　110*b*
Bone
　development of, 5–8, 7*f*
　　ossification, 5–8
　function of, 1
　normal' radiographic
　　appearances of, 9–11, 10*f*
　structure of, 1–5, 3*f*
　　blood supply, 5
　　bone marrow, 4
　　cancellous bone, 4
　　compact bone, 2–5
　　nerve supply, 5
　terminology, 11–13
　　elevations and projections,
　　　11–13
　　holes or depressions, 12
　　terms associated with
　　　teeth, 13
　types of, 8–9
　　flat bones, 9
　　irregular bones, 9
　　long bones, 8
　　sesamoid bones, 9
　　short bones, 8–9
Bone cells, 1, 5
Bone density
　increase in, 33–37
　　osteonecrosis, 35–37
　　Paget's disease, 33–35
　loss of, 30–33
　　osteomalacia and rickets,
　　　30–33
　　osteoporosis, 30
Bone destruction, 33
Bone growth, 37–39
　ankylosing spondylitis, 38–39
Bone marrow, 4–5
Bone matrix, 2
Bone metastases, 47*f*

Bone poverty, 30
Bone production process, 1
Bone tissue, 5
Bone tuberculosis, 56
Bone tumours, 40, 49–51
  benign, 33
  lytic metastasis from breast
    cancer, 50f
  malignant, 33
  metastases, 50f
  sclerotic metastases from
    prostate cancer, 49f
Bony articular surfaces
  of AC joint, 122
  of ankle joint, 180–181
  of atlantooccipital joints, 277
  of carpometacarpal joint, 97
  of costotransverse joints, 283
  of costovertebral joints, 283
  of distal tibiofibular joint, 178
  of elbow joint, 83
  of interphalangeal joints and
    metatarsophalangeal
    joints, 192
  of intertarsal joints, 188–189
  of intervertebral joints, 278
  of knee joint, 165
  of median atlantoaxial joint, 277
  of MTPJs and IPJs, 99
  of proximal tibiofibular
    joint, 178
  of sacroiliac joints, 217
  of SC joint, 124
  of shoulder joint, 113
  of vertebral arches joints, 281
  of wrist joint, 91
Bony labyrinth, 316
Brodie's abscess, 57
Brown's tumours, 54
Buccal/labial, definition of, 13
Buckle fracture of ulna, 74
  fractures, 74b
'Bunion', 164
Bursae, 16
Burst fracture, 286b–287b
  of L1, 291f

C
Calcaneal tuberosity, 152
Calcaneocuboid joint, 188
Calcaneofibular ligament, 182
Calcaneus, 151–153, 155
  fractures, 162, 162b
  right calcaneum, 153f
Calcitonin, 6, 53
Calcium, 6
Canal, definition of, 12
Canaliculi, 2–4
Cancellous bone, 2, 4, 9
Canines, 354
Capitate, 77–78, 77b
Capitulum of humerus, 65
Capsular ligaments, 14–15
Capsule, fibrous, 277
Caries, dental, 356
Carotid canal, 315
Carotid sulcus, 319
Carpal bones, 77–78
Carpometacarpal joints (CMC
    joints), 97–99
  fractures, 98b
  Rolando fracture, 98f
  type, 97–99
    blood supply, 98
    bony articular surfaces, 97
    fibrous capsule, 97
    movements, 97–98
    nerve supply, 98–99
    supporting ligaments, 97
    synovial membrane, 97
Carrying angle of elbow joint,
    86–87
Cartilage, 14
  cells, 7
Cartilaginous joints, 14,
    19–20
  types of, 19–20
    symphyses, 19–20
    synchondroses, 19
Cement, teeth, 353
Central Haversian canal, 2
Cerebral surface, 319
Cervical curve, 275

Cervical rib, 237
  bilateral, 237f
Cervical vertebrae, 245–257
  1st (atlas), 251–252, 251f
    ossification, 252
  2nd (axis), 252–254
    ossification, 253–254
  3rd to 6th (typical), 245–247
  7th (vertebra prominens), 257
  cervical spine, 250f
  fifth cervical vertebra, 249f
  lateral projection, 248f
  paediatric cervical
    spine, 251f
  sagittal T2W MRI, 249f
  third to seventh, 247f
  upper, 254f, 255f
  upper cervical spine, 256f
Chondrocytes, 14, 20
Chondroitin, 20
Chondrosarcoma, 45–48
Circumduction, 16
Circumferential lamellae, 4
Clavicle, 102–105
  ossification, 103–105
    primary centres, 103
    secondary centres,
      103–105
  radiographic appearances
    of, 103
    left clavicle, 103f
    left clavicle fracture, 104f
    right clavicle fracture, 104f
  right clavicle, 103f
Cleft palate, 326
Clinoid process
  anterior, 319
  middle, 319
Clivus, 313, 319
Closed fracture, 22
Closed manipulation, 24
CMC joints. See
    Carpometacarpal joints
    (CMC joints)
Coccyx, 270–275, 273f
Cochlea, 316

Colles' fracture of wrist joint, 95, 95*b*

Comminuted fracture, 22
  of patella, 139

Compact bone, 2–5

Compound (open) fracture, 22

Compression fracture, 22

Computed tomography (CT), 27, 41, 110, 132–134, 203, 226, 286, 322

Conchae, nasal, 341

Condylar fossa, 313

Condylar process, 349

Condyle, definition of, 11

Connective tissue membrane, 8

Conoid tubercle of clavicle, 102

Coracoacromial ligament, 122

Coracoclavicular ligaments, 122

Coracohumeral ligament, 114

Coracoid process, 110, 110*b*
  of scapula, 107

Coronal suture, 310

Coronoid fossa of humerus, 65

Coronoid process, 349
  of ulna, 72

Cortex, 9

Cortisol, 54

Costal cartilages, 232–233

Costal tuberosity of clavicle, 102

Costoclavicular ligament, 125

Costotransverse joints, 283–284, 285*f*

Costotransverse ligament, 283

Costovertebral joints, 283–284, 284*f*, 285*f*

Cranial bones, 324*f*

Cranial fractures, 322
  comminuted depressed skull fracture, 322*f*
  depressed skull fracture with extradural haematoma, 323*f*

Cranium, 299
  individual bones of, 308–324

Crest, definition of, 11

Cribriform plate, 321

Crista galli, 321

Crown, teeth, 353

Cuboid, 151, 153–155

Cuneiform bones, 153

Curvatures, vertebral, 275–277

Cushing's syndrome, 56

Cusps, definition of, 13

Cysts, bone, 43, 45*f*

D

Deciduous teeth, 355

Degenerative disc disease, 294*b*–297*b*, 294*f*, 295*f*

Degenerative joint disease, 59

Deltoid tuberosity of humerus, 65

Dense bone. *See* Compact bone

Dental caries, 356

Dental formulae, 355–356

Dental pulp, teeth, 353

Dentine, teeth, 353

Dentition, 355

Depressed fracture, 22

Descending process of lacrimal bones, 331

Destructive diseases, 30

Development, of bones, 5–8

Developmental dysplasia of hip (DDH), 214–216, 215*f*

Diabetic foot complications, 164

Diaphysis, 6, 7*f*

Diarthroses. *See* Synovial joints

Dislocation
  of AC joint, 123
  of elbow, 85*b*
  of shoulder joint
    anterior, 116–118
    posterior, 118–119
    recurrent, 116
  of vertebral column, 240*b*
  of wrist, 16*b*

Dislocation, 27

Distal, definition of, 12–13

Distal epiphysis of tibia, 143

Distal row, 153–155

Distal surface of radius, 71

Distal tibiofibular joint, 178–179, 179*b*
  type, 178–179
    blood supply, 179
    bony articular surfaces, 178
    movements, 178
    nerve supply, 179
    strengthening ligaments, 178

Dorsal, definition of, 12

Dorsal and palmar (pvolar) radioulnar ligaments, 93

Dorsal radiocarpal ligament, 93

Dorsal sacral foramina, 269

Dorsal sacroiliac ligament, 218

Dorsal surface, 269–270

Dorsoradial ligament, 97

Dorsum sellae, 319

Down's syndrome, 330

Dual-energy X-ray absorptiometry (DXA/DEXA), 30

E

Elastic cartilage, 20

Elbow dislocation, 89
  trauma, 89*b*

Elbow joint, 83–91, 84*f*
  left elbow joint, 84*f*, 85*f*, 87*f*
  right elbow, 88*f*
    dislocation, 90*f*
  type, 83–87
    blood supply, 86
    bony articular surfaces, 83
    carrying angle, 86–87
    fibrous capsule, 85
    intracapsular structures, 85–86
    movements, 86
    nerve supply, 86
    supporting ligaments, 86
    synovial membrane, 85

Ellipsoid joints, synovial, 17

Enamel, teeth, 353

Enchondroma, 41

Endocrine, 51–56
Endosteum, 4–5
Ensthesophytes, 37
Epicondyle, definition of, 11
Epinephrine, 54
Epiphyseal cartilage, 5
Epiphyseal plate, 7, 9
Epiphyses, 7
Ethmoid bone, 299, 318,
    320–324, 321f, 336
  cribriform plate, 321
  ethmoidal labyrinths, 321–322
  ossification, 322–324
  perpendicular plate, 321
Ethmoidal air cells, 321
Ethmoidal process, 331
Ethmoidal sinuses, 344
Ewing's sarcoma, 44–45, 48f
Exostosis, 37
Extension, 16
Extensor hoods, 99
External, definition of, 12
External rotation, 16
External surface
  of frontal bone, 309
  ilium, 200
  of mandible, 349
  of nasal bones, 329
  of occipital bone, 311
  of parietal bones, 310
Extradural hematoma, 317

F
Fabella, 5, 169
Face, 299
  individual bones of, 324–336
Facet, 241
  definition of, 11
  for first costal cartilage of
      clavicle, 102
  joint osteoarthritis, 294b–297b
  of patella
    for lateral condyle of
        femur, 136
    for medial condyle of
        femur, 136

Facial bones, 299–300
  imaging appearances of,
      333–336
  occipitomental projection, 333f
  3D CT image, 334f
Fall on outstretched hand
    (FOOSH), 67
Femoral head, necrosis of, 35
Femur, 127–136
  features of distal end of, 129
  features of proximal end of,
      127–130
    right femur, 128f
  features of shaft (diaphysis)
      of, 129
  ossification, 129–130, 130f
    fractures, 132b
    left femur, 130f, 131f, 132f
    neck of right femur
        fracture, 133f
    right femur midshaft
        fracture, 136f
    subtle neck, 134f
Fibroblastic granulation tissue, 26
Fibrocartilage, 16, 20
Fibrous capsule, 14–15, 15f
  of AC joint, 122
  of ankle joint, 181
  of atlantooccipital joints, 277
  of carpometacarpal joint, 97
  of costotransverse joints, 283
  of costovertebral joints, 283
  of elbow joint, 85
  of interphalangeal and
      metatarsophalangeal
      joints, 192
  of knee joint, 165
  of median atlantoaxial joint, 278
  of MTPJs and IPJs, 99
  of proximal tibiofibular joint, 178
  of sacroiliac joints, 217
  of SC joint, 125
  of shoulder joint, 113
  of sternocostal joints, 233
  of vertebral arches joints, 281
  of wrist joint, 91

Fibrous connective tissue
    membranes, 5
Fibrous gomphosis joints, 353
Fibrous joints, 18–19
  types of, 18–19
    gomphoses, 18–19
    sutures, 18
    syndesmoses, 19
Fibrous sutures, 299
Fibula, 144–150
  features of distal end of, 144
  features of proximal
      end of, 144
  features of shaft of, 144
  ossification, 144–145
    fractures, 147b–148b
    lateral tibial plateau fracture,
        148f, 149f
    left tibia and fibula, 145f,
        146f
Fibular collateral ligament, 168
Fibular notch of tibia, 143
First carpometacarpal joint,
    97–99
Fissure
  definition of, 12
  pterygoid, 320
Flail chest, 236
Flat bones, 9
Flexion, 16
Focal bone destruction, 33
Foot, 150–164
  individual bones, 151–153
    ossification, 155
  metatarsal bones, 150–164
    ossification, 156
  phalanges, 156–158
    ossification, 157
  right foot, 150f
  tarsal bones, 151–153
Foramen, definition of, 12
Foramen lacerum, anterior
    border of, 319
Foramen magnum, 311
Foramen ovale, 319
Foramen rotundum, 319

Foramen spinosum, 319
Foramen transversarium,
     1st (atlas) cervical
     vertebrae, 252
Foramina, 321
Forefoot, 150
Foreign bodies, in fractures, 26
Fossa, definition of, 12
Fossa for lacrimal sac, 331
Fovea of femur, 127
Fractures, 21–22, 67b
  acetabulum, 203b
  ankle joint, 184b
  carpometacarpal joint, 98b
  causes, 22
  of clavicle, 104b
  compound (open), 22
  cranium, 322b–323b
  describing traumatic injuries, 28
  dislocation, 289b–293b
  of femur, 132b
  fibula, 147b–148b
  healing, 26–27
    factors influencing rate of
      healing, 26–27
  joint/soft tissue injuries, 27–28
  mandible, 351b
  orbital cavity, 338b
  orthopaedic management
    of, 23–26
    diagnosis, 23
    immobilisation, 24
    reduction, 24
    rehabilitation, 24
  patella, 139b
  phalanges, 162b
  of scapula, 110b
  simple (closed), 22
  sternum, 226b
    minimally displaced
      transverse sternal
      fracture, 226f
  tarsometatarsal joints, 190b
  types of, 22–23, 22b
  of ulna, 68b
  vomer, 334b–335b

Fractures *(Continued)*
  wrist joint, 91–97
  of zygomatic arch, 99
Frontal bone, 299, 308–310,
    308f, 309f, 321, 324, 336
  ossification, 309
Frontal crest, of frontal bone, 322
Frontal process, 325
Frontal process of zygomatic
    bones, 327
Frontal sinuses, 309, 341, 343
Funnel chest. *See* Pectus
    excavatum
Fused epiphyseal plate, 9
Fusion, of bones, 8

G
Galeazzi fracture-dislocation of
    ulna, 76, 76f
Giant cell tumour, 43
Gigantism, 53
Glabella, of frontal bone, 309
Glenohumeral ligaments, 114
Glenoid cavity of scapula,
    105, 107
Glenoid labrum, 114
  abnormal, 116b
  tears of shoulder joint,
    118f, 119
Gliding, 16, 281
Gluteal surface, ilium, 200
Gluteal tuberosity of femur, 129
Gomphoses, 18–19
Gout, 61, 62f, 192, 192b
Granular foveolae, of frontal
    bone, 322–323
Greater cornua, hyoid bone, 361
Greater pelvis, 194
Greater sciatic notch, 199
Greater trochanter of femur, 128
Greater tuberosity of humerus, 63
Greater wings, of ethmoid bone,
    319–320
Greenstick fracture, 22
Greenstick fracture, of ulna, 74
  of humerus, 74b

Groove
  definition of, 12
  horizontal, 311
  for ulnar nerve, 65
  vertical, 322
Growth, of bones, 2
Growth hormone, 6

H
Haematogenous
    spread, 57
Haematopoiesis process, 4
Haemopneumothorax, 234
Haemothorax, 234
Hallux valgus, 164
Hamate, 77–78, 77b
Hamulus
  definition of, 11
  pterygoid, 320
Hand, 77–83
  carpal bones, 77–78
  fracture of, 79b
  metacarpal bones, 78–79
  phalanges, 79–81
Hangman's fracture of C2 (axis)
    vertebra, 286b–287b,
    288f, 289f
Haversian canal, 2, 3f
Haversian systems, 2–4, 26
Head
  of femur, 127
  of fibula, 144
  of humerus, 63
  of mandible, 349
  of radius, 68
  of scapula, 105
  of ulna, 71–72
Hemipelvis, 194
Hindfoot, 150
Hinge joints, synovial, 17
Hip bone, 198–206
  acetabulum, 201
  ilium, 198–199
  ischium, 200
  ossification, 201–206
  pubis, 200–206

Hip joint, 206–217, 208*f*
blood supply, 208
bony articular surfaces, 206
fibrous capsule, 206–207
imaging appearances of,
209–217
left hip joint, anteroposterior
projection, 209*f*
left hip joint, lateral
projection, 209*f*
left hip joint, T1W axial
MRI, 210*f*
left hip joint; 11 T1W coronal
MRI, 210*f*
intracapsular structures,
207–208
left hip joint, 207*f*
movements, 208
nerve supply, 209
supporting ligaments, 207
synovial membrane, 207
HLA-B27, 38
Hoffa's fat pad, 168
Horizontal groove, 311
Horizontal plate of palatine
bones, 328–329
anterior border, 328
lateral border, 328
medial border, 329
nasal surface, 328
palatine surface, 328
posterior border, 328
Hormone disturbances
adrenal glands, 54–56
parathyroid glands, 54
pituitary gland, 53
thyroid gland, 53
Humerus, 63–68
features of distal end of, 65
features of proximal end
of, 63–65
features of shaft (diaphysis)
of, 63–65
right humerus, 64*f*
Hyaline cartilage, 5, 14, 19–20,
233

Hydroxyapatite, 2, 6
Hyoid bone, 300, 361–362
3DCT image, 362*f*
imaging appearances of, 362
ossification, 361–362
Hyperparathyroidism, 54,
54*f*, 55*f*
Hypertrophy, 7
Hypoglossal canal, 313
Hypothyroidism, 53

I

Iliac crest, 199
Iliac fossa, 200
Iliac tuberosity, 200
Iliofemoral ligament, 207
Iliopubic eminence, 200
Ilium, 198–199
left hip bone, 198*f*, 199*f*
Imaging appearances of bones
of cranium, 322
Immobilisation, of fractures,
23–24, 26
Impacted fracture, 22
Incisors, 354
Incus, 315
Individual bones, 151–153
distal row, 153–155
intermediate row, 153–155
proximal row, 151–153
Infection, in fractures, 26
Inferior, definition, 12
Inferior angle of scapula, 105
Inferior articular facets, 241
1st (atlas) cervical
vertebrae, 252
3rd to 6th (typical) cervical
vertebrae, 246
L1-L4 (typical) lumbar
vertebrae, 263
T2-T8 (typical) thoracic
vertebrae, 258
Inferior articular processes,
typical vertebra, 242
Inferior articular surface of
tibia, 143

Inferior border, 329
of inferior nasal conchae,
332
of lacrimal bones, 331
of nasal bones, 330
of vomer, 333
Inferior lateral angle, 270
Inferior meatus, 341
Inferior nasal conchae, 299, 324,
331–332, 341
lateral aspect, 332*f*
ossification, 332
Inferior orbital fissure, 336
posterolateral border of, 319
Inferior ramus, 201
Inferior surface, 152
of vomer, 333
Inferior thoracic aperture, 221
Inferior tibiofibular joint, 19
Infraglenoid tubercle of
scapula, 107
Infraorbital groove, 336
Infrapatellar bursae, 166
Infrapatellar fat pad, 168
Infraspinatus tendon, 114
Infraspinous fossa of scapula, 105
Infratemporal surface of
Maxillae, 325
Inner ear, 316
Innominate bones. *See*
Hip bone
Inorganic mineral salts, 2
Inorganic mineralized
component, 1
Interchondral joints, 233
articular surfaces, 233
movements, 233
Interclavicular ligament, 125
Intercondylar notch/fossa of
femur, 129
Intercuneiform joints, 189
Intermediate cuneiform, 151
Intermediate row, 153–155
Intermediate sacral crests, 269
Intermetatarsal ligaments,
190, 192

Internal, definition of, 12
Internal mammary arteries, 125
Internal occipital crest, 311
Internal rotation, 16
Internal surface
    of frontal bone, 309
    ilium, 200
    of mandible, 349
    of nasal bones, 329
    of occipital bone, 311
    of parietal bones, 310
Interosseous border
    of fibula, 144
    of radius, 71
    of tibia, 143
    of ulna, 72
Interosseous talocalcaneal
        ligament, 189
Interphalangeal joints (IPJs),
        99–100, 100f, 192–193
    trauma, 100b–101b
    type, 99–100, 192–193
        blood supply, 100
        bony articular surfaces,
            99, 192
        fibrous capsule, 99, 192
        movements, 99–100, 193
        nerve supply, 100, 193
        supporting ligaments, 99,
            192–193
        synovial membrane, 99, 192
        volar plate avulsion
            fracture, 101f
Interpubic fibrocartilage disc, 220
Interspinous ligaments, 281
Interstitial lamellae, 4
Intertarsal joints, 188–190
    type, 188–190
        blood supply, 189
        bony articular surfaces,
            188–189
        joint capsules, 189
        movements, 189
        nerve supply, 189
        supporting ligaments, 189
Intertransverse ligaments, 281

Intertrochanteric crest of
        femur, 128
Intertrochanteric fracture of femur,
        132b, 134–135, 135f
Intertrochanteric line of
        femur, 128
Intertubercular sulcus of
        humerus, 63
Intervertebral disc, 278
Intervertebral disc herniation,
        294b–297b
Intervertebral foramen, 3rd to
        6th (typical) cervical
        vertebrae, 246
Intervertebral foramina, 243
Intervertebral joints, 278–280, 280f
Intra-articular fracture, 22
Intra-articular ligament, 283
Intracapsular structure
    of AC joint, 122–123
    of elbow joint, 85–86
    of intervertebral joints, 278
    of knee joint, 168
    of SC joint, 125
    of shoulder joint, 114
    of wrist joint, 93
Intracartilaginous ossification, 6–8
Intramembranous ossification,
        8, 309, 311
Intrinsic ligaments, 92–93
Irregular bones, 9
Ischial ramus, 200
Ischial spine, 200
Ischial tuberosity, 200
Ischiofemoral ligament, 207
Ischium, 200

J
Jefferson fracture. *See* Burst
        fracture
Joint capsules
    of intertarsal joints, 189
    of tarsometatarsal joints, 190
Joint cavity, 9
Joint space narrowing, 59–60
Joint structures, 15–16

Joints, 14
    cartilaginous joints
        (amphiarthroses), 19–20
    fibrous joints (synarthroses),
        18–19
    synovial joints (diarthroses),
        14–16
Joints, movements of, 16–18
Jugular foramen, 302f
Jugular notch, 221–222, 313
Jugular process, 313
Jugular tubercle, 313

K
Kienbock's disease, 35
Knee joint, 17, 164–178, 165b
    advanced osteoarthritis, 175f
    left knee joint, 167f
    osteochondritis dissecans,
        176f
    right, 165f, 166f, 171f, 172f,
        173f, 174f
        anteroposterior projection,
            169f
    right tibia, 167f
    type, 164–169
        blood supply, 169
        bony articular surfaces, 165
        fabella, 169
        fibrous capsule, 165
        intracapsular structures,
            168
        movements, 168–169
        nerve supply, 169
        supporting ligaments and
            tendons, 168
        synovial membrane,
            165–168
Kyphosis, 275

L
Labial, definition of, 13
Labrum, 16
Lacrimal bones, 300, 320, 324,
        331, 336
    ossification, 331

Lacrimal groove, 336
Lacrimal hamulus, 331
Lacrimal process, 331
Lacunae, 2
Lambda, of parietal bones, 311
Lambdoid suture, 310–311
Lamellae, 2
Lamellar, 44–45
Lamina, 3rd to 6th (typical) cervical vertebrae, 246
Lamina, definition of, 11
Lamina dura, 354
Laminae, L1-L4 (typical) lumbar vertebrae, 262
Laminae, T2-T8 (typical) thoracic vertebrae, 258
Laminae, typical vertebra, 242
Lateral, definition of, 12
Lateral (axillary) border of scapula, 105
Lateral border, 270
  of nasal bones, 330
Lateral collateral ligament, 99, 182, 192
Lateral compression injury, 205–206
  of pelvis, 205f
  3D CT image, 206f
Lateral condyle
  of femur, 136
  of tibia, 143
Lateral cuneiform, 151
Lateral epicondyle
  of femur, 129
  of humerus, 65
Lateral ligaments, 358
Lateral longitudinal arch, 157
Lateral malleolus of fibula, 144
Lateral masses, 1st (atlas) cervical vertebrae, 252
Lateral sacral crests, 269
Lateral semilunar cartilage, 168
Lateral supracondylar line of femur, 129
Lateral supracondylar ridge of humerus, 65

Lateral surfaces, 152
  of femur, 129
  of inferior nasal conchae, 331
  of lacrimal bones, 331
  of radius, 71
  of tibia, 143
  of zygomatic bones, 326
Lateral tibial plateau of tibia, 143
Legg-Calve-Perthes disease, 35, 216
Lesser cornua, hyoid bone, 361
Lesser pelvis, 194–196
Lesser sciatic notch, ischium, 200
Lesser trochanter of femur, 128
Lesser tuberosity of humerus, 63
Lesser wings, of ethmoid bone, 320
  inferior surfaces, 320
  superior surfaces, 320
Ligament of head of femur, 207
Ligamentum flavum, 281
Ligamentum nuchae, 281
Limb
  lower
    ankle joint, 179–188
    distal tibiofibular joint, 178–179
    femur, 127–136
    fibula, 144–150
    foot, 150–164
    intertarsal joints, 188–190
    knee joint, 164–178
    metatarsophalangeal and interphalangeal joints, 192–193
    patella, 136–140
    proximal tibiofibular joint, 178
    tarsometatarsal joints, 190–192
    tibia, 140–144
  upper
    elbow joint, 83–91
    first carpometacarpal joint, 97–99
    hand, 77–83

Limb (Continued)
    humerus, 63–68
    metacarpophalangeal and interphalangeal joints, 99–100
    radius, 68
    ulna, 71–77
    wrist joint, 91–97
Line, definition of, 11
Linea aspera of femur, 129
Lingual/glossal, definition of, 13
Lipohaemarthrosis, 27, 149
Lisfranc fracture dislocation, 190, 191f
Lisfranc ligament, 190
Lister's tubercle of radius, 71
Long bones, 8
Longitudinal fracture, 22
Longitudinal fractures of patella, 139
Looser's zones fractures, 33
Lordosis, 275
Lower limb
    ankle joint, 179–188
    distal tibiofibular joint, 178–179
    femur, 127–136
    fibula, 144–150
    foot, 150–164
    intertarsal joints, 188–190
    knee joint, 164–178
    metatarsophalangeal and interphalangeal joints, 192–193
    patella, 136–140
    proximal tibiofibular joint, 178
    tarsometatarsal joints, 190–192
    tibia, 140–144
Lumbar curve, 275
Lumbar vertebrae, 262–268, 264f, 265f, 266f
    L1-L4 (typical), 262–263
    L5, 263–264
    lumbar spine, 267f
    third lumbar vertebra, 266f
Lunate, 77, 77b

M

Magnetic resonance imaging (MRI), 37, 132, 286
Malignant bone tumours, 40, 49
Malleolar fossa of fibula, 144
Malleus, 315
Malunion, of fracture, 26
Mamillary process, 262
Mandible, 300, 344
    fracture, 351
    left, 348f
    mandible fracture, 352f
    ossification, 349–350
    radiographic appearances of, 350–353
        3D CT image of left lateral aspect, 350f
        panoramic tomogram/ orthopantomogram, 350f
    ramus, 349
Mandibular canal of mandible, 349
Mandibular foramen of mandible, 349
Mandibular fossa, of temporal bone, 313–314
Manubrium sterni, 221–222
March fracture, 162b
Mastoid angle, of parietal bones, 311
Maxilla, 336
Maxillae, 324–326
    left maxilla, 325f
    ossification, 326
Maxillae bones, 299, 320
Maxillary border of zygomatic bones, 327
Maxillary process, 331
Maxillary sinuses, 342
Meatus
    definition of, 12
    inferior, 341
    middle, 322, 341
    superior, 321, 341
Mechanical traction, 24
Medial, definition of, 12

Medial (vertebral) border of scapula, 105
Medial and lateral borders of femur, 129
Medial and lateral condyles of femur, 129
Medial border
    of nasal bones, 330
    of tibia, 143
Medial collateral ligaments, 99, 192
Medial collateral or deltoid ligament, 182
Medial condyle
    of femur, 136
    of tibia, 143
Medial cuneiform, 151
Medial epicondyle
    of femur, 129
    of humerus, 65
Medial longitudinal arch, 157
Medial malleolus of tibia, 143
Medial plate, 321
    of ethmoidal sinuses, 344
Medial semilunar cartilage, 168
Medial supracondylar line of femur, 129
Medial supracondylar ridge of humerus, 65
Medial surfaces, 152
    of femur, 129
    of inferior nasal conchae, 331
    of lacrimal bones, 331
    of tibia, 143
    of ulna, 72
Medial tibial plateau of tibia, 143
Median atlantoaxial joint, 277–278
Median sacral crest, 269
Medullary canals, 6
Medullary cavity, 9
Meniscus, torn, 174b–176b
Mental foramen of mandible, 349
Mental protuberance of mandible, 349
Mesial, definition of, 13

Metabolic disease, 51
    vitamin C deficiency, 51
    vitamin D deficiency, 51
Metacarpal bones, 78–79
Metacarpals fractures of hand, 83, 83b
Metacarpophalangeal joints (MTPJs), 99–100
    trauma, 100b–101b
    type, 99–100
        blood supply, 100
        bony articular surfaces, 99
        fibrous capsule, 99
        movements, 99–100
        nerve supply, 100
        supporting ligaments, 99
        synovial membrane, 99
Metaphysis, 7
Metastases, 40
Metatarsal bones, 150–164
    fifth metatarsal, 156
    first metatarsal, 151
    second metatarsal, 151–153
Metatarsals fractures, 162, 162b
Metatarsophalangeal joints, 192–193
    type, 192–193
        bony articular surfaces, 192
        fibrous capsule, 192
        movements, 193
        nerve supply, 193
        supporting ligaments, 192–193
        synovial membrane, 192
Metopic suture, 309
Middle ear, 315–316
Middle meatus, 322, 341
Middle nasal concha, 321, 341
Midfoot, 150
Molars, 355
Monteggia fracture-dislocation of ulna, 76–77
Multiaxial joints, 18
Multiple hereditary exostoses, 41
Myeloma, multiple, 48–49, 48f, 324

Myelomatosis, 48–49, 48*f*
Mylohyoid line of mandible, 349

N
Nails, for immobilisation, 24
Nasal bones, 299, 324, 329–331, 330*f*, 334
  ossification, 330–331
Nasal cavity, 339–342
  conchae, 341
  coronal CT image, 341*f*
  coronal section, 340*f*
  imaging appearances of, 341
  lateral wall, 339–341
  medial wall, 339
  sagittal section, 340*f*
Nasal conchae, 339–341
Nasal crest, 325
Nasal notches, of frontal bone, 309
Nasal part, of frontal bone, 309
Nasal spine, of frontal bone, 309
Nasal surface
  of lacrimal bones, 331
  of maxillae, 325
Nasolacrimal canal, 336
Navicular, 151, 153
Naviculocuneiform joints, 189
Neck, 349
  of femur, 127, 132–134, 132*b*
  of fibula, 144
  fractures of scapula, 110, 110*b*
  of radius, 68
Neoplasms, 40–51
  benign tumours, 41–43
  enchondroma, 40*f*
  malignant tumours, 43–49
  secondary bone tumours, 49–51
Nerve supply, 5
  of AC joint, 123
  of ankle joint, 179
  of carpometacarpal joint, 98–99
  of distal tibiofibular joint, 179
  of elbow joint, 86

Nerve supply *(Continued)*
  of interphalangeal and metatarsophalangeal joints, 193
  of intertarsal joints, 189
  of knee joint, 169
  of MTPJs and IPJs, 100
  of proximal tibiofibular joint, 178
  of SC joint, 125
  of shoulder joint, 115
  of sternocostal joints, 233
  of wrist joint, 93
Norepinephrine, 54
Notch, definition of, 12
Nuchal lines, 312
  highest, 312
  inferior, 312
  superior, 312
Nucleus pulposus, 278
Nutrient arteries, 5
Nutrient foramen of fibula, 144
Nutrient foramina, 5

O
Oblique fracture, 22
Oblique line of mandible, 349
Oblique popliteal ligament, 168
Obturator foramen, 201
Occipital angle, of parietal bones, 311
Occipital bones, 299, 310–313, 312*f*, 318
  basilar part, 313
  lateral part, 313
  ossification, 313
  squamous part, 311, 313
Occipital border, of parietal bones, 311
Occipital condyles, 311, 313
Occipital crest
  external, 312
  internal, 311
Occlusal, definition of, 13
Odontoid process, 251
Oestrogen, 51–52
Olecranon fossa of humerus, 65

Olecranon process of ulna, 72, 74
  fractures, 74*b*
Open fracture, 22
Open reduction, 24
Open reduction internal fixation (ORIF), 24
'Open-book' injuries, 203–204
Optic canal, 336
  of ethmoid bone, 319–320
Optic foramen, 336
Orbital border of zygomatic bones, 326
Orbital cavity, 336–339
  axial CT image, 337*f*
  bones forming, 336
  bones forming left orbit, 336*f*
  features of, 336–337
  imaging appearances of, 336
  3D CT image, 338*f*
Orbital fissure
  lateral border of superior, 319
  postero-lateral border of inferior, 319
Orbital plate, 321
  of ethmoidal sinuses, 344
Orbital process, 329
Orbital surface
  of lacrimal bones, 331
  of maxillae, 325
  of sphenoid bone, 319
  of zygomatic bones, 326
Organic collagenous protein fibres, 1
Osgood–Schlatter's disease, 176, 177*f*
Ossification, 311
  carpal bones, 78
  centres, 6
  cervical vertebrae, 252
    1st (atlas), 252
    2nd (axis), 253–254
    7th (vertebra prominens), 257
  clavicle, 103–105
  of coccyx, 271–272
  of ethmoid bone, 322–324

Ossification *(Continued)*
femur, 129–130, 130*f*
fibula, 144–145
of frontal bone, 309
hip bone, 201–206
centres of pelvis, 202*f*
primary centres, 201–202
secondary centres, 202–206
secondary ossification
centres of pelvis, 202*f*
humerus, 65–66
minimally displaced
supracondylar
fracture, 68*f*
ossification centres, 67*f*
primary centre, 65
right humerus, 66*f*
secondary centres, 65
hyoid bone, 361–362
inferior nasal conchae, 332
intracartilaginous, 6–8
fusion, 8
growth, 7
primary centre of, 6–7
secondary centres of, 7
intramembranous, 8, 311
of lacrimal bones, 331
lumbar vertebrae, 263
primary centres, 263
secondary centres, 263
mandible, 349–350
primary centres, 349
secondary centres,
349–350
of maxillae, 326
metacarpal bones, 79
metatarsal bones, 156
of nasal bones, 330–331
of occipital bone, 313
of palatine bones, 329
of parietal bones, 311
patella, 136–138
phalanges, 79–81, 157
primary centre of, 313
process, 5–8
radius, 71

Ossification *(Continued)*
primary centre, 71
secondary centres, 71
of sacrum, 270, 275*f*
scapula, 107–108
of sphenoid bone, 320
sternum, 224
temporal bone, 316
tibia, 143–144
typical ribs, 230
ulna, 72–73
Galeazzi fracture-
dislocation, 76
Monteggia fracture-
dislocation, 76–77
primary centre, 72
secondary centres, 72–73
vertebral column, 243–245
primary centres, 243
secondary centres, 243–244
of zygomatic bones, 327
Osteoarthritis (OA), 59–60, 59*f*,
60*f*, 174
causes, 59
radiological signs, 59–60
Osteoblasts, 1–2, 6
Osteochondritis dissecans,
174–176
Osteochondroma, 41, 43*f*
Osteochondrosis, 35
Osteoclastoma, 43
Osteoclasts, 2
Osteocytes, 2
Osteogenic cells, 2
Osteogenic sarcoma, 44
Osteoid, 1
Osteoid osteoma, 42, 44*f*
Osteolytic, 33
Osteoma, 37, 43
Osteomalacia, 30–33, 32*f*, 51
causes, 33
radiological signs, 33
Osteomyelitis, 33, 56–57
acute, 56*f*, 57*f*
causes, 57
radiological signs, 57

Osteonecrosis, 27, 35–37
causes, 36
early osteonecrosis, 37*f*
radiological signs, 37
of right hip, 36*f*
Osteopaenia, 30–33
Osteophytes, 37, 59
formation, 59–60
Osteoporosis, 30
causes, 30
localised 'disuse'
osteoporosis, 31*f*
metabolic disease, 51
osteoporotic vertebral body
fracture, 31*f*
radiological signs, 30
Osteosarcoma, 44, 46*f*, 47*f*
Osteosclerosis, 33–37

P
Paget's disease, 33–35, 34*f*, 35*f*,
44, 51, 324
causes, 35
radiological signs, 35
Palatine bones, 299, 320, 324,
327–329, 336
left, 328*f*
ossification, 329
Palatine process, 325
Palmar (volar) radiocarpal
ligament, 92
Palmar (volar) ulnocarpal
ligament, 92
Palmar ligament, of first
carpometacarpal
joint, 99
Paranasal sinuses, 342–348
and associated structures,
342*f*, 343*f*
axial CT images, 346*f*
coronal CT images, 345*f*
ethmoidal sinuses, 344
frontal sinuses, 343–344
imaging appearances of,
345–348
maxillary sinuses, 342–343

Paranasal sinuses *(Continued)*
  sagittal CT image, 345*f*
  sphenoidal sinuses, 344–345
Parathormone, 6
Parathyroid glands, 54
Parathyroid hormone (PTH), 54
Parietal bones, 299, 310–311, 318
  left, 310*f*
  ossification, 311
Parietal margin, of frontal
    bone, 309
Pars interarticularis
  L1-L4 (typical) lumbar
      vertebrae, 263
  typical vertebra, 242
Partial dislocation, of
      acromioclavicular joint, 27
Patella, 5, 136–140
  ossification, 136–138
    bipartite patella, right
        knee, 138*f*
    fractures, 139*b*
    left patella, 137*f*
    right knee, 139*f*
    right patella, 138*f*
    transverse right patella
        fracture, 140*f*
Patellar articular surface of
    femur, 129
Patellar tendon, 168
Pathological fracture, of femur, 22
Pathology, 29
  causes of, 39–61
    arthritis, 57–61
    endocrine, 51–56
    infections, 56–57
    metabolic disease, 51
    neoplasms, 40–51
  changes caused by, 29–39
    focal bone destruction, 33
    increase in bone density,
        33–37
    loss of bone density, 30–33
    new bone growth, 37–39
  ethmoid bone, 324*b*
    Paget's disease of skull, 324*f*

Pathology *(Continued)*
  hip joint, 214*b*–216*b*
  interchondral joints, 237*b*
  phalanges, 164*b*
  sacroiliac joints, 219*b*
  shoulder joint, 121*b*
  sphenoidal sinuses, 347*b*
  sternum, 227*b*–228*b*
  symphysis pubis, 220*b*
  tarsometatarsal joints, 192*b*
  teeth, 356*b*
Pectus carinatum, 228, 228*f*
Pectus excavatum, 227, 227*f*
Pedicles
  3rd to 6th (typical) cervical
      vertebrae, 246
  L1-L4 (typical) lumbar
      vertebrae, 262
  T2-T8 (typical) thoracic
      vertebrae, 258
  typical vertebra, 242
Pelvic brim, 194–196
Pelvic cavity, 195
Pelvic curve, 275
Pelvic girdle
  hip bone, 198–206
    ilium, 198–199
    ischium, 200
    pubis, 200–206
  hip joint, 206–217
    trauma, 211*b*–212*b*
  pelvis, 194–198
    male and female pelvis, 197*t*
  SIJ, 217–220
    pathology, 220*b*
  symphysis pubis, 220
    pathology, 220*b*
Pelvic inlet, 195
Pelvic outlet, 195
Pelvic sacral foramina, 269
Pelvic surface, 200, 269
Pelvis, 194–198
  female, 195*f*, 196*f*
  greater, 194
  imaging appearances of,
      196–198

Pelvis *(Continued)*
  lesser, 194–196
  male, 195*f*, 196*f*, 197*f*
Periodontal ligament, 18–19
Periodontal membrane, teeth, 354
Periosteum, 4–5, 7
Permanent teeth, 355
Perpendicular plate, 321
  of palatine bones, 329
Perthes disease, 35
Phalanges, 79–81, 156–158,
      162, 162*b*
  arches of foot, 157–158
    ossification centres of
        foot, 161*f*
    right foot, 158*f*, 159*f*, 160*f*
  fracture of neck, 83*f*
  fractures, 162*b*
  hand, dorsal (posterior)
      aspect, 80*f*
  pathology, 164*b*
  right wrist, 81*f*, 82*f*
Phalanges fractures of hand,
      83, 83*b*
Pharyngeal tubercle, 313
Pigeon chest. *See* Pectus
      carinatum
Pin, for immobilisation, 24
Pisiform, 77–78, 77*b*
Pituitary fossa, 53
Pituitary gland, 53
Pivot joints, synovial, 18
Plane joints, synovial, 18
Plantar calcaneonavicular
      ligament, 189
Plantar plate, 192
Plaster of Paris bandages, for
      immobilisation, 24
Plastic bowing fracture of
      ulna, 74
  fractures, 74*b*
Plates, for immobilisation, 24
Pneumothorax, 234
Popliteal sulcus of femur, 129
Popliteal surface of femur, 129
Popliteal tendon, 168

Positron emission tomography (PET), 49
Posterior, definition of, 12
Posterior arch, 1st (atlas) cervical vertebrae, 252
Posterior atlantooccipital membrane, 277
Posterior border, 199
  of fibula, 144
  of lacrimal bones, 331
  of radius, 71
  of ulna, 72
  of vomer, 333
Posterior cruciate (PCL), 168
Posterior dislocation
  of hip joint, 211–212, 211*f*
  of shoulder joint, 116*b*, 118–119, 118*f*
Posterior inferior iliac spine (PIIS), 199
Posterior longitudinal ligament, 279
Posterior malleolus of tibia, 143
Posterior oblique ligament, 97
Posterior sternoclavicular ligaments, 125
Posterior superior iliac spine (PSIS), 199
Posterior surface, 65, 152
  of radius, 71
  of tibia, 143
  of ulna, 72
Posterior talofibular ligament, 182
Posterior tubercle, 252
Postero-inferior border of zygomatic bones, 327
Postero-medial border of zygomatic bones, 327
Prefixes, 12
Premolars, 354–355
Prepatellar bursa, 166
Primary neoplasm, 40
Primary OA, 59

Prolapsed disc. *See* Intervertebral disc herniation
Pronation, 86
Protuberance
  external occipital, 312
  internal occipital, 311
Provisional callous, 26
Proximal, definition of, 13
Proximal end centres, 65
  greater tuberosity, 65
  humeral head, 65
  lesser tuberosity, 65
Proximal epiphysis of tibia, 143
Proximal row, 151–153
Proximal tibiofibular joint, 178
  type, 178
    blood supply, 178
    bony articular surfaces, 178
    fibrous capsule, 178
    movements, 178
    nerve supply, 178
    supporting ligaments, 178
    synovial membrane, 178
Pseudo fractures, 33
Pterion, 317
Pterygoid fissure, 320
Pterygoid hamulus, 320
Pterygoid plate
  lateral, 320
  medial, 320
Pterygoid processes, 320
  lateral pterygoid plate, 320
  medial pterygoid plate, 320
  pterygoid fissure, 320
  pterygoid hamulus, 320
Pubic arch, 195
Pubic crest, 201
Pubic tubercle, 201
Pubis, 200–206
Pubofemoral ligament, 207
Pulp cavity, teeth, 353
Pyramidal process, 329

Q
Quadriceps femoris, 168

R
Radial artery, 100
Radial collateral ligament, 86, 93
Radial fossa
  definition of, 11
  of humerus, 65
Radial head of ulna, 74
  fractures, 74*b*
Radial notch of ulna, 71–72
Radial styloid process of radius, 71
Radial tuberosity of radius, 68
Radiate ligament, 283
Radiographs, 307
Radius, 68
  features of distal end of, 71
  features of proximal end of, 68–71
    right radius, 69*f*, 70*f*
  features of shaft of, 71
Ramus, 349
Recurrent dislocation, of shoulder joint, 116*b*–119*b*
Red bone marrow, 4
Reduction, of fractures, 23–24
Rehabilitation, of fractures, 23–24
  late radiographic signs of femoral fracture, 25*f*
  radiographic signs of provisional callous, 25*f*
Remodelling process, 6
Renal osteodystrophy, 54
Rheumatoid arthritis, 33, 60–61, 60*f*, 61*f*
  causes, 61
  radiological signs, 61
Rhinosinusitis, 347
  chronic rhinosinusitis, 347*f*
Ribs, 221, 228–232
  atypical ribs, 230–232
  fractures, 234–236
    with associated pneumothorax and subcutaneous emphysema, 235*f*

Ribs *(Continued)*
  flail chest, 235*f*
  multiple rib fractures, 234*f*
  radiographic appearances
    of, 232
    anterior ribs, 232*f*
    posterior ribs, 232*f*
  typical, 229–230, 229*f*
Rickets, 30–33
  adult, 51
  causes, 33
  metabolic disease, 51
  osteomalacia, 32*f*
  radiological signs, 33
Root, teeth, 353
Rotation
  external, 16
  internal, 16
Rotator cuff tears of shoulder
    joint, 116*b*, 118*f*, 119
Rugger-jersey' sign, 54

S
Sacral canal, 270
Sacral cornua, 269
Sacral fracture, 293*f*
Sacral hiatus, 269
Sacrococcygeal curve. *See*
    Pelvic curve
Sacroiliac joints (SIJs), 217–220
  accessory ligaments, 218
  bony articular surfaces, 217
  fibrous capsule, 217
  movements, 218
  orientation, 217–218
  radiographic appearances of,
    218–220
    posteroanterior projection,
    218*f*
  supporting ligaments, 218
  synovial membrane, 217
  type, 217–220
Sacropelvic surface,
    ilium, 200
Sacrospinous ligament, 218
Sacrotuberous ligament, 218

Sacrum, 268, 268*f*, 272*f*, 273*f*,
    274*f*
  apex, 270
  and coccyx, 269*f*, 273*f*
  dorsal surface, 269–270
  fracture, 289*b*–293*b*
  lateral surface, 270
  ossification, 270
  pelvic surface, 269
Saddle joints, synovial, 17–18
Sagittal border, 310
  of parietal bones, 310
Sagittal suture, 310
Scaphoid, 77, 77*b*
  fracture of wrist joint,
    95, 95*b*
Scapula, 105–112
  anterior aspect, 107
  lateral aspect, 105–107
    left scapula, 106*f*
  notch of scapula, 107
  ossification, 107–108
    floating shoulder, 111*f*
    fractures, 110*b*
    right shoulder joint and
      scapula, 109*f*
    selected scapula ossification
      centres, 110*f*
    shoulder joint and scapula,
      108*f*
  posterior aspect, 105
Scapulothoracic joint of
    scapula,
    105
Scoliosis, 294*b*–297*b*
Screws, for immobilisation, 24
Scurvy, 51, 52*f*
Secondary bone tumours,
    49–51
Secondary neoplasms/
    tumours, 40
Secondary OA, 59
Sella turcica, 319
Semicircular canals, 316
Septic arthritis, 56
Sesamoid bones, 5, 9

Shaft
  of clavicle, 102
  fracture, 67
    of humerus, 67*b*
  of tibia and/or fibula,
    147–148
Sharpey's fibres, 278
Short bones, 8–9
Short plantar ligament, 189
Shoulder girdle
  AC joint, 122–124
  clavicle, 102–105
  SC joint, 124–126
  scapula, 105–112
  shoulder joint, 112–122
Shoulder joint, 112–122
  calcific tendinopathy, 121*b*,
    121*f*
  full thickness tear, 120*f*
  pathology, 121*b*
  right shoulder joint, 112*f*,
    113*f*, 115*f*
  trauma, 116*b*
  type, 113–115
    blood supply, 115
    bony articular surfaces, 113
    fibrous capsule, 113
    intracapsular structures, 114
    movements, 114–115
    nerve supply, 115
    strengthening ligaments, 114
    synovial membrane,
      113–114
    tendons, 114
Simple (closed) fracture, 22
Simple bone cysts, 43
Singular arthrosis, 14
Singular bursa, 16
Sinuses
  of bone, 6
  paranasal, 342
Skull, 299–308
  base of skull fractures, 323
  features in base of, 303*f*
  features of, 301*f*, 302*f*
  foramina in base of, 304*f*

Skull *(Continued)*
  imaging appearances of,
    305–308
    axial CT images of
      cranium, 306*f*
    lateral projection, 305*f*
    3D CT images, 307*f*
  individual bones of cranium,
    308–324
    ethmoid bone, 320–324
    frontal bone, 308–310
    occipital bone, 311–313
    parietal bones, 310–311
    sphenoid bone, 318–320
    temporal bone, 313–316
  individual bones of face,
    324–336
    hyoid bone, 361–362
    inferior nasal conchae,
      331–332
    lacrimal bones, 331
    mandible, 344
    maxillae, 324–326
    nasal bones, 329–331
    nasal cavity, 339–342
    orbital cavity, 336–339
    palatine bones, 327–329
    paranasal sinuses, 342–348
    teeth, 353–357
    TMJ, 357–362
    vomer, 332–336
    zygomatic bones, 326–327
  position of bones of, 300*f*, 301*f*
Slipped upper femoral epiphysis
  (SUFE), 216, 216*f*, 217*f*
Slipped' disc. *See* Intervertebral
  disc herniation
Soft tissue tumour, 46*f*
Soleal line of tibia, 143
Spheno-ethmoidal recess, 341
Sphenoid bone, 299, 310,
  318–320, 318*f*, 336
  ethmoid bones, 318
  frontal bones, 318
  occipital bones, 318
  ossification, 320

Sphenoid bone *(Continued)*
  parietal bones, 318
  vomer bones, 318
  zygomatic bones, 318
Sphenoidal angle, of parietal
  bones, 311
Sphenoidal crest, 319
Sphenoidal process, 329
Sphenoidal rostrum
  process, 319
Sphenoidal sinuses, 319,
  344–345
Sphenomandibular ligament, 358
Sphenopalatine notch, 329
Sphenosquamosal suture, 319
Spine
  definition of, 11
  of scapula, 105
Spinoglenoid notch of
  scapula, 105
Spinous process
  3rd to 6th (typical) cervical
    vertebrae, 246
  L1-L4 (typical) lumbar
    vertebrae, 263
  T2-T8 (typical) thoracic
    vertebrae, 258
  typical vertebra, 242
Spinous tubercles, 269
Spiral fracture, 22
Spiral groove of humerus, 65
Spiral line of femur, 129
Splints, for immobilisation, 24
Spondylitis, 219
Spondylolisthesis, 294*b*–297*b*,
  298*f*
Spondylolysis, 294*b*–297*b*, 297*f*
Spondylosis, 294*b*–297*b*
Spongy bone, 4
Squamosal border, of parietal
  bones, 310
Squamosal suture, 310
Squamous, definition of, 11
Stapes, 315
Staphylococcus infection, 56
Sternal end of clavicle, 102

Sternoclavicular joint (SC joint),
  124–126
  type, 124–126
    blood supply, 125
    bony articular surfaces, 124
    fibrous capsule, 125
    intracapsular structure, 125
    movements, 125
    nerve supply, 125
    supporting ligaments, 125
    synovial membrane, 125
Sternocostal joints, 233
  articular surfaces, 233
  blood supply, 233
  fibrous capsule, 233
  movements, 233
  nerve supply, 233
Sternum, 221–228
  body, 222
  imaging appearances of,
    224–228
  manubrium sterni, 221–222
  ossification, 224
  ossification centres, 225*f*
  posteroanterior projection, 224*f*
  primary centres, 224
  sagittal CT image, 225*f*
  xiphoid process, 222–224
Strengthening ligaments
  of distal tibiofibular joint, 178
  of shoulder joint, 114
Stress fractures, 162, 162*b*
Styloid process
  of fibula, 144
  of temporal bone, 361
Stylomandibular ligament, 358
Stylomastoid foramen, 302*f*
Sub-acute/chronic sign, 57
Sub-trochanteric/shaft of femur,
  132*b*, 135
Subacromial bursa, 113
Subchondral sclerosis, 59–60
Subcutaneous emphysema,
  234*b*–236*b*
Sublingual fossa of
  mandible, 349

Subluxation, 27
of AC joint, 123
Submandibular fossa of
mandible, 349
Subscapular bursa, 113
Subscapular fossa
definition of, 11
of scapula, 107
Subscapularis tendon, 114
Subtalar joint, 188
Sulcus
definition of, 12
for superior sagittal venous
sinus, 311
Sulcus calcanei, 152
Sulcus tali, 152
Superciliary arches, of frontal
bone, 309
Superior, definition of, 13
Superior angle of scapula, 105, 221
Superior articular facets, 241
1st (atlas) cervical vertebrae,
252
3rd to 6th (typical) cervical
vertebrae, 246
L1-L4 (typical) lumbar
vertebrae, 263
T2-T8 (typical) thoracic
vertebrae, 258
Superior articular processes
L1-L4 (typical) lumbar
vertebrae, 262
typical vertebra, 242
Superior border
of inferior nasal conchae,
331–332
of lacrimal bones, 331
of nasal bones, 330
of scapula, 107
of vomer, 333
Superior meatus, 321, 341
Superior nasal concha, 321, 341
Superior orbital fissure, 336
lateral border of, 319
superior border of, 320
Superior pubic ligament, 220

Superior ramus, 201
Superior surface, 152
of vomer, 333
Superior thoracic aperture, 221
Superior tibiofibular joint, 18
Supination, 86
Supporting ligaments
of AC joint, 122
of ankle joint, 182
of carpometacarpal joint, 97
of elbow joint, 86
of interphalangeal joints and
metatarsophalangeal
joints, 192–193
of intertarsal joints, 189
of MTPJs and IPJs, 99
of proximal tibiofibular joint,
178
of SC joint, 125
of tarsometatarsal joints, 190
and tendons of knee joint, 168
of wrist joint, 92–93
Supracondylar fractures, 67
of humerus, 67b
Supracondylar ridge, definition
of, 11
Supraglenoid tubercle of
scapula, 107
Supraorbital foramen, 309, 336
Supraorbital margins, of frontal
bone, 309
Suprapatellar bursa, 165–166
Suprascapular artery, 123, 125
Supraspinatus tendon, 114
Supraspinous fossa of
scapula, 105
Supraspinous ligament, 281
Surgical neck of humerus, 63, 67
fractures, 67b
Suspected physical abuse, 236,
236f
Sustentaculum tali, 152
Sutural ligament, 18
Sutures, 18
Symphyses, 19–20
Symphysis menti of mandible, 349

Symphysis pubis, 220, 220f
bony articular surfaces, 220
intracapsular structures, 220
movements, 220
radiographic appearances
of, 220
supporting ligaments, 220
type, 220
Synchondroses, 19
Syndesmophytes, 37
Syndesmoses, 19
Synostoses, 18–19
Synovial bicondylar joint, 357
Synovial cavity, 14–15, 15f
Synovial fluid, 14–15
Synovial joints, 14–16, 15f, 16b
accessory joint structures,
15–16
features of, 14–15
movements of joints, 16–18
types of, 17–18
synovial ball and socket
joints, 18
synovial bicondylar joints, 17
synovial ellipsoid joints, 17
synovial hinge joints, 17
synovial pivot joints, 18
synovial plane joints, 18
synovial saddle joints, 17–18
Synovial membrane, 14–15, 15f
of AC joint, 122
of ankle joint, 181–182
of atlantooccipital joints, 277
of carpometacarpal joint, 97
of costotransverse joints, 283
of costovertebral joints, 283
of elbow joint, 85
of interphalangeal and
metatarsophalangeal
joints, 192
of knee joint, 165–168
of median atlantoaxial
joint, 278
of MTPJs and IPJs, 99
of proximal tibiofibular
joint, 178

Synovial membrane *(Continued)*
  of sacroiliac joints, 217
  of SC joint, 125
  of shoulder joint, 113–114
  of vertebral arches joints, 281
  of wrist joint, 92
Synovial saddle joint, 97

T
Talocalcaneonavicular joint, 188
Talonavicular joint, 188
Talonavicular ligament, 189
Talus, 151–152, 152*f*, 155
Tarsal bones, 151–153, 151*b*
Tarsometatarsal joints, 190–192
  fractures, 190*b*
  pathology, 192*b*
  type, 190
    joint capsules, 190
    movements, 190–192
    supporting ligaments, 190
Tarsometatarsal ligaments, 190
Tarsus, 151
Teeth, 353–357
  dental formulae, 355–356
  dentition, 355
  lower premolar tooth, 354*f*
  permanent, 355*f*
  radiographic appearances of,
    356–357
  terms associated with, 13
  types of, 354–355
    canines, 354
    incisors, 354
    molars, 355
    premolars, 354–355
Temporal bones, 299, 310,
    313–316
  imaging appearances of,
    316–318
    axial CT images of superior
      and inferior aspect of
      petrous part, 316*f*
    left temporal bone, 317*f*
  inner ear, 316
  lambdoid suture, 313

Temporal bones *(Continued)*
  left temporal bone, 314*f*
  mandibular fossa, 315
  mastoid part, 315
    mastoid notch, 315
    mastoid process, 315
  middle ear, 315–316
  ossification, 316
  petrous part, 315
    anterior surface, 315
    apex, 315
    carotid canal, 315
    internal acoustic meatus,
      315
    jugular fossa, 315
    posterior surface, 315
  sphenosquamosal
    suture, 313
  squamosal suture, 313
  squamous part, 313–314
  temporal surface, 314
  tympanic part, 315
  zygomatic bone, 313
  zygomatic process, 314
Temporal border of zygomatic
    bones, 327
Temporal process of zygomatic
    bones, 327
Temporal surface of zygomatic
    bones, 326
Temporomandibular joint (TMJ),
    17, 357–362
  blood supply, 358
  bony articular surfaces, 357
  fibrous capsule, 357
  imaging appearances
    of, 359
    left temporomandibular joint,
      360*f*
  intracapsular structure, 358
  left temporomandibular
    joint, 358*f*
  movements, 358
  nerve supply, 358
  supporting ligaments, 358
  synovial membrane, 357

Tendons, 16
  sheaths, 16
  of knee joint, 168
  of shoulder joint, 114
    infraspinatus, 114
    subscapularis, 114
    supraspinatus, 114
    teres minor, 114
Teres minor tendon, 114
Terminology, for bones, 11*b*
Testosterone, 6
Thoracic cage, 221
Thoracic curve, 275
Thoracic vertebrae, 257–262,
    261*f*, 262*f*
  imaging appearances of, 289
  T1, 259
  T2-T8 (typical), 258–259
  T9, 259
  T10, 259
  T11 and T12, 259–260
  typical, 258*f*, 259*f*
Thoracoacromial artery, 123
Thorax
  costal cartilages, 232–233
  interchondral joints, 233
  ribs, 228–232
  sternocostal joints, 233
  sternum, 221–228
  thoracic cage, 222*f*
Thyroid gland, 53
Thyroxine, 6, 53
Tibia, 140–144
  features of proximal end of,
    143–144
  features of shaft of,
    143–144
  left, 141*f*, 142*f*
  ossification, 143–144
Tibial collateral ligament, 168
Tibial condyles of fibula, 148
Tibial tuberosity of tibia, 143
Tibiofibular joint
  inferior, 145*f*
  superior, 145*f*
Tophi, 61

Torus fracture of ulna, 74
  fractures, 74*b*
Transfacial fractures (Le Fort
    fractures), 335, 335*f*
Transverse acetabular
    ligament, 207
Transverse fracture, 22
  of patella, 139
Transverse humeral ligament, 114
Transverse metacarpal
    ligaments, 99
Transverse process, 229
  1st (atlas) cervical vertebrae, 252
  3rd to 6th (typical) cervical
      vertebrae, 246
  L1-L4 (typical) lumbar
      vertebrae, 262
  L5 lumbar vertebrae, 263
  T2-T8 (typical) thoracic
      vertebrae, 258
  typical vertebra, 242
Transverse ridges, 269
Transverse tubercles, 270
Trapezium, 77–78, 77*b*
Trapezoid, 77–78, 77*b*
Trapezoid line of clavicle, 102
Trauma, 89*b*
  AC joint, 123*b*
  hip joint, 211*b*–212*b*
  interchondral joints, 234*b*–236*b*
  of MTPJs and IPJs, 100*b*–101*b*
  shoulder joint, 116*b*
Triiodothyronine, 53
Tripod fractures, 334–335
Triquetral, 78
Triquetrum, 77, 77*b*
Trochanter, definition of, 11
Trochanteric fossa of
    femur, 129
Trochlea, 83
  definition of, 12
  of humerus, 65
Trochlear articular surface, 152
Trochlear notch
  definition of, 11
  of ulna, 72

Tubercle
  definition of, 12
  of intercondylar eminence, 143
  tuberosity of humerus, 63
Tuberculosis, 56
Tuberculum sellae, 319
Tuberosity, definition of, 12
Tumours, 40
  benign, 41–43
  Ewing's sarcoma, 44–45
    simple bone cyst, 45*f*
  giant cell, 43
  of hyaline cartilage, 45–48
  malignant, 43–49
  secondary bone, 49–51
Turbinates, 341
Tympanic part, of temporal
    bone, 315
Typical vertebra, 241–245,
    241*f*, 242*f*. See also
    Cervical vertebrae
  anteroposterior projection of
      lumbar spine, 244*f*
  imaging appearances of, 244
  lateral projection of lumbar
      spine, 244*f*
  sagittal CT image of lumbar
      spine, 245*f*

U
Ulna, 71–77
  features of distal end of, 72
    fractures, 74*b*
    immature skeleton, 75*f*
    left forearm, 73*f*
    Monteggia fracture-
        dislocation, 76*f*
  features of proximal end
      of, 71–72
  features of shaft of, 72
Ulnar artery, 100
Ulnar collateral ligament, 86, 93
Ulnar notch of radius, 71
Ulnar styloid process of ulna, 72
Ulnar tuberosity of ulna, 72
Upper cervical vertebrae, 254*f*

Upper limb
  elbow joint, 83–91
  first carpometacarpal
      joint, 97–99
  hand, 77–83
  humerus, 63–68
  metacarpophalangeal and
      interphalangeal joints,
      99–100
  radius, 68
  ulna, 71–77
  wrist joint, 91–97
Upper teeth, 324

V
Vacuum phenomenon, 294
Vaginal processes, of
    sphenoid, 319
Ventral, definition of, 13
Ventral sacroiliac ligament, 218
Vertebra prominens, 257
Vertebrae
  cervical, 245–257
  lumbar, 262–268
  thoracic, 257–262
  typical, 241–245, 241*f*, 242*f*,
      244*f*, 245*f*
Vertebral arches
  joints of, 281–282
  typical vertebra, 242, 258
Vertebral body, typical vertebra,
    242, 258
Vertebral column, 238
  cervical vertebrae,
      245–257
  coccyx, 270–275
  joints of, 277–284
  lateral view, 239*f*
  lumbar vertebrae, 262–268
  ossification, 243–245
  pathology, 294
  sacrum, 268
  sagittal T1W MRI, 240*f*
  thoracic vertebrae, 257–262
  typical vertebra, 241–245,
      241*f*, 242*f*

Vertebral curvatures, 275–277
  development of secondary
    curves, 275–277
  foetus, 275
Vertebral endplates, superior and
  inferior, 242
Vertebral foramen
  1st (atlas) cervical
    vertebrae, 252
  3rd to 6th (typical) cervical
    vertebrae, 246
  L1-L4 (typical) lumbar
    vertebrae, 262
  T2-T8 (typical) thoracic
    vertebrae, 258
  typical vertebra, 242
Vertebral notches; superior and
  inferior, 243
Vertical groove, of frontal
  bone, 322
Vertical shear injury, 204–205
  axial CT image, 205f
  of pelvis, 204f
Vestibule, 316

Vitamin C deficiency, 51
Vitamin D deficiency, 51
Vitamin deficiencies, 51
Volar plate, 99
Volkmann's canals, 4
Vomer, 300, 324, 332–336
  bones, 318, 320
  ossification, 333–336

W
Wedge compression fracture.
    See Anterior compression
    fracture
Woven bone, 26
Wrist joint, 91–97
  Colles fracture right wrist, 96f
  fractures, 95b
  left wrist joint, 92f
  right wrist joint, 91f, 94f
  scaphoid fracture right wrist, 96f
  type, 91–94
    blood supply, 93
    bony articular surfaces, 91
    fibrous capsule, 91

Wrist joint *(Continued)*
    intracapsular structures, 93
    movements, 93
    nerve supply, 93
    supporting ligaments, 92–93
    synovial membrane, 92
  wrist ossification centres, 95f

X
Xiphoid process, 221–224

Z
Zygoma, 314
Zygomatic arch fractures, 327
Zygomatic bones, 299, 318, 324,
    326–327, 336
  left zygomatic bone, 327f
  ossification, 327
Zygomatic process, 325
  of frontal bone, 309
  of temporal bone, 315
Zygomaticomaxillary complex
    fracture (ZMC fracture),
    334–335, 335f